SP Pvt. Ltd.

Dedicated To Parents

Phytocompounds
Sources and Bioactivities

Mallappa Kumara Swamy
and
Gudepalya Renukaiah Rudramurthy
Department of Biotechnology
East West First Grade College
No. 63, off Magadi Road, Vishwaneedam
Post, Anjana Nagar, Bengaluru
Karnataka – 560 091

2019

Studium Press (India) Pvt. Ltd.

Phytocompounds
Sources and Bioactivities

ISBN: 978-93-85046-43-8

Published by:

Studium Press (India) Pvt. Ltd.
4735/22, 2nd Floor, Prakash Deep Building
(Near Delhi Medical Association),
Ansari Road, Darya Ganj, New Delhi-110 002
Tel.: + 91-11-43240200-15 (15 lines); Fax: 91-11-43240215
E-mail: pubdir@studiumpress.in

Printed at India

Foreword

Higher plants have been used as the primary source of medicines by humans since the ancient times. Even today, several health problems are addressed using plant products all over the world. Medicinal plants possess several bioactive compounds like alkaloids, glycosides, tannins, terpenoids, polyphenols, saponins, resins, and oils that are therapeutically effective in solving many human health problems. The plant-derived compounds are the main source of many traditional medicinal systems, including the Ayurveda, Siddha, Unani, and Homoeopathy medicines. Importantly, plant compounds help in maintaining the health and vitality of individuals without any side effects. In fact, the medicinal plants are easily available, cheaper and possess no toxicity as compared to the chemotherapy drugs. More recent survey shows that there is a surge in research regarding the use of plant metabolites as potential leads for the drug discovery. Several plant secondary metabolites directly involve in the plant growth and development, and are very crucial for the plant to adapt to the environmental challenges. Some of them are recognized to be useful as bioactive compounds for human use as herbal medicines.

At present, new drug discovery is challenged by the reduction in the number of new drug approvals in addition to the high cost involved in research. The advancement of combinatorial chemistry has been found to be effective in discovering novel lead molecules. However, the success rate of it is hampered due to many reasons. Alternatively, plant resources are very promising, because plant compounds, either in pure form or crude extracts offer unlimited opportunities in obtaining new drug lead molecules due to their unmatched chemodiversity. The primary step in the discovery of a plant-derived drug involves the identification of new chemical entities that are isolated from a specific medicinal plants *via* bioassay-guided fractionation. In this case, it is important to identify the right candidate plants, which is mainly done based on tribal non-documented uses, the traditional documented uses, and all-inclusive literature survey. Biological activity guided fractionation of the identified medicinal plant might help to standardize the plant extract or its pure bioactive compounds as a novel drug. Thus, the right source of plants is critical in improving the drug discovery process with limited cost and high success rates. Thus, research focus towards the cutting-edge analytical techniques and instrumentations that are involved in the extraction, isolation and characterization of bioactive compounds from plant sources are very important to speed up the drug discovery process. Plant bioactive principles exhibit many therapeutic properties and provide unlimited opportunities of drug leads discovery. Further, plant metabolites are exceptionally useful as lead molecular scaffolds and offer the possibility of synthetic modifications to enhance their biological activity.

The present book on "*Phytocompounds: From sources to bioactivities and applications*", includes 13 chapters contributed by the potential researchers/scientists. The first chapter presents the information on the role of flavones in combating different types of cancers with more emphasis on the molecular aspects of anticancer activity. The second chapter discusses on the mode of action of a bioflavonoid, luteolin in the treatment of colorectal cancer. In the third chapter, the nanoformulations of the phytocompound, curcumin is discussed in treating glioblastoma. This is followed by the chapter four, where different plant-based drugs and their role in treating neurological disorders are documented in detail. The botanical, phytochemical and pharmacological aspects of medicinal herbs, such as *Averrhoa carambola*, *Cinnamomum zeylanicum, Chlorophytum borivilianum, Terminalia chebula* and *Lantana camara* are discussed comprehensively in the chapter number five, six, seven, eight and nine, respectively. Several potential anticancer plants are summarized in the chapters, ten and eleven. Also, in these chapters, the important methods to validate any herbs for their potential anticancerous properties are highlighted. In the chapter number twelve, rosmarinic acid's chemical structure, sources, biosynthesis and its production through biotechnological approaches are discussed in detail. In addition, this chapter highlights on various biological activities of rosmarinic acid. The final chapter discusses on the electrochemical aspects of phytochemicals derived from natural products.

The chapters included in this book show that different plants and their phytocompounds can be effective in treating many human health problems in a different manner. Some of these compounds act as antioxidants, function as immunomodulators, stimulates the patient's immune response, inhibit inflammations, microbial pathogens, fight against cancer cells, etc. The information provided in this book will be very useful for researchers to further explore their biomedical potentials in near future. The plant-based drug discovery process necessitates the involvement of integrated approaches, interdisciplines and advanced analytical tools and instruments. This edited book discusses different aspects of medicinal plants, phytocompounds and their biological activities. I congratulate the editors for their noble academic efforts spent on bringing out this volume.

Prof. Uma Rani Sinniah
Professor
Department of Crop Science, Faculty of Agriculture, Universiti Putra Malaysia, 43400 Serdang, Selangor, Malaysia

About the Editors

Dr. Mallappa Kumara Swamy

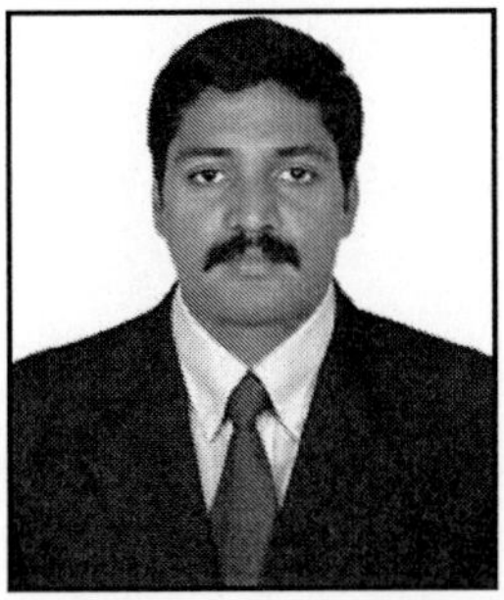

Dr. Mallappa Kumara Swamy; Working as an Associate Professor, Department of Biotechnology at East West First Grade College, Bengaluru, India. He has completed his Postdoctoral Research at the department of Crop Science, Faculty of Agriculture, Universiti Putra Malaysia (UPM), Serdang, Selangor, Malaysia. Before that, he had worked as an Associate Professor and Head, Department of Biotechnology, Padmashree Institute of Management and Sciences, Bangalore University, Bengaluru, India. He obtained his PhD (Biotechnology) from Acharya Nagarjuna University, Guntur, India in 2013. He is having more than 15 years of teaching and research experience in the fields of plant biotechnology, secondary metabolites production, phytochemistry and bioactive studies. To his credit, he has published more than 80 research publications in peer- reviewed journals and 16 book chapters in reputed book publishers. Recently, he has edited 4 books, published by Springer Nature Singapore Pte Ltd., Singapore in 2018 and 3 books are in preparation to be published by Springer Nature Singapore Pte Ltd., Singapore. He is also serving as the Editorial board member and reviewer for few high impact international Journals. Presently, he is working in the area of natural products research, plant cell and tissue culture technology for bioactive compounds production and evaluation of their bioactivities. Also, his research is focused on nanobiotechnology for medical applications.

Dr. Gudepalya Renukaiah Rudramurthy

Dr. Gudepalya Renukaiah Rudramurthy; Working as a Professor and Head, Department of Biotechnology at East First Grade College, Bengaluru, India. He has obtained his PhD (Biotechnology) from

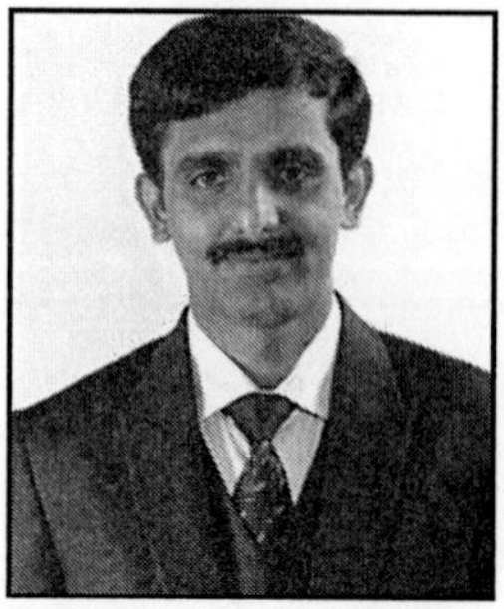

Jawaharlal Nehru Technological University, Hyderabad (JNTUH), Telangana, India in 2016. He has more than 17 years of teaching and research experience in the fields of molecular diagnostics, natural product and nanoparticles research. To his credit, he has published more than 30 research and review publications in peer- reviewed international and national journals.

Preface

Herbal medicines are the most suitable and safe to be used as an alternative medicine compared to the synthetic drugs. Since the time immemorial, plants have significantly improved the survival rate of humans. More than 25 % of the currently available modern drugs are being derived from the traditionally documented medicinal plants. Typically, all rich traditional medicinal practices such as Ayurveda, Kampo, Traditional Chinese Medicine, and Unani rely upon plant products. In recent times, herbal medicines are highly valued due to their wide ranging pharmacological activities, safety, and low cost, adding to their high demand. This has led to the overexploitation of medicinal plants, and lead to the extinction of some species. Hence, adopting novel strategies, including plant cell, tissue and organ culture, and other biotechnological approaches are highly preferred for producing major plant bioactive compounds without cultivation. Some of the majorly recognized and isolated phytocompounds include rosmarinic acid, curcumin, resveratrol, catechin, taxol, podophyllotoxins, camptothecin, vinblastine, vincristine, etc. With the proper knowledge and exploration of these isolated molecules could provide an alternative source to reduce health risks. Further, a detailed understanding of the plant sources, occurrence in different plant organs, chemistry, and pharmacological activities of phytocompounds will certainly benefit researchers to develop novel drug leads. The enlightenment of molecular mechanisms of the biosynthesis of bioactive molecules and their biological actions provides an overview to understand and apply in medicinal uses including targeted drug therapies. Natural products research has become a trusted area among scientists aimed towards understanding the chemistry, analytical methodologies, biosynthetic mechanisms, and pharmacological activities of several phytocompounds.

Phytocompounds: Sources and Bioactivities, is a very timely effort in this direction. This book with 13 chapters discusses about various types of medicinal plants and their bioactive compounds with pharmacological properties. We hope that this book will be helpful for graduate students, teachers, researchers and industry persons who are functioning in the fields of natural product chemistry, drug discovery, pharmacology, health care, and medicinal plant research.

We are highly grateful to all our contributors for readily accepting our invitation and sharing their knowledge to compose the chapters, enduring editorial suggestions to finally produce this interesting book. We greatly appreciate their commitment. We are also thankful to Prof. Uma Rani Sinniah for her suggestions and writing the foreword for this volume. We, also thank the team of Studium Press (India) Pvt. Ltd, and special thanks to Prof. J.N. Govil for generous support and cooperation at every stage in the publication of this book.

We express our respect to our family members for understanding the importance of the work during preparation of this book and extending extra time for this work. We, thank our workmates, well wishers and friends for their direct or indirect cooperation during the preparation this book.

Bengaluru, Karnataka
India

Mallappa Kumara Swamy
Gudepalya Renukaiah Rudramurthy

Table of Contents

1

Flavones Combat Cancer *via* Multidimensional Molecular Approaches

RITU RAINA[1] AND ARIF HUSSAIN[1]*

ABSTRACT

Carcinogenesis is a multistep, multiple-stage process that includes a sequence of events including genomic and epigenetic alterations leading to the development of cancers. Chemoprevention refers to the use of natural, synthetic or biological compounds or their combinations to disturb the progression of cancer development. Chemoprevention by an increased ingesting of vegetables and fruits is the most encouraged and affordable strategy to prevent and decrease the incidence of cancer. Flavonoids are the natural polyphenols that are ubiquitously found in plant-derived foodstuffs, such as vegetables and fruits. Over the last few decades, more than 10,000 flavonoids occurring in plants have been identified and characterized. They are comprised of numerous subclasses including flavonols, flavan-3-ols, flavones, flavanones, isoflavones anthocyanins, and proanthocyanidins. Flavones such as apigenin, luteolin, baicalein, chrysin have shown their chemopreventive outcome by targeting various hallmarks of cancer due to their ability to modulate multiple key proteins which are involved in the regulation of cellular proliferation, differentiation, apoptosis, signal transduction pathways, angiogenesis or metastasis and modulation of epigenetic alterations. However, their precise molecular mechanism is yet to be explored to use them for a better cancer treatment. The current knowledge on the function of flavones in cancer prevention can be used further to develop more effective treatment strategies.

[1] School of Life Sciences, Manipal Academy of Higher Education, Dubai, UAE
**Corresponding author*: E-mail: dr.arifhussain@yahoo.co.in

Key words: Luteolin, Chrysin, Cancer hallmarks, Anticancer, Chemoprevention.

1. INTRODUCTION

Cancer is a multistep, multifactorial disease which is caused due to the buildup of epigenetic and genetic alterations within a cell that leads to a gradual abnormal cellular appearance, altered cell growth, and finally, the formation of carcinoma (Busch *et al.*, 2015). The multistep nature of carcinogenesis expedites a strong basis for cancer prevention as a potential therapeutic approach to arrest, reverse or block the carcinogenesis. The dietary agents mediated chemoprevention approach is one such strategy in cancer prevention and treatment which acts by targeting various molecular events involved in cancer, thereby significantly decrease the incidence and mortality of cancer. Many scientific reports indicate that the regular consumption of fruits and vegetables has the ability to inhibit the process of cancer progression and development. This anticancer potential of dietary agents is mediated by some valuable chemical constituents present in them. For instance, polyphenols are found in various fruits and vegetables in a significant amount (Nema *et al.*, 2015; Hoensch and Ortel, 2015). Most polyphenols such as curcumin, genistein, resveratrol, apigenin, fiesten, luteolin, etc., have shown their anti-neoplastic action through inducing apoptosis, inhibition of cell proliferation, evading metastases and angiogenesis, and the modulatory action on cell signaling pathways (Shukla *et al.*, 2013; Nema *et al.*, 2015; Shi *et al.*, 2015; Koosha *et al.*, 2016; Souza *et al.*, 2017) in various type of cancers. Hence, their therapeutic potential are gaining more interest in recent times for the development of a better cancer treatment regimen.

Flavonoids, a subclass of polyphenols are ubiquitously present in fruits and vegetables, and other plant derived sources. They are considered as potential chemo-preventive agents due to their better availability, cheaper price and higher specificity against cancer cells as compared to the traditional cancer treatment regime (Sak *et al.*, 2014; Kasala *et al.*, 2015; Hoensch and Oertel, 2015; Nema *et al.*, 2015; Shankar *et al.*, 2017; Souza *et al.*, 2017). Study reports have indicated that flavonoids, such as apigenin, fisetin, luteolin, etc., have a profound modulatory effect on various cancer cells, and they act by targeting various molecular targets. Many studies have shown their ability to modulate the abnormal behavior of the cancer cells and sensitize them to cell death and reverse the deregulation of cell cycle, cause cell cycle arrest at G1/S phase or G2/M phase, exert anti-proliferative activity by modulating different cell-signaling pathways like as PI3K/AKT/m TOR pathway, Nf-kB pathway, and JAK/STAT pathway (Fig. 2 and 3)

(Shukla *et al.*, 2013; Shehzad *et al.*, 2016; Koosha *et al.*, 2016; Tuorkey, 2016). So, flavonoids are being studied extensively for their preventive cancer properties (Nema *et al.*, 2015). Flavonoids have a basic 15-carbon phenylpropanoid core (C6-C3-C6 system), and can be further sub-grouped, into several groups like flavanones, flavones, isoflavones, 3-deoxy flavonoids, flavonols and anthocyanins (Hoensch and Oertel, 2015; Jiang *et al.*, 2016; Koosha *et al.*, 2016; Souza *et al.*, 2017; George *et al.*, 2017).

Scientific studies suggest that flavones have an enormous potential in the prevention and treatment of cancer as they act as antioxidative, antiproliferative, pro-apoptotic, cell cycle regulators and epigenetic modifiers. This chapter describes in detail the scientific investigations, supporting these studies.

2. SOURCES OF FLAVONES, THEIR CHEMICAL STRUCTURES AND ANTICANCER ACTIVITIES IN ANIMAL MODELS

Flavones such as apigenin, chrysin, tangeretin, luteolin, baicalein, nobiletin are derived from various plants or plant's parts (fruits, vegetables, leaves, roots, etc.), and have gained scientific and public interest for their chemo-preventive potential in cancer treatment (Khoo *et al.*, 2010; Jiang *et al.*, 2016; Koosha *et al.*, 2016; Sung *et al.*, 2016; Souza *et al.*, 2017). Some of the major flavones chemical structures are shown in the Fig. 1. Flavones have shown to act at all stages of cancer development by up-or down-regulating the multiple key proteins involved in the modulation of cellular proliferation, differentiation, programmed cell death, different signal transduction pathways, angiogenesis or metastasis, hence targeting various hallmarks of cancer (Nema *et al.*, 2015) (Figs. 2 and 3). The major flavones exhibiting anticancer activities and their mode of action are discussed in the following sections.

2.1. Apigenin

Apigenin is a major flavonoid with a chemical formula of $C_{15}H_{10}O_5$ and a molecular weight of 270.236 g/mol. It is present profusely in a variety of natural sources, like fruits, vegetables, green teas etc. It is found in parsley, celery, onions, oranges, oregano, chamomile, artichoke, and vine spinach (Sung *et al.*, 2016; Souza *et al.*, 2017). Both in cell lines and in animal models apigenin has demonstrated diminution of cancer cell proliferation in a variety of human cancers, like ovarian, prostate, colon, lung, breast, and leukemia by the modulation of different cell survival pathways (Souza *et al.*, 2017).

The chemopreventive effect of apigenin has been discovered in at least a dozen *in vivo* studies. Apigenin (20 and 50 μg/mice), when given orally for

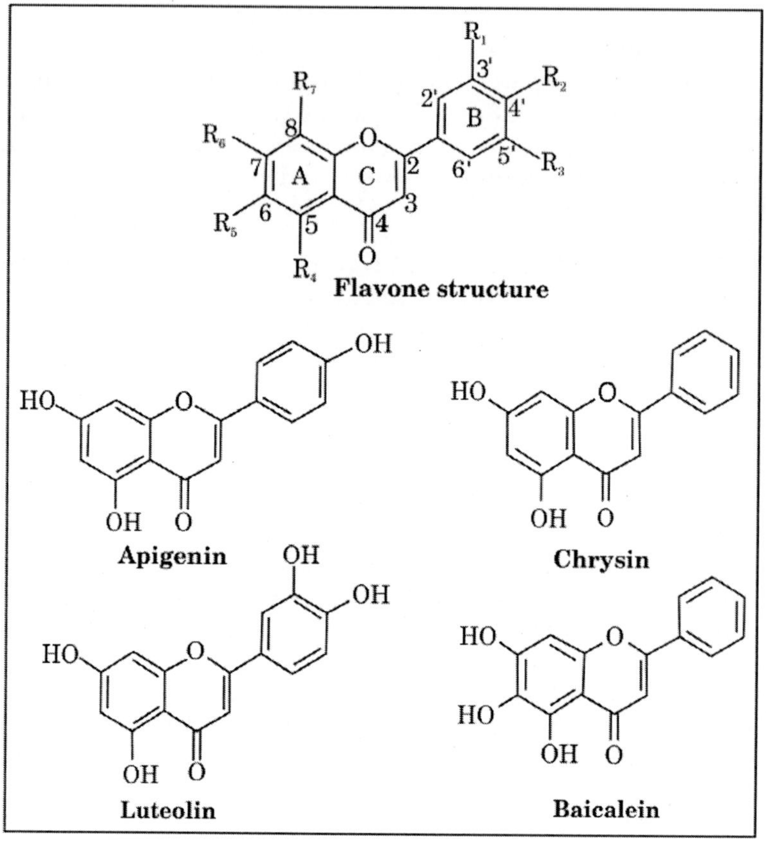

Fig. 1: Chemical Structure of Flavones.

20 weeks decreased tumor volumes and completely abolished the prostate adenocarcinoma in a mouse (TRAMP) model by inhibiting the (PI3K)/Akt/ Forkhead box O-signaling pathway and inhibited angiogenesis and metastasis by the inhibition of insulin-like growth factor (IGF)-I/IGF binding protein-3 signaling pathway (Khoo *et al.*, 2010; Zhang *et al.*, 2016). In addition, apigenin (2.5 mg/kg) when given orally for 20 weeks in hamsters reduced 2,4-Dimethoxybenzaldehyde (DMBA) induced tumor volume in oral carcinogenesis (Sung *et al.*, 2016).

2.2. Chrysin

Chrysin is a naturally occurring flavonoid belongs to apigenin family with a chemical formula of $C_{15}H_{10}O_4$ and a molecular weight of 254.241 g/mol. Chrysin, also known as 5, 7-dihydroxyflavone is found in many plants species, propolis (or bee resin) and in honey. At present, chrysin is commercially available in the form of capsules as a dietary supplement for increasing the

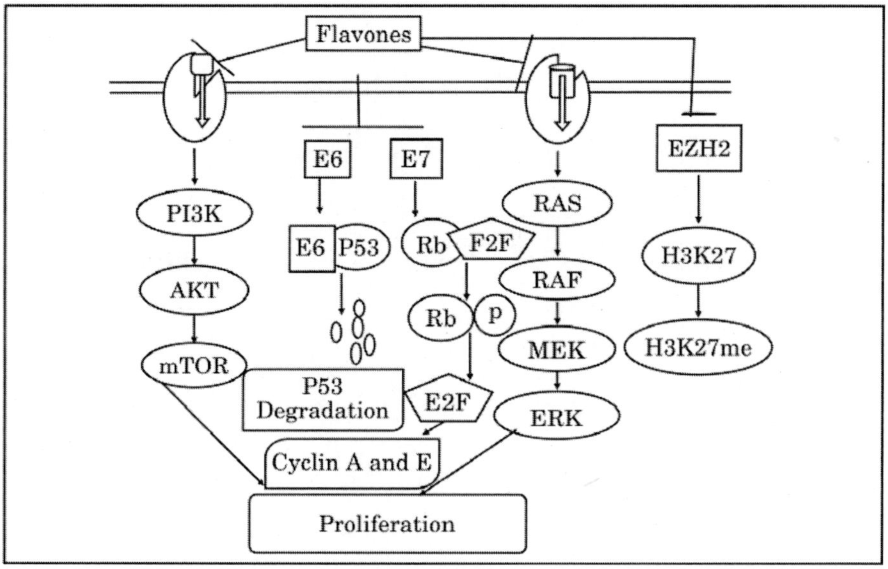

Fig. 2: Flavones act through various molecular targets.

lean body mass, and as a testosterone uplifting agent. It has been reported to have anti-bacterial, anti-oxidant, anti-allergic, anti-inflammatory and anti-cancer action (Kasala *et al.*, 2015; Zhang *et al.,* 2016; Chyliñska-Wrzos *et al.,* 2017). *In vivo* evaluation of chrysin has shown its chemopreventive effects in male rats with colonic cancer induced by azoxymethane (AOM) as well as in wistar rats by induction of DNA Fragmentation and apoptosis and inhibition of COX-2 and NF-IL-6 (Koosha *et al.*, 2016).

2.3. Luteolin

Luteolin (3,4,5,7-tetrahydroxy flavone) is yellow crystalline, solid in pure form has a molecular weight of 286.24g/mol, and a chemical formula of $C_{15}H_{10}O_6$. It is found in vegetables like parsley, carrots, artichoke, onion, broccoli, celery, green pepper several spices like thyme, oregano (Attoub *et al.,* 2011; Ham *et al.*, 2014; Tuorkey, 2016). Interestingly, Koosha and coworkers have demonstrated that luteolin to exhibit anti-cancer effect in BALB/c mice by modulating COX2, MMP2 and MMP9 (Koosha *et al.,* 2016).

2.4. Baicalein

Baicalein is a flavone with a chemical formula of $C_{15}H_{10}O_5$ and a molecular weight of 270.24 g/mol. It is present in the root extracts of the plant, *Scutellaria baicalensis* and is used in the Chinese medicine as a bioactive

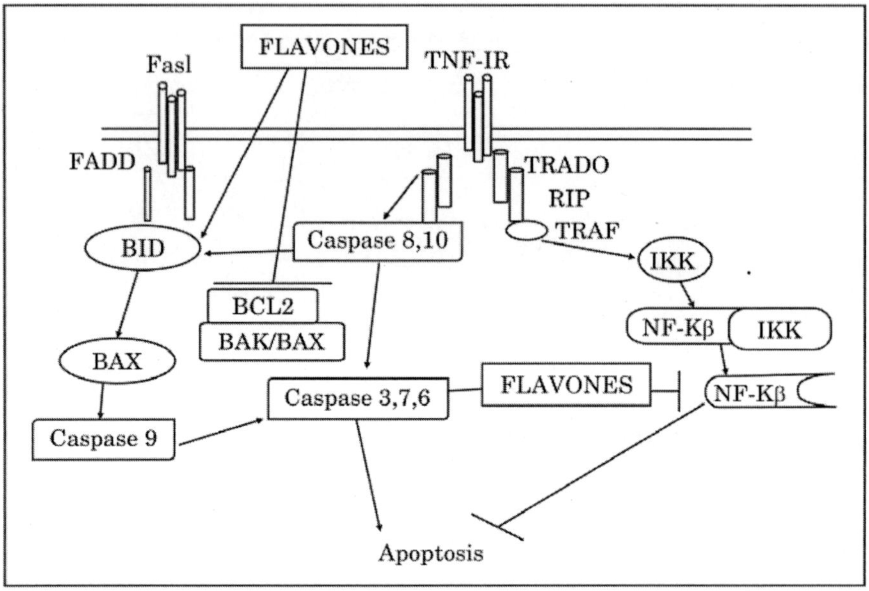

Fig. 3: Flavones induce apoptosis.

agent. Numerous studies have reported that baicalein possess numerous biological functions like anti-oxidant, anti-pyretic, anti-viral, anti-inflammatory and antitumor properties (Koosha *et al.*, 2016; Liu *et al.*, 2016). Also, its chemopreventive effect has been documented in AOM induced cancer in mice by inhibiting PI3K/Akt, iNOS, NFkB; increasing caspase-3 and -8; attenuating Bcl-2 and MMP-2 and -9; inducing Bax.

3. FLAVONES DETER CELL GROWTH IN HUMAN CANCERS

Cancer is marked by an uncontrolled proliferation of cells and accumulation of cells due to the disruption of balance between the rate of cell death and rate of cell proliferation. *In vitro* and *in vivo* studies have shown that flavones, such as apigenin, chrysin, luteolin, baicalein, exhibit a strong growth inhibitory action towards the tumor growth and development.

3.1. Apigenin

Apigenin has revealed a selective time-and dose-dependent cytotoxic effect in all HPV16 and HPV18 cervical cancer cell lines, such as HeLa, CaSki, C33A and SiHa, but not in HaCaT (Immortalized nontumorigenic human epidermal cell line) (Souza *et al.,* 2017). Several studies have demonstrated the inhibition of cell multiplication and initiation of apoptosis, and autophagy by apigenin (Sung *et al.,* 2016; Souza *et al.*, 2017). Apigenin is the inhibitor of casein kinase 2 (a serine/threonine-selective protein kinase) that regulates the proliferation and NFkβ activation in glioma cells (George *et al.,* 2017). It has shown anti-cancer effect on various colon, prostate and bladder cancer cells, like HT-29, HCT-116, CaCo-2, SW480, HT1376, T24, PC-3 cells in time-and dose-dependent manner by the modulation of different molecular targets (Shi *et al.,* 2015; Koosha *et al.,* 2016; Shankar *et al.,* 2017). Apigenin prevents the phosphorylation of Akt/PKB by stimulating binding of FoxO3a to p27/Kip1, thereby improving its apoptotic ability, and inhibiting the proliferation in human prostate cancer cells (PC-3 and LNCaP) and the transgenic adenocarcinoma of the mouse prostate (TRAMP) model (Shukla *et al.,* 2013).

3.2. Chrysin

Chrysin inhibits the proliferation of many types of cancer cells tested including leukemia, gastric carcinoma (NCI-N87), colon carcinoma HCT-116 and SW480), and esophageal squamous cancer (KYSE-30) cells (Chyliñska-Wrzos *et al.,* 2017). Zhang *et al.* (2016) reported that chrysin can suppress the cell multiplication and trigger apoptosis against HeLa cancer cells, and also inhibited various colon cancer cells like LoVo, HT-5 5 and HCA-7 cell lines with IC_{50} values of 0.8 mM, for Lovo and 0.4 mM for the other two cancer cells. In addition, DNA synthesis within the cells was also inhibited, and the IC_{50} values were found to be 1.8, 2.5, and 4.2 mM for LoVo cells, HT-55 and HCA-7 respectively (Zhang *et al.,* 2016), and it was shown to considerably repress a primary ovarian cancer (Caov-3) cells multiplication (Wang *et al.,* 2015; Koosha *et al.*, 2016). The cell viability of cancer cell lines like HCT116, DLD1, SW837 diminished with the exposure of chrysin at 100 µM and 50 µM concentrations (Chyliñska-Wrzos *et al.,* 2017). The activity of chrysin may be improved by combining it with other flavonoids or by altering its chemical structure. Chrysin inhibited HeLa cells with an IC_{50} of 14.2 µM and U937 cells with an IC_{50} of 16 µM. While, breast carcinoma cells (MDA-MB-231), glioma cells (U87-MG and U-251), and prostate cancer cells (PC3) were inhibited at an IC_{50} of 100 µM. A human esophageal squamous cell carcinoma cell line, KYSE-510 was inhibited with an IC_{50} value of 63 µM (Khoo *et al.*. 2010). Likewise, it has been reported that a combination of apigenin and chrysin could decrease cell multiplication and cell invasion effectively in MDA-MB-231 and HepG2 when compared to free chrysin (Chyliñska-Wrzos *et al.,* 2017). Also, chrysin nanoparticles and pure chrysin inhibited two human breast cancer cell lines; MCF7 and T47D (Anari *et al.*, 2015). It was also found that nanochrysin upregulated BRCA1 gene expression and down regulated the hTERT and FTO genes in the T47D cell line (Chyliñska-Wrzos *et al.,* 2017).

3.3. Luteolin

Luteolin has shown cytotoxicity towards all colon cancer cells (COLO-320DM, HT-29, CaCo-2, and HCT-15) that were evaluated (Koosha *et al.,* 2016). The doses of luteolin ranging between 25 and 200 μM have shown a significacnt cytotoxicity towards various breast (MDA-MB231, MDA-1833, and MCF7/6), lung (LNM35), colon (HT29), and liver (HepG2) cancer cell lines (Attoub *et al.,* 2011). Luteolin has the potent activity against cancers, inflammation, and oxidation, and it can reverse multidrug resistance (MDR) in many types of cancer cells (Park *et al.,* 2012; Ou *et al.,* 2013; Chen *et al.,* 2014; Jeon *et al.,* 2014; Khan *et al.,* 2014; Tuorkey, 2016). Luteolin acts as a strong anticancer agent against many types of malignancies including breast, squamous carcinoma, esophageal, lung, colon, liver and prostate cancers, and it exhibits antiproliferative, antioxidative and anti-inflammatory properties (Pandurangan and Esa, 2014). According to them, luteolin induces apoptosis in colon cancer cells by modulating the expressions of Bcl-2, Bax, and caspase 3 (Pandurangan and Esa, 2014). Luteolin activated death receptors, Fas and FADD in HeLa cells by repressing E6 expression (Ham *et al.,* 2014). Various researchers have reported that in HT-29 colon cancer cells, luteolin induces apoptosis by activating caspase 3 pathway. Luteolin showed cytotoxicity towards A549 lung adenocarcinoma cells through pro-apoptotic and anti-migration effects. The cytotoxicity was observed to be in a time- and dose-dependent manner (Meng *et al.,* 2016).

3.4. Baicalein

Baicalein inhibited various cancers like hepatic, pancreatic, breast, bladder, and colorectal cancer by interacting with various molecular targets. The anticancer activities of baicalein are attributed to its capacity to inhibit MAPK, (Akt), MMP2/MMP9 and activating caspases 3/9 (Liu *et al.,* 2016). It suppressed the proliferation and invasion of breast cancer cell line MDA-MB-231 in *vitro* and *in vivo* by inhibition of EMT *via* down regulation of SATB1 and Wnt/β-catenin pathway (Ma *et al.,* 2016).

4. FLAVONES INHIBIT HUMAN CANCERS *VIA* INDUCING APOPTOSIS

Cancer cells show resistance to cell death and initiation of self-programmed death, and these are the key targets of cancer chemopreventive agents. All flavones like apegenin, luteolin, chrysin, and baicalein have shown cytotoxic effect by inducing apoptosis in various cancer cell lines and animal models.

4.1. Apigenin

Apigenein induces cancer cell death *via* apoptosis, which was triggered by the mitochondrial redox impairment in different cervical cancer cell lines. In all cervical cell lines (HeLa, SiHa, CaSki, and C33A), apigenin considerably amplified the production of reactive oxygen species leading to the induction of cancer cell death. However, the total ROS production was not changed in the HaCaT cells after exposure to apigenin (Souza *et al.,* 2017a). Both *in vitro* and *in vivo* studies have reported the chemopreventive characteristics of apigenin. Its mechanisms of action is by inducing a p53-dependent pathway, which is the most documented pathway for the stimulation of apoptosis and arresting of cell cycle (Sung *et al.,* 2016). In colon adenocarcinoma (SW480) cells, apigenin increased the expression of caspases and Bax, and inhibited Bcl-2 expression (Koosha *et al.,* 2016). Treatment of T-24 (bladder carcinoma) cells with 20- 30 μg/ml of apegenin activated the mitochondrial apoptotic pathway which is marked by the activation of Bax, PARP, and caspases, and downregulation of Bcl-2 and release of cytochrome C (Shi *et al.* 2015).

4.2. Chrysin

Chrysin has demonstrated anti-oxidant and anti-inflammatory effects, and has shown cancer chemopreventive action *via* initiation of apoptosis by modifying pro- and anti-apoptotic proteins in different types of cancers. Chrysin induced apoptosis in most of the cancer cells tested, and it may proceed *via* different pathways. For instance, in C6 glioma cells, it was due to the increase of p21WAF/CIP1 expression and not p53 expression, while it inhibited leukemic U937 cell lines through AKT inactivation and caspase stimulation mediated apoptosis (Khoo *et al.,* 2010: Zhang *et al.,* 2016). In HCT116 cells, chrysin induced apoptosis by mitochondrial pathway that is marked by upregulation of BID, Bax, and caspase-3 and down-regulation of Bcl-2 (Chyliñska-Wrzos *et al.,* 2017). Chrysin activated TNF pathway in different cell lines like lung (A549), rectal (SW837), and colon (DLD1, and HCT116) cancer cells by the activation of TNFα and TNFβ gene expressions (Chyliñska-Wrzos *et al.,* 2017). Chrysin prompted Caov-3 cells apoptosis after 48 h treatment by upregulating PARP and caspases (Wang *et al.,* 2015). Gamut reports indicate that combination of chrysin with different chemotherapeutic drugs decreased the toxicity of the drugs and increased the effectiveness of the drugs — like combination of chrysin and cisplatin was found to be highly toxic to cancer cells like Hep-G2 which is mediated by the activation of pro-apoptotic proteins, such as P53, Bax, caspases 8, 9, DR5, and inactivation of Bcl 2 also combination of chrysin with DOX decreased the IC50 values of DOX in different cell lines likes 78% in H460, 47% in H157 and H1975 cells and 43% in A549 cells ,indicating that chrysin worked synergistically with DOX to induce cancer cell death. Interestingly in A549 cells, the combination of chrysin and docetaxel (DTX) increased the induction of apoptosis by DTX, and diminished the toxicity of DTX (Chyliñska-Wrzos *et al.,* 2017).

4.3. Luteolin

Luteolin can induce apoptosis by both pathways, namely intrinsic and extrinsic in numerous cancer cell lines, and thus activates the expression of caspases 3, 7, 8, tumor related apoptosis inducing ligand (TRAIL), death receptors, such as DR4, DR5, and Fas/FasL, and cause inequity of the Bax/Bcl-xl ratio (Ham *et al.*, 2014; Koosha *et al.,* 2016). It inhibits NF-βB thus activating TNF-α-induced apoptosis, The mechanism of action most probably is that luteolin induces production of reactive oxygen species leading to TNF-α-induced apoptosis. Reactive oxygen species generated by luteolin also activates AMPK, AMPK is a novel regulator of NFkB in luteolin-induced cancer cell death, luteolin induces apoptosis in human non-small-cell lung cancer A549cells by phosphorylating JNK, activating the mitochondrial pathways of apoptosis while inhibiting NF-κB translocation. Another mechanism of luteolin's induction of apoptosis is by accumulation and stabilizing p53 luteolin enhanced p53 expression in two cell lines CO115 an HCT15. Same was observed in animal models, it stimulated p53 production leading to enhanced cisplatin activity and reduced cytotoxicity caused by cisplatin in nude mouse xenograft model, (Tuorkey, 2016). Luteolin induces apoptosis in a variety of cancer cells like A549, MCF-7/6, AGS, LNM35, and MDA-MB231-1833 (Attoub *et al.,* 2011). Luteolin exerts anti-carcinogenic activity in HeLa cells by inhibiting the expression of E6 and E7, and thus causing inactivation of HPV-18 oncogene and activating caspases (Ham *et al.,* 2014). In lung adenocarcinoma (A549) cells, luteolin prompted apoptosis by down regulating Bcl-2, activating caspases 3, 9 and Bax expression (Meng *et al.,* 2016). Combination of luteolin with various chemotherapeutic drugs has helped in overcoming multi drug resistance in various cell lines. Luteolin inhibits Nrf2 pathway in oxaliplatin resistant cell lines and *in vivo* in non-small-cell lung cancer. Luteolin and paclitaxel activated caspase-8 and -3 and increased expression of Fas by blocking STAT3 thus luteolin can be used in combination with chemotherapeutic to enhance their therapeutic effect and decrease toxicity caused by the conventional drugs.

4.4. Baicalein

In MDA-MB-231 cells, baicalein (25–100 μM) induced apoptosis by activating caspase-9/-3 (Liu *et al.*, 2016). In HeLa, T4, and U14 cervical cancer cells, baicalein inducts cell death by increasing the expression of Bax, caspases and FasL Bcl-2 proteins, and decreasing the expression of Bcl-2 (Peng *et al.,*

2015; Liu *et al.,* 2016). Similar results were indicated in HT-29 and gastric cell line, SGC-7901. In addition, DNA fragmentation was also reported in these cell lines. *In vivo* studies in HT-29 colon tumor xenografts proved the same while in HCT116 cells, the activation of caspases was observed (Liu *et al.,* 2016). Another study in MDA-MB-231 stated that baicalein considerably diminished the expression of SATB1, SNAIL and vimentin Wnt1 and β-catenin proteins, while augmenting the expression of E-cadherin (Ma *et al.,* 2016). In pancreatic cancer (PaCa) cells, baicalein augmented the ratio of Bax/Bcl2 ratio, stimulated mitochondrial cytochrome c release, and upregulated caspases 3, 7, 9. The above results were conûrmed by *in vivo* results as well, where baicalein repressed tumor growth in human pancreatic cancer (HPAC) cell lines and mice xenograft models, while Mcl-1, a member of Bcl2 family was down regulated (Liu *et al.,* 2016). Baicalein suppressed the expression of NF-κB, c-Myc, VEGF, and, HIF-1α in ovarian cancer cell lines (OVCAR_3 and CP-70), and however, no effect was seen in the normal ovarian cell lines (IOSE-364). Baicalein decreased the expression MMP-2 and repressed the stimulation of a p-38 MAPK-dependent NF-κB signaling pathway (Liu *et al.,* 2016).

5. FLAVONES INHIBIT HUMAN CANCERS *VIA* CELL CYCLE ARREST

A regulatory process that stops progress through the cell cycle during one of the normal phases (G1, S, G2, and M). The biochemical pathways that restrain cell cycle transition and/or induce cell death after stress are known as cell cycle checkpoints. Cyclins and cyclin-dependent kinases control cell cycle progression through the different stages like G1, S, G2, and M. DNA damage can arrest cells in G2 before progressing to mitosis, and in G2, the cell can undergo DNA repair mechanisms or apoptosis similarly during G1. In cancer all the regulatory genes are inactivated leading to uncontrolled proliferation and flavones activate these genes leading to cell cycle arrest.

5.1. Apigenin

Apigenin causes apoptosis by activating p53 in various cancer cell lines, such as colorectal, oral, hepatic and pancreatic cancers. It caused cell cycle arrest at G1 phase by modulating cdk2 kinases in T4 bladder cancer cells (Sung *et al.*, 2016; George *et al.,* 2017). Apigenin caused the arrest of LNCaP cells in G0-G1 cell cycle phase, and completely arrested at G2/M phase (Shukla *et al.,* 2013). Moreover, apigenin suppressed aflatoxin B1 and CDK4 and increased p53, p21 in hepatocellular carcinoma leading to cell cycle arrest (Souza *et al.,* 2017). Apigenin upregulated p21 and p53 and downregulated cyclin B1, Cdc-25 and Cdc-2 in HCT-116 cells (Koosha *et al.,*

2016). In T24 cells, 20-40 µg/ml of apigenin increased the number of cells in sub G1 and there was a reduction of cells in G2/M, and 30 µg/ml of apigenin reduced all the cyclins, Cdc2, Cdc25 proteins (Shi *et al.,* 2015).

5.2. Chrysin

In esophageal cell line, KYSE-510, G2/M cell cycle arrest and apoptosis was induced by chrysin (80 µM) mediated by p21 upregulation, downregulation of cyclinB1, whereas the combination of chrysin and apigenin doubled cells in G2/M phase in SW480 cells (Khoo *et al.,* 2010).

5.3. Luteolin

Luteolin exerts cell cycle arrest in various cell lines by inhibiting the expression of Cyclins A, B1, CDC2, CDK2, AKT, Bcl-xL, Bcl-2, and upregulatees increased expression of caspases, Bax, and p21, and further inhibits NFkβ, thus activating TNFα induced apoptosis (Tuorkey, 2016). In HT-29 cells, luteolin arrests cells by inhibiting cyclin D and CDK2. It causes G2/M arrest in CaCo-2 and SW480 cells (Koosha *et al.*, 2016). Luteolin effectively increased the sub-G1 (apoptotic) fraction of cells through caspase-3 and -7 dependent pathways. Luteolin arrests G0/G1 cell cycle growth in neuroblastoma (SH-SY5Y) cell line (Attoub *et al.,* 2011; Tuorkey 2016). In HeLa cells, it inhibited the E6 and E7 oncogenes leading to the activation of tumor suppressors, p53 and Rb, that further excited cyclin-dependent kinase inhibitor p21 and inhibit E2F, respectively. In addition, it downregulated E2F5, which stimulates the cell cycle by activating E7 (Ham *et al.,* 2014). Luteolin inhibits the phosphorylation of histone H3 Ser10 by VRK1 and induces chromatin condensation at the G2/M phase (Ham *et al.,* 2014).

5.4. Baicalein

Baicalein induced cell cycle arrest at the G1 phase in H-29 cells (Koosha *et al.,* 2016), and also inhibited complexes of cyclins and cyclin-dependent kinases (CDKs) to regulate the cell cycle (Liu *et al.,* 2016) leading to G1/S phase arrest in T4 bladder cells, G1 arrest in HT-29 cells, S phase arrest in HCT-116 and SGS-7901 gastric cell lines, which is all related to its ability to diminish protein levels of cyclin B1 and cyclin D1 (Liu *et al.*, 2016).

6. FLAVONES INHIBIT HUMAN CANCERS *VIA* TARGETING CELL SURVIVAL SIGNALS

Cell signaling pathways like PI3K/AKT/mTOR, MAPK, and RAS-RAF pathways are seen to be upregulated in cancer. These pathways are responsible for the cell survival. Various dietary agents including flavones have shown their inhibitory effects on these signaling pathways in various ways.

6.1. Apigenin

Apigenin hinders PI3K and MAPK pathways in prostate cancer by downregulating insulin-like growth factor 1 (IGF-1) (Souza *et al.,* 2017). Apegenin induced the expression of p38 and ERK in MAPK pathway and decreased expression of AKT/mTOR in HT-29 adenocarcinoma (Koosha *et al.,* 2016) and is a potent inhibitor of PI3K-Akt, mitogen-activated protein kinases (c-Jun, ERK1/2, and p38), focal adhesion kinase and caein kinase-2 (Shukla *et al.*, 2013). Apigenin suppressed prostate cancer by PI3K/Akt/FoxO-signaling pathway (Shukla *et al.*, 2013) and can also stimulate notch 1 signaling (Chyliñska-Wrzos *et al.,* 2017).

6.2. Chrysin

Chrysin shows clampdown of the ERK/c-Fos and JNK/c-Jun signaling pathways in AGS gastric cancer cells (Chyliñska-Wrzos *et al.,* 2017), and it repressed p-mTOR, p-4EBP1 and p-AKT expression in Caov-3 cells in time and dose-dependent manner (Wang *et al.,* 2015).

6.3. Luteolin

Luteolin inhibited Wnt/β-catenin pathway in an invasive colon cancer cells, HCT-15, and PI3K/Akt, and ERK pathways in HT-29 cell lines (Pandurangan and Esa, 2014; Koosha *et al.,* 2016). It also repressed Raf and PI3K activities, and reduced the phosphorylation of MEK and Akt (Kim *et al.,* 2013; Tuorkey, 2016). Luteolin, at lower concentrations suppressed the metastatic potential of various cell lines like MDA-MB231-1833, MCF-7/6 and LNM35 cancer cells (Attoub *et al.*, 2011). Luteolin arrested the growth of colon cancer cells by downregulating the expression of Wnt/β-catenin/GSK-3β signaling (Pandurangan *et al.,* 2013). The Wnt/β-catenin/GSK-3β signaling was also inhibited *in vivo* studies (Pandurangan *et al.,* 2013; Pandurangan and Esa, 2014; Tuorkey 2016).

6.4. Baicalein

Baicalein has been observed to attenuate MAPK/AKT/mTOR signaling pathways in both *in vitro* and *in vivo* models. Its mechanism of action is attributed to the upregulation of DNA-damage-inducible transcript 4 (DDIT4) expression, which mediated the inhibition of mTOR in a breast cancer mouse model, and HT-29 cells. Because of its action on various pathways, baicaelin is been considered as a promising chemopreventive agent (Koosha *et al.,* 2016; Liu *et al.,* 2016).

7. FLAVONES INHIBIT HUMAN CANCERS *VIA* TUMOR CELL INVASION AND METASTASIS

7.1. Apigenin

Apigenin is being reported to inhibit tumor cell invasion and metastasis in different cancer cell lines. The greatest reduction in the basal migratory ability by apigenin was found to be highest for HeLa cells, followed by C33A, SiHa, and CaSki cells. For the C33A and HeLa cells, apigenin significantly inhibited cell migration (Koosha *et al.,* 2016; Souza *et al.*, 2017), and also inhibited hypoxia induced EMT by suppressing β1 and FAK phosphorylation (Tuorkey, 2016). *In vivo* studies have reported the same, and anticipated that oral administration of 20 and 50 mg/mice for 20 weeks reduced tumor volumes, and suppressed the metastasis. The complete prevention of organ metastasis was observed *in vivo* model of prostate cancer (TRAMP model), and this effect was credited to the inactivation of (PI3K)/Akt/Forkhead box O-signaling pathway (Shukla *et al.*, 2013; Sung *et al.,* 2016).

7.2. Chrysin

In MDA-MB-231 and BT-549 breast cell lines, chrysin inhibited the metastasis and cell invasion by suppressing the expression of MMP10, vimentin, snail and slug, and down-regulating E-cadherin expression (Chyliñska-Wrzos *et al.,* 2017). The co-treatment of chrysin with apigenin for 36 hrs in MDA-MB-231 cells showed a reduced cell migration. It was also reported that in AGS gastric cancer cells, chrysin inhibits ERK/c-Fos and JNK/c-Jun pathways that suppress MMP-9, thus controlling the cell invasiveness (Chyliñska-Wrzos *et al.,* 2017). *In vivo* models of colon cancer have shown the anti-metastatic effect of chrysin by decreasing the expression of MMP9 and MMP-2 as well as COX-2 and i-NOS (Pandurangan and Esa, 2014; Koosha *et al.*, 2016).

7.3. Luteolin

Luteolin showed anti-metastatic effect in breast cancer cell lines, MDA-MB-231 and 4175. Even 10 μM of luteolin inhibited VEGF factor, significantly. VEGF is a potent angiogenic and cell survival factor. Luteolin inhibited VEGF and Vasculogenic mimicry (VM) in gastric cancers (Cook *et al.,* 2017). Luteolin suppressed the expression of mdm2 and prevented the invasion of prostate cancer (PC3) cells by inhibiting mdm2 expression, and encouraged E-cadherin expression in prostate cancer cell line, PC3 (Zhou *et al.,* 2009). Whereas, in A549 cancer cells, luteolin inhibited PI3k, AKT, and NFkβ, Snail pathways, which down regulated the expression of E-cadherin, and inhibited the cell invasion and migration (Chen *et al.,* 2013; Tuorkey, 2016; Meng *et al.,* 2016). Luteolin induced pro apoptotic and anti-invasive effect by the phosphorylation of MEK, and its down-stream kinase, ERK (Pandurangan and Esa, 2014; Meng *et al.*, 2016).

7.4. Baicalein

Baicalein efficiently repressed the cell invasion and metastasis in various cell lines like MDA-MB-231 and colon cancer cells by downregulating MMP-9 and MMP-2, and suppressing AKT pathway (Shi *et al.,* 2015). *In vitro* migration assay has shown that baicalein inhibits the migration and invasion of gastric cancer cells by decreasing the expression of various molecules like vimentin, N-cadherin, ZEB1, and ZEB2, and thus inactivating TGF-β/ Smad4 pathway (Liu *et al.,* 2016). In another study, baicaelin prohibited the migration and invasion of MDA-MB-231 cells by downregulating the SATB1 and Wnt/β-catenin pathways to inhibit EMT, and also augmented the expression of E-cadherin and suppressed the expression of vimentin and Snails (a zinc finger transcription factor) (Ma *et al.,* 2016).

8. FLAVONES INHIBIT HUMAN CANCERS *VIA* EPIGENETIC MODULATION

Cancer is characterized by an aberrant epigenetic changes, and reversible nature of epigenetic changes makes it a promising target for cancer treatment and prevention. Methylation of promoter CpG islands and trimethylation of H3K27 leads to inactivation of various genes like GTSP1, TIMP, CDH1, RASSFIA, etc. Flavones have been shown to inhibit DNMTs and EZH2, and thus activating these genes (Kanwal *et al.,* 2016). Several studies have indicated that flavones like luteolin, apigenin, and chrysin inhibit DNMT activities, which was further evaluated and confirmed by molecular docking studies (Park *et al.*, 2017). Apigenin and luteolin inhibited 5-cytosine DNMT in KYSE 510 cells, and apigenin inhibited HDACs in PC3 cells, and in PC-3 xenograft model. Apigenin inhibited HDAC1 and HDAC3 at an oral dose of 20 or 50 mg/mouse for 8 weeks (Busch *et al.*, 2015; Ganai 2017). Chrysin is a histone deacetylase inhibitor, and can significantly inhibit the tumor growth (Chyliñska-Wrzos *et al.,* 2017). Luteolin significantly inhibits EZH2 and SUZ12 proteins in human prostate cancer (DU145 and 22Rv1) cells. Thus, it prevents the trimethylation of histone H3 lysine 27 (H3K27) and kills cancer cells. Molecular docking of luteolin with EZH2 showed that luteolin fitted into the catalytic site of EZH2 (Attoub *et al.*, 2011; Kanwal *et al.*, 2017). It is reported that luteolin behaves as a strong HDAC inhibitor in LNM35 cells and LNM35 tumor xenografts in athymic mice, and also it downregulated DNMT1 and caused global hypomethylation in HeLa cells (Krifa *et al.*, 2013). So, luteolin may be a promising HDAC inhibitor for cancer treatments (Attoub *et al.*, 2011; Tuorkey, 2016). Luteolin leads to an increased acetylation of H3 and causes upregulation of FAS/FASL and downregulation of c-jun expression and cell cycle regulatory molecules (Wang *et al.*, 2018).

9. CONCLUSIONS AND FUTURE PROSPECTS

Cancer is a multi-factorial, multi-step and multi-genetic process with several molecular alterations including epigenetic alterations. Most of the chemopreventive approaches against cancers are not effective and chemotherapy is associated with various adverse side effects in patients. Thus, there is a need to use bioactive compounds that are capable of targeting more than one pathway involved in cancer growth. In this regard, plant-derived phytochemicals including flavones are highly desirable as they posses high chemical diversity and exhibit superior anticancer activity with no or less side effects. Hence, they are highly preferred in the treatment of cancers in recent times.

The modulatory capabilities of various aberrant molecular pathways by flavones make them highly promising dietary chemopreventive and therapeutic agents. Further, *in vivo* and larger scale clinical trials are needed to use dietary flavones as a safe and effective anti-cancer strategy.

REFERENCES

Anari E, Akbarzadeh A, Zarghami N. Chrysin-loaded PLGA-PEG nanoparticles designed for enhanced effect on the breast cancer cell line. Artificial cells, Nanomedicine, and Biotechnology. 2016; 44(6): 1410-6.

Attoub S, Hassan AH, Vanhoecke B, Iratni R, Takahashi T, Gaben AM, Bracke M, Awad S, John A, Kamalboor HA and Al Sultan MA. Inhibition of cell survival, invasion, tumor growth and histone deacetylase activity by the dietary flavonoid luteolin in human epithelioid cancer cells. European Journal of Pharmacology. 2011; 651(1-3):18-25.

Busch C, Burkard M, Leischner C, Lauer UM, Frank J, Venturelli S. Epigenetic activities of flavonoids in the prevention and treatment of cancer. Clinical Epigenetics. 2015; 7(1):64.

Chyliñska-Wrzos P, Lis-Sochocka M, Jod³owska-Jêdrych B. Chrysin and its potential antineoplastic effect. European Journal of Biological Research. 2017; 7(3): 245-254.

Cook MT, Liang Y, Besch-Williford C, Hyder S. Luteolin inhibits metastasis of triple-negative breast cancer cells to the lungs. *In*: Proceedings of the American Association for Cancer Research Annual Meeting 2017; Apr 1-5; Washington, DC. Philadelphia

(PA): AACR; Cancer Res 2017; 77(13 Suppl): Abstract nr 4914. doi:10.1158/1538-7445.AM2017-4914

Ganai SA. Plant-derived flavone Apigenin: The small-molecule with promising activity against therapeutically resistant prostate cancer. Biomedicine and Pharmacotherapy. 2017; 85:47-56.

George VC, Dellaire G, Rupasinghe HV. Plant flavonoids in cancer chemoprevention: Role in genome stability. The Journal of Nutritional Biochemistry. 2017; 45:1-4.

Ham S, Kim KH, Kwon TH, Bak Y, Lee DH, Song YS, Park SH, Park YS, Kim MS, Kang JW, Hong JT. Luteolin induces intrinsic apoptosis *via* inhibition of E6/E7 oncogenes and activation of extrinsic and intrinsic signaling pathways in HPV-18-associated cells. Oncology Reports. 2014; 31(6):2683-91.

Hoensch HP, Oertel R. The value of flavonoids for the human nutrition: Short review and perspectives. Clinical Nutrition Experimental. 2015; 3:8-14.

Kanwal R, Datt M, Liu X, Gupta S. Dietary flavones as dual inhibitors of DNA methyltransferases and histone methyltransferases. PloS One. 2016; 11(9): e0162956.

Kanwal R, Yang X, Shankar E, Gupta S. Luteolin selectively inhibits EZH2 and blocks H3K27 methylation in prostate cancer cells. *In:* Proceedings of the American Association for Cancer Research Annual Meeting 2017; 2017 Apr 1-5; Washington, DC. Philadelphia (PA): AACR; Cancer Res 2017; 77(13 Suppl): Abstract nr 2230. doi:10.1158/1538-7445.AM2017-2230.

Kasala ER, Bodduluru LN, Madana RM, Gogoi R, Barua CC. Chemopreventive and therapeutic potential of chrysin in cancer: Mechanistic perspectives. Toxicology Letters. 2015; 233(2):214-25.

Khoo BY, Chua SL, Balaram P. Apoptotic effects of chrysin in human cancer cell lines. International Journal of Molecular Sciences. 2010; 11(5):2188-99.

Kim YS, Kim SH, Shin J, Harikishore A, Lim JK, Jung Y, Lyu HN, Baek NI, Choi KY, Yoon HS, Kim KT. Luteolin suppresses cancer cell proliferation by targeting vaccinia-related kinase 1. PloS One. 2014; 9(10): e109655.

Koosha S, Alshawsh MA, Looi CY, Seyedan A, Mohamed Z. An association map on the effect of flavonoids on the signaling pathways in colorectal cancer. International Journal of Medical Sciences. 2016; 13(5):374.

Krifa M, Alhosin M, Muller CD, Gies JP, Chekir-Ghedira L, Ghedira K, Mély Y, Bronner C, Mousli M. *Limoniastrum guyonianum* aqueous gall extract induces apoptosis in human cervical cancer cells involving p16 INK4A re-expression related to UHRF1 and DNMT1 down-regulation. Journal of Experimental and Clinical Cancer Research. 2013; 32(1):30.

Liu H, Dong Y, Gao Y, Du Z, Wang Y, Cheng P, Chen A, Huang H. The fascinating effects of baicalein on cancer: A review. International Journal of Molecular Sciences. 2016; 17(10):1681.

Ma X, Yan W, Dai Z, Gao X, Ma Y, Xu Q, Jiang J, Zhang S. Baicalein suppresses metastasis of breast cancer cells by inhibiting EMT *via* downregulation of SATB1 and Wnt/â-catenin pathway. Drug Design, Development and Therapy. 2016; 10:1419.

Meng G, Chai K, Li X, Zhu Y, Huang W. Luteolin exerts pro-apoptotic effect and anti-migration effects on A549 lung adenocarcinoma cells through the activation of MEK/ERK signaling pathway. Chemico-Biological Interactions. 2016; 257:26-34.

Nema R, Jain P, Khare S, Pradhan A. Flavonoid and cancer prevention–Mini review. Research in Pharmacy. 2015; 2(2): 46-50

Pandurangan AK, Esa NM, Luteolin, a bioflavonoid inhibits colorectal cancer through modulation of multiple signaling pathways: A review. Asian Pacific Journal of Cancer Prevention. 2014; 15(14):5501-8.

Park JE, Sun Y, Lim SK, Tam JP, Dekker M, Chen H, Sze SK. Dietary phytochemical PEITC restricts tumor development *via* modulation of epigenetic writers and erasers. Scientific Reports. 2017; 7:40569.

Peng Y, Guo C, Yang Y, Li F, Zhang Y, Jiang B, Li Q. Baicalein induces apoptosis of human cervical cancer HeLa cells *in vitro*. Molecular medicine reports. 2015; 11(3): 2129-2134.

Sak K. Cytotoxicity of dietary flavonoids on different human cancer types. Pharmacognosy Reviews. 2014; 8(16):122.

Shankar E, Goel A, Gupta K, Gupta S. Plant Flavone Apigenin: An Emerging Anticancer Agent. Current Pharmacology Reports. 2017; 3(6): 423-446.

Shehzad A, Anwar MN, Zahid H, Ravinayagam V, Al-Rumaih HS, Al-Khulaifi F, Al-Boiajan H, Al-Suhaimi EA. Multifactorial role of flavonoids in prevention and treatment of various cancers. InAnales de la Real Academia Nacional de Farmacia 2016; 82(3): 297-302.

Shi MD, Shiao CK, Lee YC, Shih YW. Apigenin, a dietary flavonoid, inhibits proliferation of human bladder cancer T-24 cells *via* blocking cell cycle progression and inducing apoptosis. Cancer Cell International. 2015; 15(1):33.

Shukla S, Bhaskaran N, Babcook MA, Fu P, MacLennan GT, Gupta S. Apigenin inhibits prostate cancer progression in TRAMP mice *via* targeting PI3K/Akt/FoxO pathway. Carcinogenesis. 2013; 35(2):452-60.

Souza RP, Bonfim-Mendonça PD, Gimenes F, Ratti BA, Kaplum V, Bruschi ML, Nakamura CV, Silva SO, Maria-Engler SS, Consolaro ME. Oxidative stress triggered by Apigenin induces apoptosis in a comprehensive panel of human cervical cancer-derived cell lines. Oxidative Medicine and Cellular Longevity. 2017; 2017: 1-18.

Sung B, Chung HY, Kim ND. Role of apigenin in cancer prevention *via* the induction of apoptosis and autophagy. Journal of Cancer Prevention. 2016; 21(4):216.

Tuorkey MJ. Molecular targets of luteolin in cancer. European Journal of Cancer Prevention. 2016; 25(1):65.

Wang SW, Chen YR, Chow JM, Chien MH, Yang SF, Wen YC, Lee WJ, Tseng TH. Stimulation of Fas/FasL-mediated apoptosis by luteolin through enhancement of histone H3 acetylation and c-Jun activation in HL-60 leukemia cells. Molecular Carcinogenesis. 2018; 57(7): 866-77.

Wang Y, Wei Z , Wang X, Ding Z, Guo C Teng D. Effect of Chrysin on the Apoptosis and Protein Kinase B (AKT) Pathway in Caov-3 Cell LineLat. American Journal of Pharmacy. 2015; 34(5): 993-8.

Zang M, Hu L, Zhang B, Zhu Z, Li J, Zhu Z, Yan M, Liu B. Luteolin suppresses angiogenesis and vasculogenic mimicry formation through inhibiting Notch1-VEGF signaling in gastric cancer. Biochemical and Biophysical Research Communications. 2017; 490(3): 913-919.

Zhang MM, Huang SS, Long D, Lin X. Anti-proliferative action of chrysin in colon cancer cells and its effects on signaling pathways. International Journal of Clinical and Experimental Medicine. 2016; 9(11):22784-92.

2

Understanding the Mechanism of Luteolin, a Bioflavonoid on Colorectal Cancer

Ashok Kumar Pandurangan[1]*, Suresh Kumar Anandasadagopan[2], Prathibha Sivaprakasam[1], Sekar Kumaran[3] and Sangeetha Naveen[4]

ABSTRACT

Colorectal cancer (CRC) is one of the major health problems in the Western part of the world, and in India, also CRCs incidence slowly raising due to the unbalanced food habits, especially, high fat diet and low fiber intake. Natural products are safe, and very effective against many cancer types. Luteolin is chemically known as (2-[3,4-dihydroxyphenyl]-5,7-dihydroxy-4-chromenone), and it is a flavonoid available as a natural form and it was highly found in certain vegetables and fruits. In this chapter, we have discussed on the anti-tumor effect of Luteolin against CRC. Further, it discusses on how Luteolin modulates the key signalings, such as phosphoinositol-3-Kinase (PI3K) / Akt / Wnt / β-catenin and NF-E2-related factor 2 (Nrf2) pathways. Luteolin may be a strong cytotoxic drug as it facilitates the apoptotic mode of cell death in different cancer models. In a nutshell, the preclinical evidences suggest that Luteolin can be developed as a chemotherapeutic drug that needs to be tested in clinical settings.

Key words: Colorectal cancer, Luteolin, Flavonoid, Signaling, Antioxidant.

[1] School of Lifesciences, B.S. Abdur Rahman Crescent Institute of Science and Technology, Vandalur, Chennai-600048, India
[2] Biochemistry and Biotechnology Laboratory, Central Leather Research Institute (CLRI), Adayar, Chennai-600025, India
[3] Department of Botany, Periyar University Constituent College of Arts & Science, Harur-636903, Dharmapuri. Tamil Nadu, India
[4] GLR Laboratories Pvt Ltd., 444 Gokulam Street, Mathur, Chennai-68, India
**Corresponding author*: ashokkumar.sls@crescent.education

1. INTRODUCTION

Colorectal cancer (CRC) is ranked the third most common cancer in the Western part of world, and also alarmingly increasing in other parts of the world as well. The incidence of CRC is in rise due to the high fat diet, less dietary fiber intake age, alcohol intake, and smoking. CRCs are localized with or without lymph node metastases. About 20% of cancer patients are found to have a metastatic CRC isolated to the liver (Haraldsdottir *et al.,* 2014). Surgery, radiation therapy and chemotherapy remain the key therapies available for CRC. Especially, chemotherapy is the mainstay of treatment to the selected CRC patients with a metastatic tumor and recurrence that can be rescued. In recent years, a considerable progress has been eminent in the treatment of metastatic CRC (Pandurangan, 2013; Pandurangan and Esa, 2013).

In cancer drug discovery, natural products contribute a major part, either as such or as its derivatives (Harvey *et al.,* 2015). Among natural products, flavonoids and alkaloids are the major categories that contribute as chemo drugs. Many plant species contain flavonoids that are biologically active compounds. So far, 5000 different flavonoids are identified and they are classified into 10 different subgroups based on their chemical nature. Flavonoids are categorized into six subgroups; flavones, flavanones, flavonols, catechins, isoflavones and anthocyanidins, which are relatively common in human diets (Kocic *et al.*, 2013; Pandurangan and Esa, 2014). Flavonoids, such as Epigallocatechin, Quercetin, Baicalein, Chrysin, Luteolin, Kaempferol, Myricetin, Hesperetin and Naringenin are majorly reported to possess anticancer property (Darband *et al.,* 2018; Garcia *et al.,* 2018). Ma *et al.* (2018) reported that Quercetin inhibits SAS oral cancer cells and induce apoptotic mode of cell death by increasing the levels of Cytochrome C (Ma *et al.,* 2018). Previous study indicated that Baicalein suppressed the lung cancer (Small Cell Lung Carcinoma) cell proliferation, cell invasion and Epithelial-Mesenchymal Transition by up-regulating the E-cadherin protein expression and down-regulated Twist1 and Vimentin protein expressions (Su *et al.,* 2018). Chrysin is flavones subclass of flavonoid, and inhibits CRC cell proliferation by activating the autophagic marker protein LC3-II (Lin and Chen, 2018). Recently, Chang *et al.* (2017) reported that the administration of Naringenin, a flavonone class of flavonoid inhibits A549 lung cancer cell proliferation by suppressing the matrix metalloproteinase (MMP) 9 and 2 expressions (Chang *et al.,* 2017). In breast cancer classification, Triple-negative breast cancer (TNBC) is an aggressive form of cancer and this was because of lack of receptors hence the treatment for TNBC is highly difficult. But, administration of Myricetin to TNBC cells inhibited the growth by inducing apoptotic mode of cell death. Administration of

Myricetin generates ROS in TNBC cells and leads to apoptosis however Myricetin but was less inhibitory for non-tumorigenic cells (Knickle *et al.*, 2018). On the other hand, Berberine, Piperine, capsaicin and Paclitaxel were well known alkaloids acts as a strong antitumor agents (Qian and Yang, 2014; Greenshields *et al.*, 2015; Ingle *et al.*, 2018).

Luteolin is a strong bioflavonoid that inhibits colorectal cancer in different *in vitro* and *in vivo* models. In this book chapter, we have discussed in detail about the mechanistic action of Luteolin against colorectal cancer.

2. BENEFICIAL EFFECTS OF LUTEOLIN

Luteolin is chemically known as (2-[3,4-dihydroxyphenyl]-5,7-dihydroxy-4-chromenone) (Fig. 1), and it is a flavonoid available naturally and it is highly found in certain vegetables and fruits. Particularly, broccoli, celery, green peppers, parsley, cabbages, apple skins, onion leaves, carrots, and *chrysanthemum* flowers are rich in Luteolin (Pandurangan and Esa, 2014). This phytocompound is reported to possess many health benefits, including anti-diabetic, antibacterial, anti-inflammatory, hepatoprotective, neuroprotective, cardioprotective effects (Shanmugam *et al.*, 2016; Kim *et al.*, 2017; Ha *et al.*, 2017; Fu *et al.*, 2018; Baiyun *et al.*, 2018). Baiyun *et al.* (2018) reported that the administration of Luteolin activates PI3K/AKT/Nrf2 signaling pathway, and thereby it protects against $HgCl_2$-induced cardiac damage. It is well documented that treating Luteolin to THP-1 human monocyte cells, inhibited the high glucose (HG)-induced production of Reactive oxygen species (ROS) by activating sirtuins and forkhead box O3a molecules (Kim *et al.*, 2017).

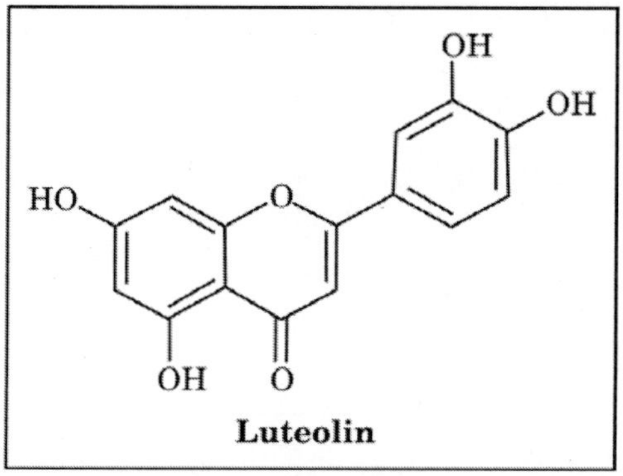

Fig. 1: 3,4,5',7'-tetra hydroxy flavone (Luteolin).

3. LUTEOLIN AND COLORECTAL CANCER

There are several reports stating that Luteolin inhibits CRC in different models. Luteolin is a strong antioxidant compound that scavenges free radicals and also increased the enzymic antioxidants (Kumar and Sudhandiran, 2008). Also, it modulates PI3K/Akt/Wnt/β-catenin, Nrf2/Keap-1 signaling pathways. The overall pathway is illustrated in Fig. 2. The role of Glycoconjugates in assembling the moieties of oligosaccharides of the glycoprotein chains is essential. It is already well documented that during the neoplastic conditions, their level is elevated. Hence, they are considered as non-specific markers of tumors (Sen *et al.,* 1983; Inagaki *et al.,* 2014). Pandurangan *et al.* (2012) revealed that in mouse induced with Azoxymethane (AOM), and subsequently administered with Luteolin reduces the glycoconjugates level. Luteolin is reported to modulate the levels of Mg^{2+} ATPase, Ca^{2+} ATPase and $Na^{+}K^{+}$ ATPase in AOM-Induced CRC in mice (Pandurangan *et al.,* 2013a). Also, the activities of mitochondrial enzymes (α-ketoglutarate dehydrogenase, succinate dehydrogenase and Isocitrate dehydrogenase) are modulated by the administration of Luteolin to AOM-induced CRC in mouse model (Pandurangan *et al.,* 2014b). The detailed mechanistic action of Luteolin against different models of CRC is depicted in Fig. 2.

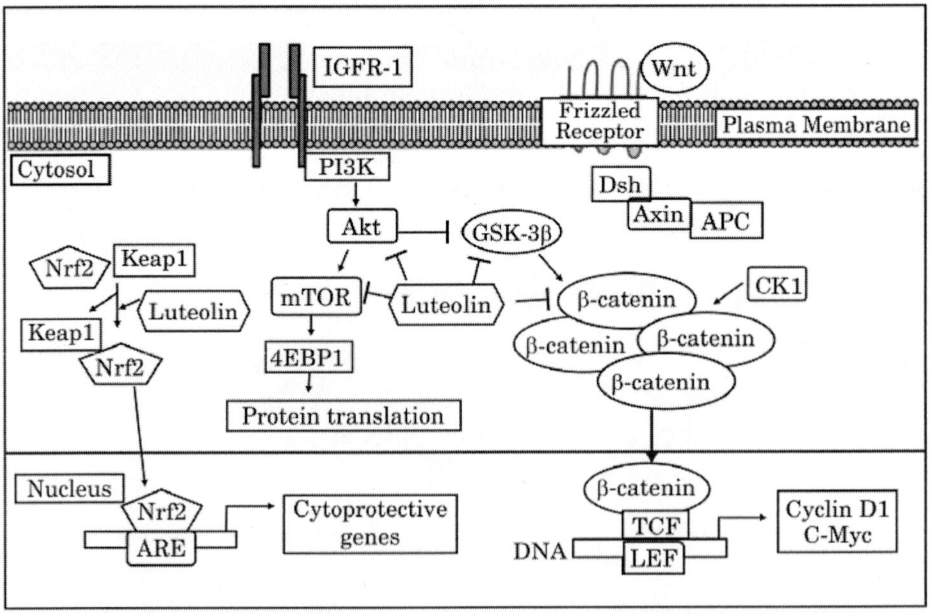

Fig. 2: Luteolin alters the key signaling pathways. It was discussed that three major pathways were regulated by Luteolin. Administration of Luteolin inhibits the Akt and β-catenin. It also activates the Nrf2 pathway thereby the downstream cytoprotective genes were transcribed.

3.1. Luteolin inhibits the expression of MDR-1

Multi-drug resistance (MDR) is a leading problem in treating CRC patients. Multi-drug resistant protein (MDR)-1 or p-glycoprotein acts as a transmembrane protein. The role of MDR-1 is inevitable in eliminating the xenobiotics, and drugs by effective efflux into the extracellular space (Kathwala *et al.,* 2015). Luteolin along with Baicalein were tested for their efficacy in Doxorubicin-resistant LoVo human colorectal cancer cell line. The results revealed that comparatively, Luteolin showed better efficacy in killing the doxorubicin resistant LoVo human colorectal cancer cells. Also, Luteolin down regulated the MDR-1 gene expression in Doxorubicin-resistant LoVo human CRC cells. These results clearly indicate that Luteolin is effective in culminating the gene responsible for the drug resistance, and it sensitizes the CRC cells (Palko-Labuz *et al.,* 2017).

3.2. Luteolin induces apoptosis in CRC

Xiao *et al.* (2017) reported that oncolytic viruses have attracted increasing interest due to their potent antitumor effects. The administration of Luteolin along with the oncolytic virus (CD55-TRAIL) showed a synergistic anti-tumor effect in HT-29, SW620 and SW480 human colorectal cancer cells. The combination therapy induced apoptosis by activating the X-linked inhibitor of apoptosis protein (XIAP), Poly (ADP-ribose) polymerase (PARP) and caspase 9 expressions. The *in vitro* results were verified with *in vivo* xenograft model of colorectal cancer. A total 24 BALB/c female nude mice were inoculated with HT-29 colorectal cancerous cell line. The above animals supplemented with Luteolin, CD55-TRAIL and both Luteolin and CD55-TRAIL. The combination group significantly decreased the tumor volume and enhanced the expression of TUNEL (Terminal deoxynucleotidyl transferase (TdT) dUTP Nick-End Labeling) staining, a marker of apoptosis.

3.3. Luteolin effect on sphingolipid metabolites in CRC

Abdel Hadi *et al.* (2015) studied the effects of Luteolin on the equilibrium, between ceramide and sphingosine -1 phosphate in Caco-2 colorectal cancer cells. These two sphingoid mediators play opposite roles on the fate of a cell (Abdel Hadi *et al.,* 2015). They also observed that Luteolin cytotoxic effects on Caco-2 cells by suppressing both sphigosine-1 phosphate biosynthesis and ceramide traffic, suggesting the involvement of Luteolin in dietary supplements as a valuable strategy to advance the current trends of treating CRC.

3.4. Luteolin inhibits the iNOS and COX-2 expressions in CRC

Pandurangan *et al.* (2014c) have shown that the administration of Luteolin suppressed the colonic inflammation by modulating the two key enzymes that mediate inflammation, namely cyclooxygenase-2 (COX-2) and inducible nitric oxide synthase (iNOS) in AOM-induced colorectal carcinogenesis. The accumulation of iNOS and nitric oxide (NO) in inflamed colon of CRC indicated the involvement of iNOS in the pathogenesis of CRC (Takahashi *et al.*, 1997; Pandurangan *et al.*, 2014c; Gunasekaran *et al.*, 2018). COX-2 is an enzyme that catalyzes the synthesis of Prostaglandins (PG). The increased accumulation of PGs in the cells triggers the inflammation. There are many reports stating that the COX-2 expression is higher in CRC. In colon, the increased COX-2 expression induces the inflammation. Both iNOS and COX-2 inhibitors, including Luteolin showed a substantial inhibition of CRC in different models (Gunasekaran *et al.*, 2018; Ghareeb *et al.*, 2018; Yang *et al.*, 2018; Gungor *et al.*, 2018).

3.5. Luteolin downregulates PI3K/Akt signaling *via* IGF-1R in CRC

Lim *et al.* (2012) reported that the supplementation of Luteolin suppressed the activation of the phosphatidylinositol 3-kinase (PI3K)/Akt and extracellular signal-regulated kinase (ERK1/2) pathways by suppressing Insulin like Growth Factor (IGF)-IR signaling in CRC cell line. The IGF actively participates in the growth of various cancers, including CRC. It has been already reported that, Luteolin exerts the anti- proliferative effect on HT-29 human colon cancer cells by inducing cell cycle arrest and apoptosis. Further, studies have shown that in HT-29 CRC cells, the administration of Luteolin blocks the secretion of pro- and mature IGF-II, and also reduce the expression of the IGF-IR precursor protein. Along with that, Luteolin reduces the activation of the Akt and ERK1/2 signaling.

3.6. Luteolin inhibits the Wnt/β-catenin pathway in CRC

Wnt/β-catenin signaling is one of the critical signaling, take parts in the cell proliferation process. Under the normal circumstances, the β-catenin molecule is associated with Adenomatous polyposis coli (APC), Glycogen syntheses kinase (GSK)-3β, Axin and Casein kinase-1 in cytosol of the cell. After, β-catenin protein is phosphorylated by the enzyme, GSK-3β, it undergoes the ubiquitantion process. In CRC, 80% were contains APC gene mutations and about 10-12% have β-catenin gene mutations (Shang *et al.*, 2018). Due to these mutations, there is a crisis in the formation of assembly in the cytosol (Jamieson *et al.*, 2014; Koch, 2017). Thus, non-phosphorylated β-Catenin enters into nucleus, and binds with T-Cell factor (TCF) and Lymphocyte enhancer factor (LEF), and transcribes the cell proliferation genes, namely Cyclin D1 and C-Myc (Sebio *et al.,* 2014; Song *et al.,* 2015). Although, it is known that targeting Wnt/β-catenin inhibits the CRC, and many drugs that downregulate Wnt/β-catenin signaling have been proved experimentally to be effective (Ashokkumar and Sudhandiran, 2011; Li *et al.*, 2018; Wang *et al.,* 2018; Reabroi *et al.,* 2018). Luteolin was reported to suppress the Wnt/β-catenin pathway *in vitro* and *in vivo* models. Luteolin, time dependently and dose dependently inhibited the Wnt/β-catenin pathway in HCT-15 colon adenocarcinoma cells (Pandurangan *et al.*, 2013). The translocation of cytosolic free β-catenin protein to nucleus is the crucial event in CRC, and the administration of Luteolin effectively blocked the β-catenin protein translocation into the nucleus (Ashokkumar and Sudhandiran 2011; Pandurangan *et al.*, 2013).

Baskar *et al.* (2011) investigated that Luteolin-7-O-glucoside (LUT7G) obtained from the leaves of *Ophiorrhiza mungos* Linn. exhibit the anticancer effect on Colo320 DM cells through apoptosis, DNA fragmentation, free radical scavenging and expression of β-catenin (Porter and Vaillancour 2004). Previous studies have shown a positive correlation between β-catenin accumulation and cancer cell proliferation, including colon carcinoma (Derksen *et al.,* 2004; Saldanha *et al.*, 2004; Calvisi *et al.*, 2004). The chemo preventive efficacy on rats induced with Dimethyl Hydrazine (DMH) for four weeks consecutively and treating with three different doses (LUT7G) for 16 weeks was tested. The results show that LUT7G inhibits the DMH-induced Aberrant Crypt Foci (ACF) formation in colon of rats, and also it suppressed the β-catenin mutation. Hence, LUT7G may be used as a potential candidate for anti-carcinogenic agent (Baskar *et al.,* 2011).

3.7. Luteolin inhibits the expressions of MMP 9 and 2 in CRC

The formation of new blood vessels from the microvasculature to supply nutrients and oxygen to the tumor is called angiogenesis. The tumor acquired with an angiogenic phenotype and numerous signaling molecules facilitate the angiogenic factors. Matrix metalloproteinases (MMPs) are the key regulating factors, which performs the matrix remodeling activity required for spout formation and vessel growth. The MMPs are involved in the role of degrading extracellular matrix (ECM), and they belong to the family of Zn^{2+} binding, Ca^{2+}-dependent endopeptidases (Millauer *et al.,* 1993; Brooks *et al.*, 1994; Coussens *et al.,* 1996; Bergers *et al.,* 2000). Administration of 1.2 mg/kg body weight of Luteolin lowers the expressions of MMP-9 and 2. Real Time-Polymerase Chain Reaction analysis of the gene, *tissue inhibitor of matrix metalloproteinase (TIMP)-2* was downregulated in the mouse model of AOM-induced CRC, and the administration of Luteolin increased the *TIMP-2* gene expression (Pandurangan *et al.,* 2014a).

Qiu *et al.* (2013) studied the Luteolin encapsulation with the self-assembled Monomethoxypoly(ethylene glycol)-poly(å-caprolactone) (MPEG-PCL) micelles to create the water-soluble Luteolin/MPEG-PCL micelle. The advantages of MPEG-PCL micelles for drug delivery are nontoxic, biocompatible, biodegradable, amphiphilic and stable in blood. Luteolin/MPEG-PCL showed a significant *in vitro* cytotoxicity in C-26 CRC cell line, and also sustained the release of Luteolin from micelles. Lu/MPEG-PCL micelles or Luteolin (Luteolin at the dose of 30 mg/kg body weight) micelles administered intravenously to rats enhanced the systemic circulation of Luteolin *in vivo*, and inhibited the cancer cell growth. The results of their studies showed that encapsulating with micelles can be a promising application in cancer treatment.

3.8. Luteolin prompts cell cycle arrest at G2/M phase in CRC

Wang *et al.* (2004) studied seven apigenin analogs (chrysin, luteolin, quercetin, kaempferol, naringenin, myricetin and acacetin) against Caco-2 and SW480 human colonic carcinoma cell lines. Their study results showed that G2M phase cell cycle arrest when treated with all of the apigenin analogs except myricetin and naringenin in a dose dependent manner. There was a significant decrease in the cell viability during treatment with Luteolin and other flavonoid derivatives at the dose of 60–80 µM. These results suggest that when the cells are treated with high doses, cytotoxicity is induced. However, at low doses, the cell number is decreased by cytostatic effects. The collective observations from this study reveals that the inductions of cell-cycle arrest in G2/M phase by five of seven apigenin analogs confirmed the synergistic arrest of cell cycle at lower concentrations. In a nutshell, apigenin analogs are good candidates to be used as a chemotherapeutic agent.

Lim *et al.* (2007) reported that the Luteolin modulates cell cycle progression, and induces apoptotic mode of cell death in HT-29 human CRC cells. The administration of Luteolin to human HT-29 colorectal cancer cells promoted both G2/M and G1 phase cell cycle arrest. Luteolin inhibited cells within 2 hrs of treatment through the activities of cyclin dependent kinase (CDK) 4 and CDK2 leading to G1 and G2/M cell-cycle arrest. In addition, Luteolin promoted apoptosis through down-regulation of few anti-apoptotic proteins, namely survivin, Bcl-xL, Mcl-1, p21, and MDM2. This study provides a strong reason for using Luteolin as a possible anti-tumorigenic agent.

3.9. Luteolin modulates the Nrf2 signaling in CRC

Nrf2 is a transcription factor, and belongs to the Cap-N-collar family. Generally, it is bound with its regulator, Keap1 that undergo proteosomal degradation (Dinakova - Kostova *et al.,* 2005; Furukawa and Xiong, 2005). When a cell encounters oxidative stress, the Nrf2 loses its contact from keap1, and facilitates the nuclear translocation and activates the antioxidative genes. It is documented that the administration of Luteolin to AOM-induced BALB/c mice enhanced the Nrf2 expression and downstream targets, such as UDP-GT and GST (Pandurangan *et al.,* 2014b).

3.10. Luteolin scavenges the ROS and restored the enzymic antioxidants in CRC

Manju and Nalini (2007) showed that Luteolin treatment inhibits the colon tumor incidence and decreases the levels of Mucinase and β-glucuronidase at the initiation and post initiation levels during Dimethyl hydrazine (DMH) induced carcinogenesis in rats. Luteolin, possibly prevents CRC by decreasing the levels of bacterial Mucinase and β-glucuronidase, thereby, it prevents the recycling of glucuronide-conjugated carcinogens in the lower part of the intestine. According to their observations, it is recommended that the administration of Luteolin is very effective in the initiation stage than the post initiation stage of carcinogenesis. Also, they have shown that administering Luteolin intragastrically inhibits colorectal cancer by decreasing the levels of thiobarbituric acid reactive substances (TBARS), activities of the enzymic antioxidants superoxide dismutase (SOD), catalase (CAT), elevated levels of reduced glutathione (GSH), glutathione peroxidase (GPx), glutathione–S-transferase (GST) and glutathione reductase (GR), and nonenzymic antioxidants vitamin C and vitamin E. The outcome of their study shows the potential application of Luteolin as a chemo preventive mediator for individuals at risks of colon cancer development (Manju *et al.*, 2005; Ashokkumar and Sudhandiran, 2008).

3.11. Luteolin sensitizes CRC cells and induces TNF-α-mediated apoptosis

Shi *et al.* (2004) investigated that Luteolin sensitizes Tumor Necrosis Factor (TNF)-α-mediated apoptosis significantly in two different human CRC cell lines, namely COLO205 and HCT116. This sensitization of CRC cells were achieved by the inhibition of NF-κB expression. It resulted in the inhibition of anti-apoptotic genes, such as A20 and cellular inhibitor of apoptosis protein-1(c-IAP1) that are well known as NF-κB-regulated anti-apoptotic genes. On the other hand, pre-treatment of Luteolin to CRC cells resulted to inhibit the prolonged activation of JNK that is induced by the TNF-α. This is the important process in the sensitization of Luteolin on TNF-α-mediated apoptosis. TNF-α play a dual role in cancers, *i.e.,* simultaneously it activates cell survival and cell death. In cancer prevention, the inhibition of NF-κB activation is the reliable strategy to enhance the sensitivity, because the majority cancer cells are resistant to TNF-α-induced apoptosis (Baldwin, 2001; Yamamoto and Gaynor, 2001). Their results show that Luteolin sensitizes TNF-α-induced apoptosis *via* its inhibitory effect on the NF-κB signaling pathway. Post treatment of Luteolin did not exert any sensitization effect. Luteolin enhanced caspase 8 activation through anti-apoptotic genes. They found that TNF-α induced the expressions of both A20 and c-IAP1 significantly, and this up-regulation was diminished when the CRC cells were treated with Luteolin. Several reports indicated that NF-κB inhibition resulted in the prolonged JNK activation that in turn facilitates TNF-α-induced apoptotic mode of cell death (Tang *et al.* 2001; De Smaele *et al.*, 2001). The pre-treatment of Luteolin also augmented and prolonged the TNF-α-mediated activation of JNK. Alice *et al.* (2010) showed that Luteolin and Ursolic acid, common flavonoids present in fruits and vegetables are involved in DNA repair and maintaining genomic stability in Caco-2 CRC cell line when exposed to oxidative agents. The administration of Luteolin protects cells from the RO-induced DNA damage. Apart from protecting the DNA from oxidative damages, Luteolin increased the DNA repair activity.

4. CONCLUSIONS

In conclusion, Luteolin is reported to have beneficial effects against various cancer types. A number of reports have stated that Luteolin induces cytotoxicity and cell death in CRC cells. *In vivo* results have confirmed that Luteolin administration reduces the tumor formation in chemically induced colorectal cancer. Luteolin, clearly modulates the predominant signaling pathways, such as PI3K/Akt/Wnt/β-catenin and Nrf2 signaling. Based on these pre-clinical evidences, Luteolin can be tested in clinical settings for developing it as a chemotherapeutic agent.

REFERENCES

Abdel Hadi L, Di Vito C, Marfia G, Ferraretto A, Tringali C, Viani P, *et al.* Sphingosine Kinase 2 and Ceramide Transport as Key Targets of the Natural Flavonoid Luteolin to Induce Apoptosis in Colon Cancer Cells. PLoS ONE. 2015; 10(11):e0143384.

Ashokkumar P, Sudhandiran G. Protective role of luteolin on the status of lipid peroxidation and antioxidant defense against azoxymethane-induced experimental colon carcinogenesis. Biomedicine & Pharmacotherapy. 2008; 62(9): 590-7.

Ashokkumar P, Sudhandiran G. Luteolin inhibits cell proliferation during Azoxymethane-induced experimental colon carcinogenesis *via* Wnt/β-catenin pathway. Investigational New Drugs. 2011; 29(2): 273-84.

Baldwin AS. Control of oncogenesis and cancer therapy resistance by the transcription factor NF-kappa B. Journal of Clinical Investigation. 2001; 107(3): 241-6.

Baskar AA, Ignacimuthu S, Michael GP, Al Numair KS. Cancer chemopreventive potential of luteolin-7-O-glucoside isolated from *Ophiorrhiza mungos* Linn. Nutrition & Cancer. 2011; 63(1): 130-8.

Baiyun R, Li S, Liu B, Lu J, Lv Y, Xu J, Wu J, Li J, Lv Z, Zhang Z. Luteolin-mediated PI3K/AKT/Nrf2 signaling pathway ameliorates inorganic mercury-induced cardiac injury. Ecotoxicology and Environmental Safety. 2018; 161: 655-661.

Bergers G, Brekken R, Mahon GM, *et al*. Matrix metalloproteinase-9 triggers the angiogenic switch during carcinogenesis. Nature: Cell Biology. 2000; 2: 737-744.

Brooks PC, Montgomery AM, Rosenfeld M, *et al*. Integrin alpha v beta 3 antagonists promote tumor regression by inducing apoptosis of angiogenic blood vessels. Cell. 1994; 79(7): 1157-1164.

Calvisi DF, Ladu S, Factor VM, Thorgeirsson SS. Activation of β-catenin provides proliferative and invasive advantages in cmyc/TGF-a hepatocarcinogenes is promoted by phenobarbital. Carcinogenesis. 2004; 25: 901–908.

Chang HL, Chang YM, Lai SC, Chen KM, Wang KC, Chiu TT, Chang FH, Hsu LS. Naringenin inhibits migration of lung cancer cells *via* the inhibition of matrix metalloproteinases-2 and -9. Experimental and Therapeutic Medicine. 2017; 13: 739-744.

Coussens LM, Werb Z. Matrix metalloproteinases and the development of cancer. Chemical Biology. 1996; 3(11): 895–904.

Darband SG, Kaviani M, Yousefi B, Sadighparvar S, Pakdel FG, Attari JA, Mohebbi I, Naderi S, Majidinia M. Quercetin: A functional dietary flavonoid with potential chemo-preventive properties in colorectal cancer. Journal of Cellular Biology. 2018; 233: 6544-6560.

De Smaele E, Zazzeroni F, Papa S, Nguyen DU, Jin R, Jones J, Cong R, Franzoso G. Induction of gadd45b by NF-kappaB downregulates pro-apoptotic JNK signalling. Nature. 2001; 414(6861): 308-13.

Derksen PW, Tjin E, Meijer HP, *et al*. Illegitimate WNT signaling promotes proliferation of multiple myeloma cells. Proceedings of the National Academy of Sciences of the United States of America. 2004; 101: 6122–6127.

Dinkova-Kostova AT, Holtzclaw WD, Kensler TW. The role of keap1 in cellular protective responses. Chemical Research in Toxicology 2005; 8: 1779-91.

Fu J, Sun H, Zhang Y, Xu W, Wang C, Fang Y, Zhao J. Neuroprotective Effects of Luteolin Against Spinal Cord Ischemia-Reperfusion Injury by Attenuation of Oxidative Stress, Inflammation, and Apoptosis. Journal of Medicinal Food. 2018; 21(1): 13-20.

Furukawa M, Xiong Y. BTB protein Keap1 targets antioxidant transcription factor Nrf2 for ubiquitination by the Cullin 3-Roc1 ligase. Molecular and Cellular Biology. 2005; 25: 162-71.

Garcia ER, Gutierrez EA, de Melo F, Novaes RD. Flavonoids Effects on Hepatocellular Carcinoma in Murine Models: A Systematic Review. Evidence-Based Complementary and Alternative Medicine. 2018; 6328970.

Ghareeb AE, Moawed FSM, Ghareeb DA, Kandil EI. Potential Prophylactic Effect of Berberine against Rat Colon Carcinoma Induce by 1,2-Dimethyl Hydrazine. Asian Pacific Journal of Cancer Prevention. 2018; 19(6): 1685-1690.

Greenshields AL, Doucette CD, Sutton KM, Madera L, Annan H, Yaffe PB, Knickle AF, Dong Z, Hoskin DW. Piperine inhibits the growth and motility of triple-negative breast cancer cells. Cancer Letters. 2015; 357: 129-140.

Gunasekaran S, Venkatachalam K, Namasivayam N. Anti-inflammatory and anticancer effects of p-methoxycinnamic acid, an active phenylpropanoid, against 1,2-dimethylhydrazine-induced rat colon carcinogenesis. Molecular and Cellular Biochemistry. 2018. doi: 10.1007/s11010-018-3398-5.

Gungor H, Ilhan N, Eroksuz H. The effectiveness of cyclooxygenase-2 inhibitors and evaluation of angiogenesis in the model of experimental colorectal cancer. Biomedicine & Pharmacotherapy. 2018; 102: 221-229.

Ha SK, Lee JA, Cho EJ, Choi I. Effects of Catechol O-Methyl Transferase Inhibition on Anti-Inflammatory Activity of Luteolin Metabolites. Journal of Food Science. 2017; 82(2):545-552.

Haraldsdottir S, Einarsdottir HM, Smaradottir A, Gunnlaugsson A, Halfdanarson TR. [Colorectal cancer - review]. Laeknabladid. 2014; 100: 75-82.

Harvey AL, Edrada-Ebel R, Quinn RJ. The re-emergence of natural products for drug discovery in the genomics era. Nature Reviews: Drug Discovery. 2015; 14: 11-129.

Inagaki Y, Gao J, Song P, Kokudo N, Nakata M, Tang W. Clinicopathological utility of sialoglyco conjugates in diagnosing and treating colorectal cancer. World Journal of Gastroenterology. 2014; 20(20): 6123-32.

Ingle SG, Pai RV, Monpara JD, Vavia PR. Liposils: An effective strategy for stabilizing Paclitaxel loaded liposomes by surface coating with silica. European Journal of Pharmaceutical Sciences. 2018; 122: 51-63.

Jamieson C, Sharma M, Henderson BR. Targeting the β-catenin nuclear transport pathway in cancer. Seminars in Cancer Biology. 2014; 27: 20-9.

Kathawala RJ, Gupta P, Ashby CR Jr, Chen ZS. The modulation of ABC transporter-mediated multidrug resistance in cancer: A review of the past decade. Drug Resistance Updates. 2015; 18: 1-17.

Kim A, Lee W, Yun JM. Luteolin and fisetin suppress oxidative stress by modulating sirtuins and forkhead box O3a expression under *in vitro* diabetic conditions. Nutrition Research and Practice. 2017; 11: 430-434.

Koch S. Extrinsic control of Wnt signaling in the intestine. Differentiation. 2017; 97: 1-8.

Kocic B, Kitic D, Brankovic S. Dietary flavonoid intake and colorectal cancer risk: Evidence from human population studies. Journal of B.U.ON.: official journal of the Balkan Union of Oncology 2013; 18: 34-43.

Knickle A, Fernando W, Greenshields AL, Rupasinghe HPV, Hoskin DW. Myricetin-induced apoptosis of triple-negative breast cancer cells is mediated by the iron-dependent generation of reactive oxygen species from hydrogen peroxide. Food and Chemical Toxicology. 2018; 118: 154-167.

Li T, Zhang L, Huo X. Inhibitory effects of aesculetin on the proliferation of colon cancer cells by the Wnt/β-catenin signaling pathway. Oncology Letters. 2018; 15(5): 7118-7122.

Lin YM, Chen CI. Chrysin Attenuates Cell Viability of Human Colorectal Cancer Cells through Autophagy Induction Unlike 5-Fluorouracil/Oxaliplatin. International Journal of Molecular Sciences. 2018; 1763.

Lim DY, Cho HJ, Kim J, Nho CW, Lee KW, Park JH. Luteolin decreases IGF-II production and downregulates insulin-like growth factor-I receptor signaling in HT-29 human colon cancer cells. BMC Gastroenterology. 2012; 23: 12:9.

Lim DY, Jeong Y, Tyner AL, Park JH. Induction of cell cycle arrest and apoptosis in HT-29 human colon cancer cells by the dietary compound luteolin. American Journal of Physiology Gastrointestinal Liver Physiology. 2007; 292(1): G66-75.

Ma YS, Yao CN, Liu HC, Yu FS, Lin JJ, Lu KW, Liao CL, Chueh FS, Chung JG. Quercetin induced apoptosis of human oral cancer SAS cells through mitochondria and endoplasmic reticulum mediated signaling pathways. Oncology Letters 2018; 15: 9663-9672.

Manju V, Balasubramaniyan V, Nalini N. Rat colonic lipid peroxidation and antioxidant status: the effects of dietary luteolin on 1,2-dimethylhydrazine challenge. Cell Molecular Biology Letters. 2005; 10(3): 535-51.

Manju V, Nalini N. Protective role of luteolin in 1,2-dimethylhydrazine induced experimental colon carcinogenesis. Cell Biochemistry Function. 2007; 25(2): 189-94.

Millauer B, Wizigmann-Voos S, Schnurch H, *et al.* High affinity VEGF binding and developmental expression suggests Flk-1 as a major regulator of vasculogenesis. Cell. 1993; 72: 835–846.

Palko-Labuz A, Sroda-Pomianek K, Uryga A, Kostrzewa-Suslow E, Michalak K. Anticancer activity of baicalein and luteolin studied in colorectal adenocarcinoma LoVo cells and in drug-resistant LoVo/Dx cells. Biomedicine & Pharmacotherapy 2017; 88: 232–241.

Pandurangan AK. Potential targets for prevention of colorectal cancer: A focus on PI3K/Akt/mTOR and Wnt pathways. Asian Pacific Journal of Cancer Prevention. 2013; 14: 2201-2205.

Pandurangan AK and Ganapasam S. Luteolin, a bioflavonoid attenuates Azoxymethane-induced effects on mitochondrial enzymes in Balb/c mice. *Asian* Pacific Journal of Cancer Prevention. 2013, 14(11), 6669-6672.

Pandurangan AK, Anandha Sadagopan SK, Dharmalingam P, Ganapasam S. Inhibitory effect of luteolin on the status of membrane bound ATPases against azoxymethane-induced colorectal cancer. Journal of Chemical and Pharmaceutical Research, 2013b; 5(6): 123-127.

Pandurangan AK, Ananda Sadagopan SK, Dharmalingam P, Ganapasam S. Luteolin, a bioflavonoid inhibits Azoxymethane-induced colorectal cancer through Nrf2 signaling. Toxicology Mechanisms & Methods. 2014; 24(1): 13-20.

Pandurangan AK, Esa NM. Dietary non-nutritive factors in targeting of regulatory molecules in colorectal cancer: An update. Asian Pacific Journal of Cancer prevention. 2013; 14: 5543-5552.

Pandurangan AK, Dharmalingam P, Ananda Sadagopan SK, Ramar M, Munusamy A Ganapasam S. Luteolin induces growth arrest in colon cancer cells through the involvement of Wnt/β-catenin/GSK-3β signaling. Journal of Environmental Patholoigy, Toxicology Oncology 2013a; 32(2): 131-139.

Pandurangan AK, Esa NM. Luteolin, a bioflavonoid inhibits colorectal cancer through modulation of multiple signaling pathways: a review. Asian Pacific Journal of Cancer Prevention. 2014; 15: 5501-5508.

Pandurangan AK, Dharmalingam P, Anandasadagopan SK Ganapasam S. Inhibitory effect of Luteolin on the status of membrane bound ATPases against Azoxymethane-induced colorectal cancer. Journal of Chemical and Pharmacetical Research. 2013a; 5(6): 123-127.

Pandurangan AK, Dharmalingam P, Anandasadagopan SK, Ganapasam S. Effect of Luteolin on the levels of Glycoproteins during Azoxymethane-induced colon carcinogenesis in mice. Asian Pacific Journal of Cancer Prevention. 2012; 13(4): 1569-73.

Pandurangan AK, Dharmalingam P, Sadagopan SK, Ganapasam S. Luteolin, a Bioflavonoid, Attenuates Azoxymethane-Induced Effects on Mitochondrial Enzymes in Balb/c Mice. Asian Pacific Journal of Cancer Prevention. 2014b; 14 (11): 6669-6672

Pandurangan AK, Dharmalingam P, Sadagopan SK, Ganapasam S. Luteolin inhibits matrix metalloproteinase 9 and 2 in azoxymethane-induced colon carcinogenesis. Human & Experimental Toxicology. 2014a; 33(11): 1176-85.

Pandurangan AK, Kumar SA, Dharmalingam P, Ganapasam S. Luteolin, a bioflavonoid inhibits azoxymethane-induced colon carcinogenesis: Involvement of iNOS and COX-2. Pharmacognosy Magazine. 2014c; 10(Suppl 2): S306-10.

Porter AC, Vaillancourt. Tyrosine kinase receptor-activated signal transduction pathway which lead to oncogenesis. Oncogene. 1998; 17: 343–1352.

Qian P, Yang XW. Five new alkaloids from Coptidis Rhizoma-Euodiae Fructus couple and their cytotoxic activities against gastrointestinal cancer cells. Fitoterapia 2014; 93:74-80.

Qiu JF, Gao X, Wang BL, Wei XW, Gou ML, Men K, Liu XY, Guo G, Qian ZY, Huang MJ. Preparation and characterization of monomethoxypoly (ethylene glycol)-poly(å-caprolactone) micelles for the solubilization and *in vivo* delivery of luteolin. International Journal of Nanomedicine. 2013; 8: 3061-9.

Ramos AA, Pereira-Wilson C, Collins AR. Protective effects of ursolic acid and luteolin against oxidative DNA damage include enhancement of DNA repair in Caco-2 cells. Mutatation Research. 2010; 692: 6-11.

Reabroi S, Chairoungdua A, Saeeng R, Kasemsuk T, Saengsawang W, Zhu W, Piyachaturawat P. A silyl andrographolide analogue suppresses Wnt/β-catenin signaling pathway in colon cancer. Biomedicine & Pharmacotherapy. 2018,101, 414-421.

Saldanha G, Ghura V, Potter L, and Fletcher A: Nuclear β-catenin in basal cell carcinoma correlates with increased proliferation. British Journal of Dermatology 2004; 151: 157–164.

Sebio A, Kahn M, Lenz HJ. The potential of targeting Wnt/β-catenin in colon cancer. Expert Opinion in Therapeutic Targets. 2014; 18(6):611-5.

Sen U, Guha S, Chowdhury JR. Serum fucosyltransferase activity and serum fucose levels as diagnostic tools in malignancy. Acta Med Okayama. 1983; 37: 457-62.

Shang S, Hua F, Hu ZW. The regulation of β-catenin activity and function in cancer: therapeutic opportunities. Oncotarget. 2017; 8(20): 33972-33989.

Shanmugam S, Thangaraj P, Lima BDS, Chandran R, de Souza Araújo AA, Narain N, Serafini MR, Júnior LJQ. Effects of luteolin and quercetin 3-β-d-glucoside identified from *Passiflora subpeltata* leaves against acetaminophen induced hepatotoxicity in rats. Biomedicine & Pharmacotherapy. 2016; 83: 1278-1285.

Shi RX, Ong CN, Shen HM. Luteolin sensitizes tumor necrosis factor-alpha-induced apoptosis in human tumor cells. Oncogene. 2004; 23(46): 7712-21.

Song L, Li ZY, Liu WP, Zhao MR. Crosstalk between Wnt/β-catenin and Hedgehog/Gli signaling pathways in colon cancer and implications for therapy. Cancer Biololgy Therapeutics. 2015; 16(1):1-7.

Su G, Chen H, Sun X. Baicalein suppresses non small cell lung cancer cell proliferation, invasion and Notch signaling pathway. Cancer Biomarkers: section A of Disease markers. 2018; 22: 13-18.

Takahashi M, Fukuda K, Ohhata T, Sugimura T, Wakabayashi K. Increased expression of inducible and endothelial constitutive nitric oxide synthase in rat colon tumors induced by azoxymethane. Cancer Research. 1997; 57: 1233-1237.

Tang G, Minemoto Y, Dibling B, Purcell NH, Li Z, Karin M, Lin A. Inhibition of JNK activation through NF-kappaB target genes. Nature. 2001; 414(6861): 313-7.

Wang W, Li Y, Chen Y, Chen H, Zhu P, Xu M, Wang H, Wu M, Yang Z, Hoffman RM, Gu Y. Ethanolic Extract of Traditional Chinese Medicine (TCM) Gamboge Inhibits Colon Cancer *via* the Wnt/Beta-Catenin Signaling Pathway in an Orthotopic Mouse Model. Anticancer Research. 2018, 38(4), 1917-1925.

Wang W, VanAlstyne PC, Irons KA, Chen S, Stewart JW, Birt DF. Individual and interactive effects of apigenin analogs on G2/M cell-cycle arrest in human colon carcinoma cell lines. Nutrition & Cancer. 2004; 48(1): 106-14.

Xiào, Qin Y, Ying C, Ma B, Wang B, Long F, Wang R, Fang L, Wang Y. Combination of oncolytic adenovirus and luteolin exerts synergistic antitumor effects in colorectal cancer cells and a mouse model. Molecular Medicine Reports. 2017; 16: 9375-9382.

Yamamoto Y, Gaynor RB. Therapeutic potential of inhibition of the NF-kappaB pathway in the treatment of inflammation and cancer. Journal of Clinical Investigations. 2001; 107(2): 135-42.

Yang JY, Zhong X, Kim SJ, Kim DH, Kim HS, Lee JS, Yum HW, Lee J, Na HK, Surh YJ. Comparative Effects of Curcumin and Tetrahydrocurcumin on Dextran Sulfate Sodium-induced Colitis and Inflammatory Signaling in Mice. Journal of Cancer Prevention. 2018; 23(1): 18-24.

3

Curcumin Nanoformulations in Glioblastoma Therapy

SUBHAMOY BANERJEE[1]*

ABSTRACT

Glioblastoma is one of the most aggressive types of cancer that affects the central nervous system. Due to the presence of blood brain barrier and glioma cell's reputation of being notoriously drug resistant, the conventional anticancer drugs have a limited success in killing these cells or stopping their recurrence. Many of the therapeutic approaches include the use of conventional drugs, targeted small molecule inhibitors, monoclonal antibodies and some plant derived molecules. Curcumin is a plant derived natural compound, which exhibits a cytotoxic effect against different cancers including glioma. But, its therapeutic usage is limited owing to its poor water solubility, low bio-distribution and poor residence time. The alternative approaches have been undertaken to overcome these limitations are the encapsulation in nanoparticle, making nanoformulations, etc. Despite some limitations and challenges, the curcumin loaded nanoparticles or curcumin nanoformulations alone or in combination with other approved drugs have shown a promising result.

Key words: Glioblastoma, Curcumin nanoparticle, Nanoparticle mediated therapy, Polymeric nanoparticle, Drug delivery.

[1] School of Life Science, B S Abdur Rahman Crescent Institute of Science and Technology, Vandalur, Chennai-600048

**Corresponding author*: subhamoy.sls@crescent.education; bsubhamoy@gmail.com

1. INTRODUCTION

Glioma is a collection of tumors arising from glia. Different types of gliomas account for nearly 80% of all brain tumors in the adults (Lo, 2010). Glioblastoma multiformae (GBM), commonly called as glioblastoma is the most aggressive form of gliomas, and stage IV cancer (Carlsson *et al.*, 2014). Despite the significant developments on different types of cancer therapies, it is one of the cancer, which has a median survival rate of 12 months (Louis *et al.*, 2007). Even after 11 years, the survival rate has not increased significantly (http://www.abta.org/brain-tumor-information/types-of-tumors/glioblastoma.html). Typically, the age adjusted occurrence of glioblastoma is $3.19/10^5$ people. It is more common in males ($3.97/10^5$ people), and increases with the age. Different therapeutic strategies have been used with a limited success to treat GBM. In this book chapter, underlying molecular signaling pathways, treatment options and future therapeutic strategies have been discussed with a special emphasis on the natural compound, curcumin.

2. INSIGHT ON GLIOBLASTOMA

Every type of cancer has some commonalities and few unique properties. It varies in site of occurrence, progression rate, specific gene mutation, over expression of specific cell signaling pathways etc. Similarly, glioblastoma also has some signatures, which is different from other types of cancers. The signaling pathways, diagnostic procedures, etc. have been discussed in this section.

2.1. Modified signaling pathway

As the name suggest, glioblastoma is a multiforme, both genetically as well as histological point of view. It is a highly heterogenic structure with necrotic and hemorrhage regions, polymorphic nuclei and microvascular proliferation (Holland, 2000). Multiple mutations and chromosomal aberrations are found in glioblastoma. Also, different studies have shown deregulation of Receptor Tyrosine Kinase (RTK) based growth factor signaling pathways, *e.g.*, epidermal growth factor receptor family, hepatocyte growth factor/ mesenchymal epithelial transition (HGF/MET) (Cruickshanks *et al.*, 2017; Mao *et al.*, 2012; von Achenbach *et al.*, 2018), constitutive activation of pro-proliferative Phosphatidylinositol 3-OH Kinase (PI3K) pathway (Langhans *et al.*, 2017; Westhoff *et al.*, 2014) and inhibition of tumor suppressor pathways regulated by p53 (Biasoli *et al.*, 2014; England *et al.*, 2013) and retinoblastoma (Rb) (Biasoli *et al.*, 2013). All these changes armor glioblastoma to be resistant towards therapeutic intervention.

2.2. Diagnostic procedure

Early and accurate diagnosis of cancer plays a major role in overall survival of patients. Glioblastoma pose major challenges, both in the early diagnosis and accuracy of diagnosis, thus it is identified much late. Owing to its origin inside the brain, glioblastoma often left unidentified, because of the absence of any visible signs in the body. Generally, glioblastoma starts with the astrocyte cells in the cerebrum. Magnetic resonance imaging (MRI) and computerized tomography (CT) scan are the major techniques used to determine glioblastoma. Usually, MRI produces a very detailed image of the brain. For MRI, a dye is used as a contrasting agent to discriminate between the tumor and normal brain tissue. The second stage of confirmation is the surgical biopsy. A small tissue sample from the tumor area is surgically excised to check the molecular and histopathological signature of glioblastoma. As glioblastom grows at a rapid rate, the tumor puts pressure on the brain. As a result, vomiting, seizures, constant headache, etc., are the initial signs of glioblastoma. There are several therapeutic biomarkers available for glioblastoma. Among several markers, a few are as follows; ~87% of all diagnosed cases p53 signaling pathway got altered, MDM2 over expression found in 14% cases, RTK/Ras/PI3 signaling over activated in 88% cases, etc. (Szopa *et al.*, 2017).

3. THERAPEUTIC APPROACHES AGAINST GLIOMA

As the mortality rate of glioma is very high, thus different therapeutic approaches have been undertaken. In Table 1, the therapeutic modalities are summarized. The standard treatment for glioblastoma is similar to other cancer treatments. The treatments include surgery, radiotherapy and chemotherapeutics(Clarke *et al.*, 2010). Different therapeutic approaches are discussed in the following section.

Table 1: Different types of therapy commonly undertaken to treat glioblastoma multiforme.

Therapeutic modalities	*Assisted therapy*
Surgery	Chemotherapy
Radiotherapy	Surgery, chemotherapy
Chemotherapy	Surgery, radiotherapy

3.1. Surgery

Glioblastoma is an intracranial neoplasia. Thus, discrimination between normal and cancerous cell mass and successful resection of cancer tissues determine the success in surgery (Laraeither-Velazquez *et al.*, 2017). Thus, following contemporary techniques are successfully applied or under development to demarcate the tumor and normal cells in the brain (Lara-Velazquez *et al.,* 2017); (i) Confocal Intraoperative Microscopy, (ii) Fluorescence Guided Surgery, (iii) Laser Interstitial Therapy, (iv) Intraoperative Mass Spectrometry and (v) Optical coherence tomography. More information on those techniques are mentioned in Table 2. These surgical approaches are meant to remove the cancerous mass of glial cells. But due to its highly recalcitrant nature, recurrence of glioblastoma often pose a major challenge to the doctors and limits the therapeutic options (Weller *et al.,* 2013).

Table 2: Different types of surgical procedures with brief methodology.

Surgical procedures	*Methodology*	*References*
Confocal intraoperative microscopy	Usually operated by using fluorophores which fluoresce at Near Infra-Red wavelength (*e.g.*, -indocyanine green). It increases the sensitivity of tumor cell positioning. It also gives an array of information like micro vasculature, necrotic cells and many more complex information.	Martirosyan *et al.* (2011); Pavlov *et al.* (2016); Lara-Velazquez *et al.* (2017)
Fluorescence guided surgery	Surgery of brain tumor is guided by 5-Aminolevulinic acid (5-ALA) induced porphyrin fluorescence. It Works in the visible range of light (375-nm 475 nm) and reported for high selectivity and sensitivity. But use is limited due to side effects.	Hefti (2013); Hadjipanayis *et al.* (2015)
Laser interstitial therapy	Laser induced thermal ablation of cancerous cells are achieved by selectively targeting cells. It can be improvised to use with magnetic and thermo responsive nanoparticles.	Mohammadi and Schroeder (2014); Sharma *et al.* (2016)
Intraoperative mass spectrometry	Mass spectrometry is used to analyze the GBM specific molecular markers and metabolites through desorption specific electrospray ionization.Then it is combined with stereotaxis to specifically operate the cancerous cells.This technique avoids use of any external fluorophores and it is a very rapid technique.	Mohammadi *et al.* (2014); Sharma *et al.* (2016)
Optical coherence tomography	When the light beam is illuminated on the cells, different optical behavior is found in specific cell types. Generates detail image of cell mass *via* a color coded map. It is label free cell detection technique.	Papour *et al.* (2013); Parrozzani *et al.* (2013)

3.2. Radiotherapy

Generally, radiotherapy (RT) is considered as the target specific therapy. The radiotherapy, used for glioblastoma is of two types *i.e.,* external beam radiotherapy and intensity modulated radiotherapy. A number of variations of the standard RT has been used with an aim to intensify the dosage *viz.* brachytherapy, hyperfractionation, etc. General consensus for the radiation therapy includes a radiation dosage of 6000 cGy (centigray). Beyond this intensity, the toxicity takes place without adding any advantages (Barani and Larson, 2015). The brachytherapy uses the delivery of radioactive isotope to the tumor site. The isotope emits ionizing radiation. Despite it is a novel therapy, but it is used with variable success for the patients. In fact, the patient should be carefully chosen for a successful brachytherapy (Barbarite *et al.,* 2017). While, the hyperfractionation or hyperfractionated radiotherapy (HFRT) is a radiation therapy where controlled dose escalation takes place. This strategy followed by chemotherapeutic drugs showed a promising result for the specific cohort (Kaul *et al.,* 2016).

3.3. Chemotherapy

Generally chemotherapeutic regime is subdivided into two phases - initial phase and after recurrence. There are many types of chemotherapeutic agents or drugs are used to treat glioblastoma. Often, these chemotherapeutic agents are used with radiation therapy or surgery. Some major types of chemotherapeutic drugs are discussed below.

3.3.1. *Alkylating agent*

Alkylating agents are the first generation anticancer drugs that are still in use as a first line of therapy. One of the most common alkylating agent used is temozolomide (TMZ). TMZ methylates the DNA, thus induces DNA damage mediated cell death. But, often glioma cells confer resistance to temozolomide. The major cause is the role of MGMT (O6-methyl guanine DNA methyl transferase) gene that encodes a DNA repairing protein O6-alkyl guanine DNA alkyl transferase (AGT). So, in order to sensitize glioma cells, different treatment protocols have been designed. One of them suggest a frequent administration of TMZ to the patients. Another common approach is by using TMZ in combination with radiotherapy. The third protocol is by inhibiting PARP (poly (adenosine diphosphate-ribose)) with small molecule inhibitors as PARP also plays an important role in the drug resistance.

3.3.2. *Small molecule inhibitor*

With the advent of cell signaling, many cancer specific signaling pathways have been delineated. As a result, key molecules have been identified and small molecule inhibitors have been designed. In general, most of the small molecules come in the category of receptor tyrosine kinase inhibitor (RTKi).

For example, Erlotinib, an epidermal growth factor receptor (EGFR) inhibitor inactivates downstream molecules of receptor tyrosine kinase (RTK); Sonolisisb, targets phosphotidyl inositol-3 kinase (PI3K). Also, small molecule inhibitor of angiogenesis, for example, Sorafenib inhibits vascular endothelial growth factor receptor (VEGFR) (Jakubowicz-Gil *et al.,* 2017). Similarly, other family members of RTK *e.g.,* platelet derived growth factor receptor (PDGFR) targeted by Imatinib mesylate (Holdhoff *et al.,* 2005), fibroblast growth factor receptor (FGFR) are also target of small molecules *e.g.,* PD173074 (Anderson and Galileo, 2016). A large section of therapeutic monoclonal antibodies are developed against cell surface molecules which are very target specific and abrogates different cancer favoring cell signaling pathways. For example, Cetuximab, a chimeric (human/mouse) monoclonal antibody has been developed to target epidermal growth factor repector (EGFR) which is an important member of RTK and regulated cell proliferation. Cetuximab has shown a limited success against glioblastoma (Westphal *et al.,* 2017). Bevacizumab (Avastin™), a recombinant humanized monoclonal antibody is designed to target VEGFR shows promising result in slowing down tumor growth glioblastoma (Chekhonin and Gurina, 2015). Besides, a lot of studies have been conducted by inhibiting key molecules in pro-proliferative pathways, which are commonly regarded as second messengers, *e.*g., PI3K/Akt, Mitogen activated protein kinase (MAPK)/Ras/Raf, mTOR pathway, etc. Besides targeting the second messengers, histone deacetylase inhibitors are also used. Generally, small molecule inhibitors come in the second line of therapy, when the first line of therapy fails or GBM relapse. But, these inhibitors are not free of side effects, they are expensive and many of it has failed to show any significant improvements in patients. Thus, till date, despite there are variety of small molecule inhibitors in the drug market, very few are used with a significant success.

3.4. Immunotherapy

Immunotherapy may be defined as inducing ones immune system to kill the cancer cells. This therapeutic procedure is considered as silver bullet for varieties of diseases including cancer where immune cells systematically attacks and kills the cells. Glioblastoma cells pose unique immune environment in central nervous system with dedicated lymphatic vessels (Louveau *et al.*, 2015). Owing to the site specific nature of glioblastoma, efforts have been made to develop vaccines to induce active immune surveillance (Lim *et al.,* 2018). Rindopepimut (CDX110) is a peptide vaccine targeted against epidermal growth factor receptor variant III (EGFRvIII) (Weller *et al.*, 2014). Isocitrate dehydrogenase 1 (IDH1) peptide vaccine is also under investigation as IDH mutant gliomas are the major subtype of the disease (according to WHO) (Louis *et al.,* 2016; Schumacher *et al.*, 2014). Other than this, the use of different oncolytic viruses are also under investigation (Lim *et al.,* 2018). Immune checkpoint regulators are also under investigation.

3.5. Therapy using natural compounds

Few natural compounds have exhibited anticancer effects (*e.g.,* Taxol). In the last two decades, researches on natural compounds have gained considerable attention, because of its wide range of chemotherapeutic and chemopreventive activities and low side effects. There are many such natural compounds have been tested upon glioblastoma (Vengoji *et al.,* 2018). Many conventional drugs like temozolomide (TMZ) fails to penetrate blood brain barrier as well as shows poor result against cancer stem cells which are also highly drug resistance. Thus despite showing promising result in cell culture model, they fail in clinical trial. Some of the natural compounds like quercetin, resveratrol, icariin, curcumin, etc., show promising results by not only killing mature glioblastoma cells, but also decimating recalcitrant cancer stem cells. Roles of the following natural compounds have been described briefly:

3.5.1. *Quercetin*

It is a flavonoid compound isolated from plant *Allium cepa*. It shows a wide range of health protective activities. In one work, scientists have observed effect of quercetin on glioblastoma cell culture model (U251 cells) and found that it induced apoptosis *via* upregulating apoptosis inducing genes as well as blocking cell cycle at G2/M phase. Also, they observed the inhibitory effect of quercetin on cell migration and invasion (Liu *et al.,* 2017). Previously, other researchers also found that quercetin induced abrogation of glioblastoma cell migration and inhibition by modulating STAT6/IL3 signaling (Michaud-Levesque *et al.,* 2012). Quercetin also found to sensitize glioblastoma to the conventional drugs like temozolomide ((Jakubowicz-Gil *et al.*, 2013; Sang *et al.*, 2014).

3.5.2. *Resveratrol*

It is a stillbenoid (hydroxyl form of stillbene) isolated from a plant names *Vitis vinifera*. In the last 15 years, several reports suggest anti-tumor effect of reseveratrol. One report showed that it modulated matrix metallo proteinase-2 (MMP-2) activation in cultured gioma cell line (Gagliano *et al.*, 2005). Similarly, resveratrol was found to restore p53 activation thus mediated apoptosis through Notch-1 dependent pathway (Lin *et al.,* 2011). Further, different studies showed the effect of resveratrol on different cell signaling pathways *e.g.,* modulation of PI3K/Akt/NFêB pathway (Jiao *et al.,*

2015), differentiates glioma stem cells into non-cancerous cells *via* p53 activation, which further induced proteasome mediated Nanog degradation (Sato *et al.,* 2013), impairs glioma stem cells proliferation by affecting Notch signaling (Cilibrasi *et al.,* 2017), activates RhoA/Rho-associated kinase (ROCK) thus inhibit cell migration and invasion (Xiong *et al.,* 2016), inhibits Akt phosphorylation and induces p53 activation (Clark *et al.,* 2016). Thus, it plays important role in tacking glioblastoma cells. Further, different studies have indicated the role of resveratrol in combination therapy with TMZ (Filippi-Chiela *et al.,* 2013; Huang *et al.,* 2012; Li *et al.,* 2016; Yuan *et al.*, 2012; Zanotto-Filho *et al.,* 2015). To increase the accessibility of resveratrol to glioblastoma cells, liposomes have been employed as a delivery vehicle, where liposome targeted transferrin to cross blood brain barrier (Jhaveri *et al.,* 2018).

3.5.3. *Icariin*

It is a flavonoid compound extracted from *Herba epimedii*. It is a Chinese herb known to have a wide range of protective effects. It is thought to have the ability to cross blood brain barrier, thus have an advantage over other natural compounds to kill glioblastoma cells (Han *et al.,* 2015; Xu *et al.,* 2015). Although, there are not many research have done on the, but icariin was found to TMZ sensitization of glioma cells (Yang *et al.,* 2015).

3.5.4. *Curcumin*

Another natural compound, probably the most studied is curcumin. It is the major component of turmeric and responsible its characteristic color. Turmeric is used as spice in sub-continental food. It is obtained from the rhizome of *Curcuma longa*. Curcumin used to be present in *keto* and *enol* form (Fig. 1). Being a polyphenolic compound, it is highly soluble in non-polar solvents (Ethanol 10 mg/ml, Acetone 20 mg/ml, DMSO 25 mg/ml) but sparingly soluble in water (<0.1 mg/ml).

Curcumin poses wide range of therapeutic qualities including anticancer effect. Anticancer effect of curcumin has been established in varieties of

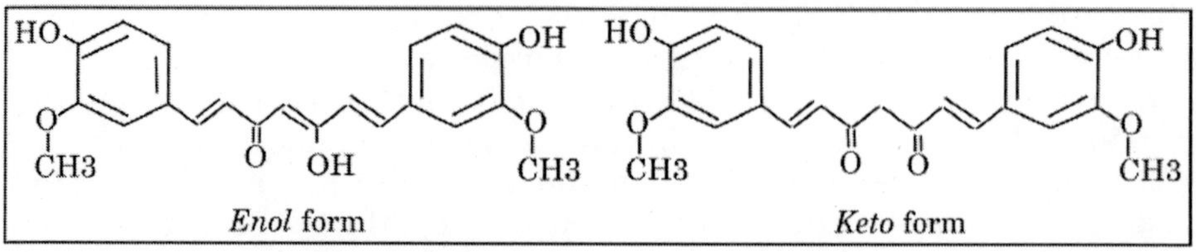

Fig. 1: Structure of curcumin- Enol and keto form.

cancer. Few important cell signaling pathways modulated by curcumin is shown in Fig. 2. Researchers have studied the effect of curcumin on glioblastoma as well and tried to establish the molecular mechanism of curcumin mediated cell death. Researchers have shown curcumin kills glioblastoma cell line T98G by activating both receptor mediated and mitochondrial pathway (Karmakar *et al.* 2006). Another study has shown chemo-suppressive effect of curcumin on AP-1 and NFkB proteins, thus sensitizes different glioblastoma cell lines to standard chemotherapeutic agents (Dhandapani *et al.,* 2007). In other work, curcumin simultaneously showed suppression of antiapoptotic signals and activation of Caspase mediated apoptosis (Huang *et al.*, 2010; Karmakar *et al.*, 2007). In U87 xenografted athymic mouse model, curcumin exhibited inhibition of tumor growth and antiangiogenic effect (Perry *et al.,* 2010) and found to affect selectively cancer cells, not the normal cells in mice (Zanotto-Filho *et al.,* 2012). The effect of curcumin is on the cell signaling molecules are further investigated in different research. Curcumin is found to play role in epigenetic modification through upregulation of receptor activator of NFκB (RANK) gene expression (Wu *et al.*, 2013), which is found to be silenced in gliomas. Curcumin abrogates AKT/mTOR pathway and induces ROS, thus sensitizes U87MG cells to TMZ (Yin *et al.*, 2014). In another work curcumin

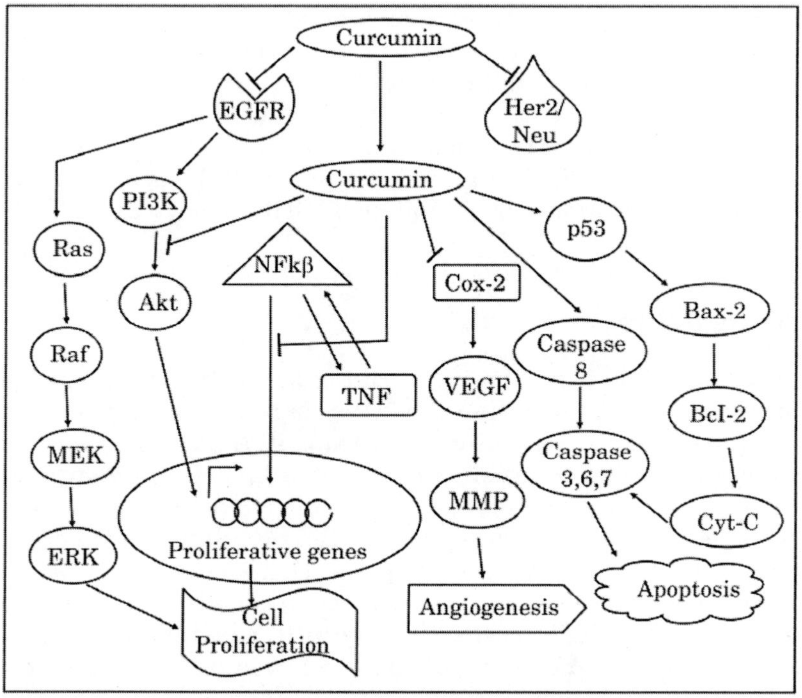

Fig. 2: Different cell signaling pathways modulated by curcumin in cancer cells.

adduct was formed for intra-nasal delivery to mouse model. It was found that curcumin adduct affected the polarity of tumor associated microglia population (Mukherjee *et al.,* 2016), thus kills glioblastoma cells. In this work, curcumin adduct was found to activate microglial NFkB and STAT-1. Curcumin in combination with TMZ inhibits autophagy, thus sensitizes the cells (Zanotto-Filho *et al.,* 2015). In one work, researchers have isolated glioma stem cells (GSCs) from resected samples. The stem cells were grown in neurosphere media and then curcumin was administered. Curcumin induced reactive oxygen species (ROS) and abrogate STAT-1 pathway (Gersey *et al.,* 2017). A recent report showed that glioblastoma cell line A172, upon exposure to curcumin exhibited endoplasmic reticulum (ER) vessel formation, presence of few specific microRNAs which indicated that curcumin induced paraptosis (another form of cell death) (Garrido-Armas *et al.*, 2018). Other than directly killing glioma cells, sensitization of glioma cells to known anti-cancer drugs have also been investigated as an alternative approach. New drugs or new therapeutics takes a long time to come to the market, whereas common drugs with well documented pathways can be used readily. So, sensitization of the resistant cells to common drugs has been investigated in different labs. In our lab, we have transfected U87MG cell line with IκBα gene. Then, common anticancer drug 5-Fluorouracil (5-FU) and curcumin nanoparticle was administered. This combination therapy was found to be effective (Banerjee *et al.,* 2014a). Few other micro RNA based work also showed promising results. Later, it was showed that NFêB inhibiting micro RNA miR-146a is involved in the elevated sensitization of glioblastoma cell line U87MG that were treated with curcumin and TMZ (Wu *et al.,* 2015). In another study, researchers have showed miR-378 enhances anticancer effect of curcumin (Li *et al.*, 2017). In another work, miR-326 sensitized glioma cells to curcumin treatment by inhibition of SHH/Gli1 pathway (Yin *et al.*, 2018).

3.5.5. *Drug delivery*

As the location of glioblastoma is difficult to access by free drugs as blood brain barrier acts as a major limiting factor, *in vivo* results of glioblastoma therapies are strikingly poor as compared to *in vitro* data. Thus, nanocarriers and liposomes have been investigated as potential delivery vehicle for one or co-delivery of more than one drugs. In order to deliver single drug *via* nanoparticles, Dhami *et al.* (2014) synthesized a cisplatin loaded protamine impregnated poly (lactide-co-glycolide) (PLGA) nanoparticle. This nanoparticle showed higher trafficking through bovine brain and enhanced cytotoxicity towards U87MG cells. Also, recently, paclitaxel (Ptx) have been encapsulated in substance P modified (which was used to increase intra-molecular di-sulfide bonds) human serum albumin (HSA) and delivered to the glioma cells. Better efficiency was observed (Ruan *et al.,* 2018).

Photosensitizers have also been tested against human glioblastoma cells U87MG and LN229 cells. In this work, multiple strategies were obtained to make it target specific and photo-tunable. Gold nanoparticles (AuNPs) were synthesized, loaded with a photosensitizer phthalocyanine 4 (Pc 4) and functionalized with two peptides EGF and Tf, targeted against epidermal growth factor receptor (EGFR) and transferrin receptor (TfR). Thus the AuNPs becomes target specific. Further, photodynamic therapy with a certain wavelength of light was shone on the cells. Thus, selectively, glioblastoma cells were killed in a controlled fashion (Dixit *et al.,* 2015). In another such photothermal therapy based approach, recently indocyanine green (ICG) was loaded in silk fibroin nanoparticle (SFNPs). ICG loaded SFNPs were targeted against C6 glioma xenograft nude mouse model. At the near infra-red wavelength (NIR), ICG showed better phototoxicity over free ICG as because SFNPs gives higher stability to ICG *in vivo* (Xu *et al.,* 2018). Most of the cancers including glioblastoma require more than one drugs for treatment purpose. In another work, lipid nanodisk was synthesized and functionalized with D-A7R peptide. This nanodisk showed enhanced cytototoxicity and better penetration capability (Zhang *et al.,* 2018b).

Nanocarriers have been designed for delivering more than one drugs. One such approach, lipid nanoparticle was synthesized and functionalized with both tripeptide Arginine-Glycine-Aspartic acid (RGD) and lactoferrin. Hence bi-functionalized lipid nanoparticle was encapsulated with anticancer drugs temozolomide (TMZ) and vincristine and delivered in human glioma cells and BALB/c nude mice glioblastoma model. High drug encapsulation efficiency, sustained release resulted in synergistic effect of drugs. Thus, resistance of glioma cells to a single drug type can be surpassed (Zhang *et al.,* 2018a). Combined delivery of chemical drug and antisense RNA has also investigated. Potent chemotherapeutic agent bis-chloroethylnitrosourea (BCNU) and small interfering RNA (siRNA) designed against vascular endothelial growth factor (VEGF) was simultaneously delivered in 3 Arginine and 6 valine based amphiphilic self-assembled micelle towards C6 glioma cells and showed a heightened anticancer effect (Yi *et al.*, 2014). As temozolomide is a potent drug against glioblastoma cells but many times the cells show tolerance towards TMZ, thus result in TMZ insensitivity and higher side effects due to elevated dosage. In one approach, PEG-PLGA nanoparticle was synthesized and antisense microRNAs (antagomiR-21 and antagomiR-10b) were encapsulated. These miRs were found to pre-sensitize glioblastoma cells before TMZ treatment (Malhotra *et al.,* 2018). siRNA is also an effective therapeutic strategy against cancer. But free siRNA has some limitations when used to treat glioblastomas. So, Srimanee *et al.* (2018) has designed cell penetrating peptide based siRNA delivery vehicle for effective delivery. This cell penetrating peptide carrying siRNA effectively silence glioblastoma cells U87MG. Choi *et al.* (2017) attempted combined delivery of TMZ and herpes simplex virus thymidine kinase (HSV-tk) gene *via* Arginine and Leucine (R7L10) peptide micelle. Hence uploaded HSV-tk and TMZ showed much higher cytotoxicity against C6 glioma cells. Tong *et al.* (2018) has designed a polyethylenimine (PEI) capped porous silica nanoparticle for higher siRNA loading capacity and increased *in vivo* circulation time. The siRNA was designed against multidrug resistance associated protein (MRP-1) and found to inhibit glioblastoma growth. In another work, hybrid chitosan-dextran (CS-DX) - superparamagnetic iron oxide nanoparticles (SPION) was synthesized. This nanoparticle facilitates MRI guided imaging and increase retention capacity inside the tumor cells. Thus, increase the targeted drug delivery potential (Shevtsov *et al.*, 2018). The different vehicle of drug delivery and different therapeutic agents has been shown in Fig. 3.

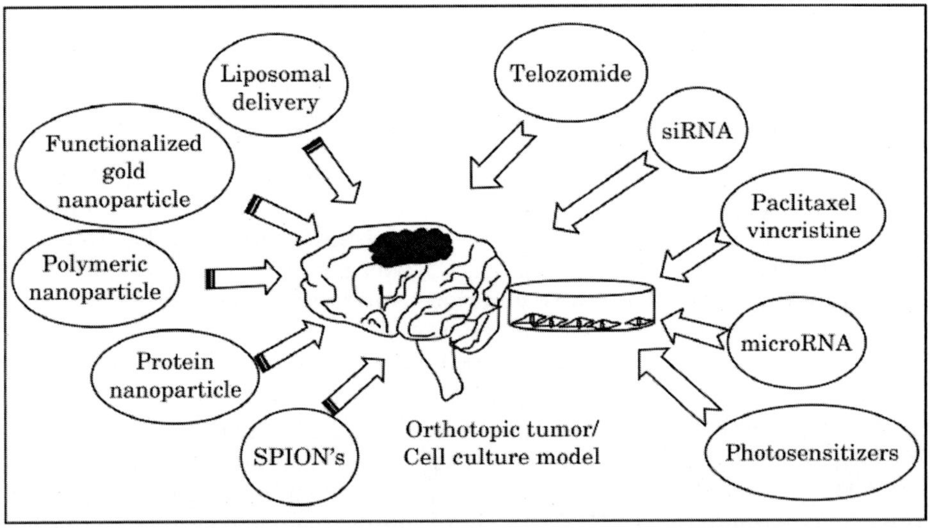

Fig. 3: Different modes of drug delivery and different agents for glioblastoma therapy.

3.6. Nanotherapy

Curcumin is a polyphenolic compound with very low water solubility. As a result, it has low residential time in physiological system which results in low bioavailability. Also, curcumin cannot cross the blood brain barrier. In order to circumvent this problem, different delivery approaches have been undertaken. Nanoparticles or nanocarriers have shown promising role in anticancer therapeutics. There are several advantages of using nanoformulation of a compound or packing it in the nano-sized delivery vehicle. The advantages are as follows; a) Particles at their nanosize has higher surface to volume ratio compared to bulk materials. Thus, nanoparticles show longer contact time during interaction with target molecules; b) Nanocarriers are small vesicles generally made up of natural or synthetic polymers. The size ranges of the nanocarriers are around 100 nm to 1 µm. Nanocarriers have several advantages like it can carry hydrophobic molecules (*e.g.,* curcumin), hydrophilic molecules (*e.g.,* biomolecules) and proteins whose solubility depends on several factors. Release of drug/bioactive molecules can be controlled based on different physico-chemical parameters, *e.g.,* pH, temperature, enzymatic activity, etc. Also, the release can be controlled in a temporal manner. Cancer microenvironment shows few unique characteristics which are absent in normal tissue condition, *e.g.,* damages blood vessels due to constant neovascularization and extracellular matrix (ECM) remodeling, low pH and high activity of ECM remodeling enzymes matrix metalloprotease (MMPs), thus render resistance towards many conventional chemotherapeutic system. As the release from the nanocarriers can be tunable, thus nanocarriers can take the advantage of otherwise hostile condition of cancer microenvironment. The pore sizes of the damaged blood vessels are bigger in tumor microenvironment and vary broadly from one types of cancer to another type. The nanocarrier size range upto 400 nm takes this advantage and shows enhanced permeation and retention (EPR) effect which is also known as passive targeting (Matsumura and Maeda, 1986; Kim *et al.,* 2015). EPR effect increases the residence time at the tumor site and hence higher drug release to the target site. Nanocarrier is an important vehicle to deliver recombinant proteins to the cancer cells. In our lab, nanocarriers have been used to deliver recombinant IκBα (63 kDa) to cervical cancer HeLa and glioblastoma cell line U87MG (Banerjee *et al.,* 2013) and prodrug converting enzyme Cytosine deaminase (Kumar Yata *et al.*, 2014). Further, fluorescent metallic gold and silver nanoparticles (nanoclusters) have been used as a theranostic agent when it was applied to the cancer cells (Sahoo *et al.,* 2014; Sahoo *et al.,* 2016; Nair *et al.,* 2017). The various types of nanocarriers are used to deliver curcumin to the target site. These approaches include curcumin delivery by micro emulsions, micelles, polymeric nanocarrier, lipid-polymer hybrid nanoparticle, protein nanoparticle, synthesis of curcumin nanoparticle etc.

3.6.1. *Nanocarrier mediated delivery of curcumin*

Despite the wide range of therapeutic advantages, the application of curcumin is limited due to its poor water solubility. There are several nanoparticle based approaches have been undertaken to treat glioma cancer cells and cancer stem cells (Pistollato *et al.,* 2016). Curcumin mixed with docosahexaenoic acid (DHA) rich oil results microemulsion. This microemulsion was delivered to the glioblastoma cells through intranasal and intravenous route (Shinde and Devarajan, 2017). Polymeric nanoparticle formulation of curcumin applied upon embryonic glioblastoma cell lines

DAOY and D283Med and spheroid culture of HSR-GBM1 and JHH-GBM14 showed marked reduction of viable cells in the cell mass (Lim *et al.*, 2011). Shao *et al.* (2011) prepared methoxy polyethylene glycol (PEG) – poly (caprolactone) (PCL) block co-polymer nanoparticles, which showed cytotoxicity on rat glioma C6 cell line. Another group has developed curcumin-loaded glyceryl monooleate (GMO) nanoparticles (NP). To increase its bioavailability, it was functionalized with the surfactant Pluronic F-68 and vitamin E D-α-tocopheryl polyethylene glycol 1000 succinate (TPGS) for delivery to the brain (Kundu *et al.,* 2012). Recently, Zhang and co-workers prepared a solid dispersion of curcumin by ball milling process with di-sodium glycyrrhizin (Na_2GA). Na_2GA formed a micelle loaded with curcumin when dissolved in water. The micelle showed higher cytotoxicity against U87MG glioblastoma cell line. Also, the micelle showed higher cell permeability and much higher bioavailability (~19 fold) than free curcumin (Zhang *et al.*, 2018c). Zhao *et al.* (2018d) synthesized a curcumin loaded nanoliposome functionalized with Rabies virus derived peptide (RDP). The RDP conjugated nanoliposome (RCL) has increased the passage through blood- brain barrier by energy dependent endocytosis process and used as a cytotoxic as well as intracranial imaging agent. Ahmadi Nasab *et al.* (2018) synthesized a pH responsive mesoporous silica nanoparticle capped with chitosan to sustained delivery of curcumin to U87MG. They have found sustained delivery at lower pH. Besides the problem of bioavailability, crossing blood brain barrier to access glioma cells. Wang *et al.* (2017) prepared a liposome made by para aminophenyl-alpha -D-mannopyranoside, which has the ability to cross blood brain barrier. The curcumin was loaded inside the nanocarrier. Also, curcumin was delivered *via* poly (lactic-co-glycolic acid) (PLGA) based hybrid polymeric nanoparticle to rat glioma C6 cell lines (Orunoglu *et al.,* 2017). Authors have found elevated cell death. Another PLGA based nanoparticle was used for dual delivery of curcumin and paclitaxel. They have synthesized PLGA based magnetic nanoparticle conjugated with transferrin targeted peptide T7. This nanoparticle showed traceability, higher blood brain barrier crossing capability and synergistic effect (Cui *et al.*, 2016). Other than dual drug delivery, our lab synthesized recombinant IκBα coated curcumin nanoparticle and observed higher U87MG cell death. Protein therapeutics is a promising field of medicine but many proteins albeit target specific, don't kill the cells directly. Instead, some drug or natural compounds show elevated cytotoxicity as a result of synergistic effect. In this work, inducible transcription factor NFkB was targeted by its cellular inhibitor IκBα and natural inhibitor curcumin, hence showed synergistic effect (Banerjee *et al.*, 2014b). Paunovi *et al.* prepared a curcumin nano-formulation and tested it upon U251 cells. The curcumin nanoparticle was synthesized by water/tetrahydrofuran solvent exchange method. Thus prepared curcumin nanoparticle was irradiated with blue light (wavelength 470 nm and power 1 W) and administered on U251 glioblastoma cells *in vitro*. The photo-excitation of curcumin nanoparticle increases the cell internalization of curcumin. Also, light induced curcumin nanoparticle activates phosphorylation of c-Jun N-terminal kinase (JNK) molecule, increases mitochondrial membrane depolarization and hence increases the cytotoxicity (Paunovic *et al.*, 2016). Besides these types of nanoparticle based approaches, which basically increase the residence time, sustained and target specific delivery, researchers have tried other approaches. One such approach is dendrimer base curcumin nanoparticle preparation and application on U251 cells. Gamage *et al.* (2016) have developed a polyamidoamine (PAMAM) based paramagnetic theranostic nanoparticle and conjugated curcumin with it. As a result, the nanoparticle showed more efficient blood brain barrier crossing capability and can be tracked by magnetic resonance relaxivity method or a MRI based technique known as Paramagnetic Chemical Exchange Saturation Transfer PARACEST. Human glioma cells U251 was grown in nude rat brain, at the normal position (orthotopic) and the hence synthesized nanoparticle was applied. MRI data showed higher localization of dendrimeric nanoparticles in the U251 cells. Also, presence of curcumin was found in serum (Gamage *et al.,* 2016). Curcumin also used as a theranostic agent. A micelle was constructed (<15 nm in diameter) and curcumin and another fluorescent nanoparticle were loaded. This construct was termed as theranostic photonic nanoparticles (TPNs), which is able to cross the blood brain barrier of orthotopic xenograft mouse model. At the NIR, curcumin acted as a donor to the fluorescent dye named as CbV. Thus, it can be monitored by imaging, also, the shrinkage of tumor can be monitored (Singh *et al.,* 2016).

Curcumin has been used directly upon the patients or on the patient sample. For the oral delivery of curcumin, N-trimethyl chitosan functionalized solid lipid nanoparticle has been proposed with a burst release capability and able to reach the brain. Higher level of encapsulated curcumin was found compared to free curcumin (Ramalingam and Ko, 2015). In order to increase the oral bioavailabilty of curcuminoid, it was loaded into micelle and administered to patients prior to their brain resection. More than usual level of curcumin was found in the patient tissue and serum of the patient (Dutzmann *et al.,* 2016). Curcuminoids are phytochemicals extracted from turmeric. These molecules also have chemopreventive activities. Such molecules found in turmeric are demethoxycurcumin and bisdemethoxycurcumin (BDMC). Some researchers showed that BDMC has increased stability and nuclear uptake (Basile *et al.,* 2009).

4. CONCLUSIONS AND FUTURE PERSPECTIVES

Natural compounds show varieties of chemotherapeutic and bio-preventive effects. Among the natural compounds, one of the most used, probably most studied molecule is curcumin. Curcumin shows a variety of activities *e.g.*, cell cycle blocker, angiogenesis inhibition, apotopsis activation, ROS scavenging etc. Also, curcumin used to have plethora of molecular targets including NFκB, TNF receptor, Cox-1, Cox-2, Histone deacetylase (HDAC) etc. to name a few. Low solubility of curcumin in water has always posed a major challenge in curcumin based therapy. The advent of polymeric and liposomal nanocarriers has opened up a new avenue for efficient curcumin delivery in the cell. Also, the distribution time and bioavailability has increased. The resultant chemotherapeutic effect of curcumin has markedly increased. Also, nanocarriers help the curcumin to cross the blood brain barrier. Some strategies include preparation and delivery of curcumin nanoparticle to the cell. The nanoparticle formation increases the stability and solubility of curcumin in water. In some therapeutic strategies, curcumin is not used as a sole therapeutic molecule but a part of combination therapy. In this type of work, curcumin sensitizes the cells so that other drugs can be effectively used. This helps in controlling aggressive chemotherapeutic protocol, thus lower the non-specific cytotoxicity. Altogether, curcumin pose a very promising role in chemotherapeutic arsenal. Also, the other molecules in curcuminoid family (other derivatives of curcumin), *e.g.*, demethoxycurcumin and bisdemethoxycurcumin are also under intensive research as chemotherapeutic agent.

There are few challenges ahead of the curcumin based therapy. One of the challenges is lower stability of the nanoparticle as a drug. Thus, therapeutic nanoaprticles used to have a low shelf life, which can't be used as a drug in market. Another challenge is non- specificity of curcumin. As it is able to bind with several cellular targets and modulate several signaling pathways, thus, may not be used as a part of targeted therapy. Nevertheless, the advent in nanoparticle research and potency of curcumin to promote cancer cell death shows the curcumin as one of the future medicine for different types of cancers including glioblastoma.

REFERENCES

Ahmadi Nasab N, Hassani Kumleh H, Beygzadeh M, Teimourian S, Kazemzad M. Delivery of curcumin by a pH-responsive chitosan mesoporous silica nanoparticles for cancer treatment. Artificial Cells, Nanomedicine, and Biotechnology. 2018; 46(1): 75-81.

Anderson HJ, Galileo DS. Small-molecule inhibitors of FGFR, integrins and FAK selectively decrease L1CAM-stimulated glioblastoma cell motility and proliferation. Cellular Oncology. 2016 Jun 1; 39(3): 229-42.

Banerjee S, Sahoo AK, Chattopadhyay A, Ghosh SS. Chemosensitization of IκBα-overexpressing glioblastoma towards anti-cancer agents. RSC Advances. 2014a;4(74): 39257-67.

Banerjee S, Sahoo AK, Chattopadhyay A, Ghosh SS. Hydrogel nanocarrier encapsulated recombinant IκBα as a novel anticancer protein therapeutics. RSC Advances. 2013;3(33): 14123-31.

Banerjee S, Sahoo AK, Chattopadhyay A, Ghosh SS. Recombinant IκBα-loaded curcumin nanoparticles for improved cancer therapeutics. Nanotechnology. 2014b;25(34): 345102.

Barani IJ, Larson DA. Radiation therapy of glioblastoma. *In:* Current Understanding and Treatment of Gliomas. 2015, pp. 49-73. Springer, Cham.

Barbarite E, Sick JT, Berchmans E, Bregy A, Shah AH, Elsayyad N, Komotar RJ. The role of brachytherapy in the treatment of glioblastoma multiforme. Neurosurgical Review. 2017;40(2): 195-211.

Basile V, Ferrari E, Lazzari S, Belluti S, Pignedoli F, Imbriano C. Curcumin derivatives: molecular basis of their anti-cancer activity. Biochemical pharmacology. 2009;78(10): 1305-1315.

Biasoli D, Kahn SA, Cornelio TA, Furtado M, Campanati L, Chneiweiss H, Moura-Neto V, Borges HL. Retinoblastoma protein regulates the crosstalk between autophagy and apoptosis, and favors glioblastoma resistance to etoposide. Cell Death and Disease. 2013;4(8): e767.

Biasoli D, Sobrinho MF, Da Fonseca AC, De Matos DG, Romao L, de Moraes Maciel R, Rehen SK, Moura-Neto V, Borges HL, Lima FR. Glioblastoma cells inhibit astrocytic p53-expression favoring cancer malignancy. Oncogenesis. 2014;3(10): e123.

Carlsson SK, Brothers SP, Wahlestedt C. Emerging treatment strategies for glioblastoma multiforme. EMBO Molecular Medicine.2014; 6: 1359-1370.

Chekhonin I, Gurina O. Trends in Malignant Glioma Monoclonal Antibody Therapy. Current Medicinal Chemistry. 2015; 11: 102-118.

Choi E, Han J, Tan X, Oh J, Lee D, Rhim T, Lee M. Combined delivery of temozolomide and the thymidine kinase gene for treatment of glioblastoma. Journal of Drug Targeting. 2017; 25: 156-162.

Cilibrasi C, Riva G, Romano G, Cadamuro M, Bazzoni R, Butta V, Paoletta L, Dalpra L, Strazzabosco M, Lavitrano M, *et al.* Resveratrol Impairs Glioma Stem Cells Proliferation and Motility by Modulating the Wnt Signaling Pathway. PloS One. 2017; 12: e0169854.

Clark PA, Bhattacharya S, Elmayan A, Darjatmoko SR, Thuro BA, Yan MB, van Ginkel PR, Polans AS, Kuo JS. Resveratrol targeting of AKT and p53 in glioblastoma and glioblastoma stem-like cells to suppress growth and infiltration. Journal of Neurosurgery. 2016; 126: 1448-1460.

Clarke J, Butowski N, Chang S. Recent advances in therapy for glioblastoma. Archives of Neurology.2010; 67, 279-283.

Cruickshanks N, Zhang Y, Yuan F, Pahuski M, Gibert M, Abounader R. Role and Therapeutic Targeting of the HGF/MET Pathway in Glioblastoma. Cancers.2017;9(7): 87. doi:10.3390/cancers9070087

Cui Y, Zhang M, Zeng F, Jin H, Xu Q, Huang Y. Dual-Targeting Magnetic PLGA Nanoparticles for Codelivery of Paclitaxel and Curcumin for Brain Tumor Therapy. ACS Applied Materials and Interfaces.2016; 8: 32159-32169.

Dhami NK, Pandey RS, Jain UK, Chandra R, Madan J. Non-aggregated protamine-coated poly (lactide-co-glycolide) nanoparticles of cisplatin crossed blood-brain barrier, enhanced drug delivery and improved therapeutic index in glioblastoma cells: *In vitro* studies. Journal of Microencapsulation 2014; 31: 685-693.

Dhandapani KM, Mahesh VB, Brann DW. Curcumin suppresses growth and chemoresistance of human glioblastoma cells *via* AP-1 and NFkappaB transcription factors. Journal of Neurochemistry 2007; 102: 522-538.

Dixit S, Miller K, Zhu Y, McKinnon E, Novak T, Kenney ME, Broome AM. Dual Receptor-Targeted Theranostic Nanoparticles for Localized Delivery and Activation of Photodynamic Therapy Drug in Glioblastomas. Molecular Pharmaceutics.2015; 12: 3250-3260.

Dutzmann S, Schiborr C, Kocher A, Pilatus U, Hattingen E, Weissenberger J, Geßler F, Quick-Weller J, Franz K, Seifert V, Frank J. Intratumoral concentrations and effects of orally administered micellar curcuminoids in glioblastoma patients. Nutrition and cancer. 2016; 68: 943-948.

England B, Huang T, Karsy M. Current understanding of the role and targeting of tumor suppressor p53 in glioblastoma multiforme. Tumour Biology. 2013; 34: 2063-2074.

Filippi-Chiela EC, Thomé MP, e Silva MM, Pelegrini AL, Ledur PF, Garicochea B, Zamin LL, Lenz G. Resveratrol abrogates the temozolomide-induced G2 arrest leading to mitotic catastrophe and reinforces the temozolomide-induced senescence in glioma cells. BMC Cancer. 2013; 13(1): 147.

Gagliano N, Moscheni C, Torri C, Magnani I, Bertelli AA, Gioia M. Effect of resveratrol on matrix metalloproteinase-2 (MMP-2) and Secreted Protein Acidic and Rich in Cysteine (SPARC) on human cultured glioblastoma cells. Biomedicine and Pharmacotherapy. 2005;59(7): 359-64.

Gamage NH, Jing L, Worsham MJ, Ali MM. Targeted Theranostic Approach for Glioma Using Dendrimer-Based Curcumin Nanoparticle. Journal of Nanomedicine and Nanotechnology. 2016;7(4): 393.

Garrido-Armas M, Corona JC, Escobar ML, Torres L, Ordóñez-Romero F, Hernández-Hernández A, Arenas-Huertero F. Paraptosis in human glioblastoma cell line induced by curcumin. Toxicology *in vitro*. 2018; 51: 63-73.

Gersey ZC, Rodriguez GA, Barbarite E, Sanchez A, Walters WM, Ohaeto KC, Komotar RJ, Graham RM. Curcumin decreases malignant characteristics of glioblastoma stem cells *via* induction of reactive oxygen species. BMC Cancer. 2017;17(1): 99.

Han H, Xu B, Hou P, Jiang C, Liu L, Tang M, Yang X, Zhang Y, Liu Y. Icaritin Sensitizes Human Glioblastoma Cells to TRAIL-Induced Apoptosis. Cell Biochemistry and Biophysics.2015; 72: 533-542.

Holdhoff M, Kreuzer KA, Appelt C, Scholz R, Na IK, Hildebrandt B, Riess H, Jordan A, Schmidt CA, Van Etten RA, Dörken B. Imatinib mesylate radiosensitizes human glioblastoma cells through inhibition of platelet-derived growth factor receptor. Blood Cells, Molecules, and Diseases. 2005;34(2): 181-185.

Holland EC. Glioblastoma multiforme: The terminator. Proceedings of the National Academy of Sciences of the United States of America.2000; 97: 6242-6244.

Huang H, Lin H, Zhang X, Li J. Resveratrol reverses temozolomide resistance by downregulation of MGMT in T98G glioblastoma cells by the NF-êB-dependent pathway. Oncology Reports.2012; 27: 2050-2056.

Huang TY, Tsai TH, HsuCW, Hsu YC. Curcuminoids suppress the growth and induce apoptosis through caspase-3-dependent pathways in glioblastoma multiforme (GBM) 8401 cells. Journal of Agricultural and Food Chemistry. 2010; 58: 10639-10645.

Jakubowicz-Gil J, Badziul D, Langner E, WertelI, Zajac A, Rzeski W. Temozolomide and sorafenib as programmed cell death inducers of human glioma cells. Pharmacological Reports. 2017; 69: 779-787.

Jakubowicz-Gil J, Langner E, B¹dziul D, Wertel I, Rzeski W. Apoptosis induction in human glioblastoma multiforme T98G cells upon temozolomide and quercetin treatment. Tumor Biology. 2013; 34: 2367-2378.

Jhaveri A, Deshpande P, Pattni B, Torchilin V. Transferrin-targeted, resveratrol-loaded liposomes for the treatment of glioblastoma. Journal of Controlled Release.2018; 277: 89-101.

Jiao Y, Li H, Liu Y, Guo A, Xu X, Qu X, Wang S, Zhao J, Li Y, Cao Y. Resveratrol inhibits the invasion of glioblastoma-initiating cells *via* down-regulation of the PI3K/Akt/NF-êB signaling pathway. Nutrients. 2015;7(6): 4383-402.

Karmakar S, Banik NL, Patel SJ, Ray SK. Curcumin activated both receptor-mediated and mitochondria-mediated proteolytic pathways for apoptosis in human glioblastoma T98G cells. Neuroscience Letters. 2006; 407(1): 53-58.

Karmakar S, Banik NL, Ray SK. Curcumin suppressed anti-apoptotic signals and activated cysteine proteases for apoptosis in human malignant glioblastoma U87MG cells. Neurochemical Research. 2007; 32: 2103-2113.

Kaul D, Florange J, Badakhshi H, Grün A, Ghadjar P, Exner S, Budach V. Accelerated hyperfractionation plus temozolomide in glioblastoma. Radiation Oncology. 2016;11(1): 70.

Kim SS, Harford JB, Pirollo KF, Chang EH. Effective treatment of glioblastoma requires crossing the blood–brain barrier and targeting tumors including cancer stem cells: The promise of nanomedicine. Biochemical and Biophysical Research Communications. 2015; 468(3): 485-589.

Kumar Yata V, Banerjee S, Ghosh S. Folic Acid Conjugated-Bio Polymeric Nanocarriers: Synthesis, Characterization and *in vitro* Delivery of Prodrug Converting Enzyme. 2014; 6(4): 388-92.

Kundu P, Mohanty C, Sahoo SK. Antiglioma activity of curcumin-loaded lipid nanoparticles and its enhanced bioavailability in brain tissue for effective glioblastoma therapy. Acta Biomaterialia. 2012; 8: 2670-2687.

Langhans J, Schneele L, Trenkler N, Bandemer H, Nonnenmacher L, Karpel-Massler G, Siegelin MD, Zhou S, Halatsch ME, Debatin KM, Westhoff MA. The effects of PI3K-mediated signalling on glioblastoma cell behaviour. Oncogenesis. 2017; 6(11):4.

Lara-Velazquez M, Al-Kharboosh R, Jeanneret S, Vazquez-Ramos C, Mahato D, Tavanaiepour D, Rahmathulla G, Quinones-Hinojosa A. Advances in brain tumor surgery for glioblastoma in adults. Brain sciences. 2017;7(12): 166.

Li H, Liu Y, Jiao Y, Guo A, Xu X, Qu X, Wang S, Zhao J, Li Y, Cao Y. Resveratrol sensitizes glioblastoma-initiating cells to temozolomide by inducing cell apoptosis and promoting differentiation. Oncology reports. 2016;35(1): 343-51.

Li W, Yang W, Liu Y, Chen S, Chin S, Qi X, Zhao Y, Liu H, Wang J, Mei X, Huang P. MicroRNA-378 enhances inhibitory effect of curcumin on glioblastoma. Oncotarget. 2017;8(43): 73938.

Lim KJ, Bisht S, Bar EE, Maitra A, Eberhart CG. A polymeric nanoparticle formulation of curcumin inhibits growth, clonogenicity and stem-like fraction in malignant brain tumors. Cancer Biology and Therapy. 2011; 11(5): 464-73.

Lim M, Xia Y, Bettegowda C, Weller M. Current state of immunotherapy for glioblastoma. Nature Reviews Clinical Oncology. 2018; 1: 1-12.

Lin H, Xiong W, Zhang X, Liu B, Zhang W, Zhang Y, Cheng J, Huang H. Notch-1 activation-dependent p53 restoration contributes to resveratrol-induced apoptosis in glioblastoma cells. Oncology Reports. 2011;26(4): 925-30.

Liu Y, Tang ZG, Lin Y, Qu XG, Lv W, Wang GB, Li CL. Effects of quercetin on proliferation and migration of human glioblastoma U251 cells. Biomedicine and Pharmacotherapy. 2017; 92: 33-8.

Lo HW. EGFR-targeted therapy in malignant glioma: Novel aspects and mechanisms of drug resistance. Current Molecular Pharmacology. 2010; 3: 37-52.

Louis DN, Ohgaki H, Wiestler OD, Cavenee WK, Burger PC, Jouvet A, Scheithauer BW, Kleihues P. The 2007 WHO classification of tumours of the central nervous system. Acta Neuropathologica. 2007; 114(2): 97-109.

Louis DN, Perry A, Reifenberger G, Von Deimling A, Figarella-Branger D, Cavenee WK, Ohgaki H, Wiestler OD, Kleihues P, Ellison DW. The 2016 World Health Organization classification of tumors of the central nervous system: A summary. Acta neuropathologica. 2016;131(6): 803-20.

Louveau A, Smirnov I, Keyes TJ, Eccles JD, Rouhani SJ, Peske JD, Derecki NC, Castle D, Mandell JW, Lee KS, Harris TH. Structural and functional features of central nervous system lymphatic vessels. Nature. 2015;523(7560): 337.

Malhotra M, Sekar TV, Ananta JS, Devulapally R, Afjei R, Babikir HA, Paulmurugan R, Massoud TF. Targeted nanoparticle delivery of therapeutic antisense microRNAs presensitizes glioblastoma cells to lower effective doses of temozolomide *in vitro* and in a mouse model. Oncotarget.2018; 9: 21478-21494.

Mao H, LeBrun DG, Yang J, Zhu VF, Li M. Deregulated signaling pathways in glioblastoma multiforme: molecular mechanisms and therapeutic targets. Cancer Investigation. 2012;30(1): 48-56.

Matsumura Y, Maeda H. A new concept for macromolecular therapeutics in cancer chemotherapy: Mechanism of tumoritropic accumulation of proteins and the antitumor agent smancs. Cancer research. 1986;46(12 Part 1): 6387-92.

Michaud-Levesque J, Bousquet-Gagnon N, Béliveau R. Quercetin abrogates IL-6/STAT3 signaling and inhibits glioblastoma cell line growth and migration. Experimental Cell Research. 2012;318(8): 925-35.

Mukherjee S, Baidoo J, Fried A, Atwi D, Dolai S, Boockvar J, Symons M, Ruggieri R, Raja K, Banerjee P. Curcumin changes the polarity of tumor associated microglia and eliminates glioblastoma. International journal of cancer. 2016;139(12): 2838-49.

Nair LV, Nair RV, Shenoy SJ, Thekkuveettil A, Jayasree RS. Blood brain barrier permeable gold nanocluster for targeted brain imaging and therapy: An *in vitro* and *in vivo* study. Journal of Materials Chemistry B. 2017;5(42): 8314-21.

Orunoglu M, Kaffashi A, Pehlivan SB, Þahin S, Söylemezoðlu F, Oðuz KK, Mut M. Effects of curcumin-loaded PLGA nanoparticles on the RG2 rat glioma model. Materials Science and Engineering: C. 2017;78: 32-38.

Paunovic V, Ristic B, Markovic Z, Todorovic-Markovic B, Kosic M, Prekodravac J, Kravic-Stevovic T, Martinovic T, Micusik M, Spitalsky Z, Trajkovic V. c-Jun N-terminal kinase-dependent apoptotic photocytotoxicity of solvent exchange-prepared curcumin nanoparticles. Biomedical microdevices. 2016;18(2): 37.

Perry MC, Demeule M, Regina A, Moumdjian R, Beliveau R. Curcumin inhibits tumor growth and angiogenesis in glioblastoma xenografts. Molecular nutrition & food research. 2010;54(8): 1192-201.

Pistollato F, Bremer-Hoffmann S, Basso G, Cano SS, Elio I, Vergara MM, Giampieri F, Battino M. Targeting glioblastoma with the use of phytocompounds and nanoparticles. Targeted oncology. 2016;11(1): 1-6.

Ramalingam P, Ko YT. Enhanced oral delivery of curcumin from N-trimethyl chitosan surface-modified solid lipid nanoparticles: Pharmacokinetic and brain distribution evaluations. Pharmaceutical Research.2015; 32: 389-402.

Ruan C, Liu L, Lu Y, Zhang Y, He X, Chen X, Zhang Y, Chen Q, Guo Q, Sun T, Jiang C. Substance P-modified human serum albumin nanoparticles loaded with paclitaxel for targeted therapy of glioma. Acta Pharmaceutica Sinica B. 2018; 8(1): 85-96.

Sahoo AK, Banerjee S, Ghosh SS, Chattopadhyay A. Simultaneous RGB emitting Au nanoclusters in chitosan nanoparticles for anticancer gene theranostics. ACS Applied Materials and Interfaces. 2013;6(1): 712-24.

Sahoo AK, Goswami U, Dutta D, Banerjee S, Chattopadhyay A, Ghosh SS. Silver nanocluster embedded composite nanoparticles for targeted prodrug delivery in cancer theranostics. ACS Biomaterials Science and Engineering. 2016;2(8): 1395-402.

Sang DP, Li RJ, Lan Q. Quercetin sensitizes human glioblastoma cells to temozolomide *in vitro via* inhibition of Hsp27. Acta Pharmacologica Sinica. 2014; 35(6): 832.

Sato A, Okada M, Shibuya K, Watanabe E, Seino S, Suzuki K, Narita Y, Shibui S, Kayama T, Kitanaka C. Resveratrol promotes proteasome-dependent degradation of Nanog *via* p53 activation and induces differentiation of glioma stem cells. Stem Cell Research. 2013;11(1): 601-10.

Schumacher T, Bunse L, Pusch S, Sahm F, Wiestler B, Quandt J, Menn O, Osswald M, Oezen I, Ott M, Keil M. A vaccine targeting mutant IDH1 induces antitumour immunity. Nature. 2014;512(7514): 324.

Shevtsov M, Nikolaev B, Marchenko Y, Yakovleva L, Skvortsov N, Mazur A, Tolstoy P, Ryzhov V, Multhoff G. Targeting experimental orthotopic glioblastoma with chitosan-based superparamagnetic iron oxide nanoparticles (CS-DX-SPIONs). International Journal of Nanomedicine. 2018;13: 1471.

Shinde RL, Devarajan PV. Docosahexaenoic acid-mediated, targeted and sustained brain delivery of curcumin microemulsion. Drug Delivery.2017; 24: 152-161.

Singh A, Kim W, Kim Y, Jeong K, Kang CS, Kim Y, Koh J, Mahajan SD, Prasad PN, Kim S. Multifunctional Photonics Nanoparticles for Crossing the Blood–Brain Barrier and Effecting Optically Trackable Brain Theranostics. Advanced Functional Materials. 2016;26(39): 7057-66.

Srimanee A, Arvanitidou M, Kim K, Hallbrink M, Langel U. Cell-penetrating peptides for siRNA delivery to glioblastomas. Peptides.2018; 104: 62-69.

Szopa W, Burley TA, Kramer-Marek G, Kaspera W. Diagnostic and Therapeutic Biomarkers in Glioblastoma: Current Status and Future Perspectives. BioMed Research International 2017; 2017: 1-13.

Tong WY, Alnakhli M, Bhardwaj R, Apostolou S, Sinha S, Fraser C, Kuchel T, Kuss B, Voelcker NH. Delivery of siRNA *in vitro* and *in vivo* using PEI-capped porous silicon nanoparticles to silence MRP1 and inhibit proliferation in glioblastoma. Journal of Nanobiotechnology. 2018; 16(1): 38.

Vengoji R, Macha MA, Batra SK, Shonka NA. Natural products: A hope for glioblastoma patients. Oncotarget. 2018; 9(31): 22194.

von Achenbach C, Weller M, Szabo E. Epidermal growth factor receptor and ligand family expression and activity in glioblastoma. Journal of Neurochemistry. 2018;doi: 10.1111/jnc.14538.

Wang Y, Ying X, Xu H, Yan H, Li X, Tang H. The functional curcumin liposomes induce apoptosis in C6 glioblastoma cells and C6 glioblastoma stem cells *in vitro* and in animals. International Journal of Nanomedicine. 2017;12: 1369.

Weller M, Cloughesy T, Perry JR, Wick W. Standards of care for treatment of recurrent glioblastoma—are we there yet?. Neuro-oncology. 2012;15(1): 4-27.

Weller M, Kaulich K, Hentschel B, Felsberg J, Gramatzki D, Pietsch T, Simon M, Westphal M, Schackert G, Tonn JC, von Deimling A. Assessment and prognostic significance of the epidermal growth factor receptor vIII mutation in glioblastoma patients treated with concurrent and adjuvant temozolomide radiochemotherapy. International journal of cancer. 2014; 134(10): 2437-47.

Westhoff MA, Karpel-Massler G, Brühl O, Enzenmüller S, La Ferla-Brühl K, Siegelin MD, Nonnenmacher L, Debatin KM. A critical evaluation of PI3K inhibition in Glioblastoma and Neuroblastoma therapy. Molecular and Cellular Therapies. 2014;2(1): 32.

Westphal M, Maire CL, Lamszus K. EGFR as a Target for Glioblastoma Treatment: An Unfulfilled Promise. CNS Drugs. 2017; 31: 723-735.

Wu B, Yao X, Nie X, Xu R. Epigenetic reactivation of RANK in glioblastoma cells by curcumin: Involvement of STAT3 inhibition. DNA and Cell Biology.2013; 32: 292-297.

Wu H, Liu Q, Cai T, Chen YD, Wang ZF. Induction of microRNA-146a is involved in curcumin-mediated enhancement of temozolomide cytotoxicity against human glioblastoma. Molecular Medicine Reports.2015; 12: 5461-5466.

Xiong W, Yin A, Mao X, Zhang W, Huang H, Zhang X. Resveratrol suppresses human glioblastoma cell migration and invasion *via* activation of RhoA/ROCK signaling pathway. Oncology Letters.2016; 11: 484-490.

Xu B, Jiang C, Han H, Liu H, Tang M, Liu L, Ji W, Lu X, Yang X, Zhang Y, Liu Y. Icaritin inhibits the invasion and epithelial to mesenchymal transition of glioblastoma cells by targeting EMMPRIN *via* PTEN/AKt/HIF 1á signalling. Clinical and Experimental Pharmacology and Physiology. 2015;42(12): 1296-307.

Xu HL, ZhuGe DL, Chen PP, Tong MQ, Lin MT, Jiang X, Zheng YW, Chen B, Li XK, Zhao YZ. Silk fibroin nanoparticles dyeing indocyanine green for imaging-guided photo-thermal therapy of glioblastoma. Drug Delivery. 2018;25(1): 364-75.

Yang L, Wang Y, Guo H, Guo M. Synergistic Anti-Cancer Effects of Icariin and Temozolomide in Glioblastoma. Cell Biochemistry and Biophysics.2015; 71: 1379-1385.

Yi N, Oh B, Kim HA, Lee M. Combined delivery of BCNU and VEGF siRNA using amphiphilic peptides for glioblastoma. Journal of Drug Targeting.2014; 22: 156-164.

Yin H, Zhou Y, Wen C, Zhou C, Zhang W, Hu X, Wang L, You C, Shao J. Curcumin sensitizes glioblastoma to temozolomide by simultaneously generating ROS and disrupting AKT/mTOR signaling. Oncology Reports. 2014;32(4): 1610-6.

Yin S, Du W, Wang F, Han B, Cui Y, Yang D, Chen H, Liu D, Liu X, Zhai X, Jiang C. MicroRNA-326 sensitizes human glioblastoma cells to curcumin *via* the SHH/GLI1 signaling pathway. Cancer Biology and Therapy. 2018; 19(4): 260-70.

Yuan Y, Xue X, Guo RB, Sun XL, Hu G. Resveratrol enhances the antitumor effects of temozolomide in glioblastoma *via* ROS dependent AMPK TSC mTOR signaling pathway. CNS neuroscience and Therapeutics. 2012; 18(7): 536-46.

Zanotto-Filho A, Braganhol E, Edelweiss MI, Behr GA, Zanin R, Schröder R, Simões-Pires A, Battastini AM, Moreira JC. The curry spice curcumin selectively inhibits cancer cells growth *in vitro* and in preclinical model of glioblastoma. The Journal of Nutritional Biochemistry. 2012;23(6): 591-601.

Zanotto-Filho A, Braganhol E, Klafke K, Figueiró F, Terra SR, Paludo FJ, Morrone M, Bristot IJ, Battastini AM, Forcelini CM, Bishop AJ. Autophagy inhibition improves the efficacy of curcumin/temozolomide combination therapy in glioblastomas. Cancer Letters. 2015;358(2): 220-31.

Zhang J, Xiao X, Zhu J, Gao Z, Lai X, Zhu X, Mao G. Lactoferrin-and RGD-comodified, temozolomide and vincristine-coloaded nanostructured lipid carriers for gliomatosis cerebri combination therapy. International Journal of Nanomedicine. 2018a;13: 3039.

Zhang M, Lu L, Ying M, Ruan H, Wang X, Wang H, Chai Z, Wang S, Zhan C, Pan J, Lu W. Enhanced Glioblastoma Targeting Ability of Carfilzomib Enabled by a DA7R-Modified Lipid Nanodisk. Molecular Pharmaceutics. 2018b; 15(6): 2437-47.

Zhang Q, Polyakov NE, Chistyachenko YS, Khvostov MV, Frolova TS, Tolstikova TG, Dushkin AV, Su W. Preparation of curcumin self-micelle solid dispersion with enhanced bioavailability and cytotoxic activity by mechanochemistry. Drug Delivery. 2018c; 25(1): 198-209.

Zhao M, Zhao M, Fu C, Yu Y, Fu A. Targeted therapy of intracranial glioma model mice with curcumin nanoliposomes. International Journal of Nanomedicine. 2018;13: 1601.

4

Drug Discovery Approaches and the Role of Plant Products in Treating Neuronal Disorders

PICHILI VIJAYA BHASKAR REDDY[1*], CHADIPIRALLA KIRANMAI[3] AND PANKAJ KALITA[1,2]

ABSTRACT

Phytotherapy plays a key role in traditional medicine system in the management of diseases. Traditional medication practices have been serving as an effective alternative source of medicine among many societies in spite of the availability of well-established drug therapy. Natural products have been playing vital role in the traditional treatment as well as in medication system for hundreds of years, in parallel with the development of the pharmaceutical industry. These natural products contain complicated mixtures of organic chemicals, which may include fatty acids, sterols, alkaloids, flavonoids, glycosides, saponins, tannins, terpenes and so forth. Use of medicinal plants against neurological disorders is an age old practice. The traditional system of utilizing medicinal plants is effectively applied to improve the brain function. The pharmacogenic plant extracts interact with the targeted signaling pathways affecting the pharmacology and thereby potentially playing a role in human disease and treatment. Neural drugs work by balancing of particular chemicals (neurotransmitters) or by selective enhancement of cerebral blood flow, cerebral oxygen usage, metabolic rate

[1] Department of Life Science and Bioinformatics, Assam University, Diphu Campus, Karbi Anglong, Assam, India.

[2] Department of Biophysics, Pub Kamrup College, Baihata Chariali, Kamrup, Assam, India.

[3] Department of Biotechnology, Vikrama Simhapuri University, Nellore, Andhra Pradesh, India

**Corresponding authors*: vpichili@gmail.com; vbreddyasuh@yahoo.com *and cerebral glucose metabolic rate in chronically impaired brain. Both G protein-coupled receptors (GPCRs) and ion channels possess important functions in the central nervous system (CNS). Plant extracts have been reported to exhibit affinity to a number of CNS receptors with a complexity of this interaction like agonist-induced activity of the human neurokinin-1 receptor, gamma amino butyric acid (GABA) receptor, N methyl D aspartate (NMDA) receptor, α-amino-3-hydroxy-5-methyl-4-isoxazolepropionic acid (AMPA) receptors etc. In the present chapter, it is aimed to document the plant based drugs and their role in treating neurological disorders and also the drug discovery approaches involved.*

***Key words*:** Phytotherapy, Pharmacogenic plant extracts, Drug targets, Side effects.

---

1. INTRODUCTION

Globalization and enhanced busy life style of the human being induces various kinds of mental stress in the daily life leading to various kinds of neurological disorders. Neurological disorders impose a major concern to the global public health scenario inclusively both in the developed and developing countries. These include headache disorders, epilepsy, dementia, multiple sclerosis, and neuro-infections and other neurological disorders associated with malnutrition, pain associated with neural problems like Parkinson's disease, stroke and traumatic brain injuries (Tapsoba and Deschamps, 2006; Nadembega *et al.,* 2011). More than 600 different health problems may affect the nervous system. It also entails a major social burden on the health care systems of the nation associated with stigma and inequity against the patient and even his/her family in the community, workplace, school and home (Zerbo *et al.,* 2013).

The brain is composed of 100 billion neurons connecting each other forming a communication networks. The neurons are specialized in different functions like thinking, learning, remembering, starring, hearing etc. to do their specialized activities. It functions to process and to store the information of the body and thus, communicating with other cells of the body. Abnormality in this coordinated system causes various neurological disorders. Thus, it is a condition of mental derangement crossing the state of normalcy and gets deranged to become the syndromes of mental disorder (Balkrishna and Misra, 2017). Mental and neurological disorders represent 13% of the burden of total morbidity in the world and in and around 13 to 49% of the world's populations develop neuropsychiatric disorders at some point in their life (Yasamy *et al.,* 2011). These pathologies affect all categories of person irrespective of sex, age and race (Poli *et al.,* 2012).

In the present chapter, an explorative explanation of different medicinally important traditional plants is supposed to be documented. Their active fraction of components and mode of actions including the drug development approaches are aimed to be mentioned in the subsequent parts of the chapters.

2. NATURAL PRODUCT AND TRADITIONAL THERAPY IN HEALTHCARE SYSTEM

Medicinal plants are an important source of new bioactive molecules with potential therapeutic importance and have been used since the ancient time (Mittal *et al.,* 2013) and remaining as a major component of health care system in spite of the availability of well-established alternatives (Casey *et al.,* 2007). Phytotherapy plays a key role in traditional medicine system in the management of diseases. In many developing countries of the world, including India, about 80% populations depend exclusively on traditional medication systems like traditional healers and medicinal plants for their primary health care needs. Traditional phytotherapy includes the practices and approaches of using different floral and faunal based natural products which include a mixture of different phytochemicals *viz.* fatty acids, sterols, alkaloids, flavonoids, glycosides, saponins, tannins, terpenes and so forth to prevent the diseases. These phytochemicals exhibit their functional activities by communicating with different mechanistic pathways and by interacting with different receptors. The human cells contain a large numbers of receptors involving the mechanistic pathways of signal transduction process for executing its functions (Ernst, 2007). Table 1 highlights the various important diseases and their corresponding receptors used for drug development and design which are the responsible drug targets in drug discovery and designing. Malfunctioning of a particular receptor/s involved in any biochemical pathway or molecular pathway or any other signal transduction cascade results in the inhibition or under-expression or over-expression of a specific protein or a gene corresponding to a specific disease condition and eventually leading to an undesirable situation in a biological system. The active component/bioactive molecule acts as agonist or antagonist to control the hypo or hyper activated receptors

Natural or synthetic neuroactive molecules like neuroleptics, antidepressants, anxiolytics are extensively used to treat these pathologies, particularly epilepsy, schizophrenia and other psychotic disorders (Starling and Feijo, 2012; Reybellet and Quio, 2015). These molecules have plant origins, traditionally used to treat different neurological disorders (Taiwe and Kuete, 2014). Moreover, different studies have documented various plant species used in these health practices. However, little research has

Table 1: List of receptors playing a role in various neurological disorders.

Disease	*Target molecule for drug*	*References*
Alzheimer's disease	Acetyl cholinesterase	Greig *et al.* (2002)
Anxiety	Corticotrophin releasing factor type 1 (CRF1)	Kehne (2007)
Delirium	Cholinesterase inhibitor	Hshieh *et al.* (2008)
Epilepsy	Gamma Amino Butyric Acid ($GABA_A$ receptor)	Rogawski and Loscher (2004)
Huntington disease	Huntingtin protein (Htt)	Lo and Hughes (2011)
Meningitis,	CD147 receptor	Bernard *et al.* (2014)
Parkinson disease	L- Dopamine (L-DOPA)	Tiziana and Sergio (2015)
Schizophrenia	N-methyl-D-aspartate (NMDA) receptor	Ghosh *et al.* (2011)
Vertigo	Dopamine receptor and calcium channel	Kariya *et al.* (1995)

approached the specific case of plants used to treat nervous system disorders. It necessitates reporting of proper documentation of disorders treated by traditional healers, medicinal plants and medical practices used for these treatments.

2.1. Role of different natural product in disease prevention

As the human population lives longer, age related diseases which are mostly related to dietary habits, continue to attack. For several thousand years, this fact had encouraged the mankind to search and include the plant based medicinal diet to prevent the deterioration in health. The use of medicinal plants as an important source of relief from illnesses can be traced back to five millennia in the form of written documents of the early civilization in China, India and Near East, but undoubtedly it is an art as old as mankind. Even today, plants are not only indispensable in health care but are expected to be ample source for safe future medicines (Anonymous, 1969; Husain *et al.,* 1988, 1992). Although years long back plants are used as a source of new drug molecule but the recent approach from combinatorial chemistry has put an end to the dominance of natural products in drug discovery. After thousands of years of bioprospecting for plant based pharmaceuticals, scientists are able to identify the most effective, relatively less harmful bioactive molecules. However, experts find that most of the plant derived natural products (molecules) that could be probably valued at billions of dollars often remain undiscovered or unexplored for their pharmacological activity. Phytomedicine has gained its popularity because it can be used as a nutraceutical and can be managed in the self-medication system. According to an estimate not less than 80 percent of the world's population uses the herbal therapy for their primary health care (Barnes and Ernst, 1998; Anonymous, 2008). The search for plant based drugs and dietary supplements have accelerated in recent years. More than a hundred active compounds currently isolated from the higher plants and widely used in different neurological disorders. For example, the discovery of the anticonvulsant properties of phenobarbitone in 1912 marked the foundation of the modern pharmacotherapy of epilepsy. Since then different AEDs like phenytoin, ethosuximide, carbamazepine, sodium valproate and a range of benzodiazepines have been regarded as antiepileptic drugs prevailing in the market among the clinicians. An intensive period of development of drugs for epilepsy throughout the 1980s and 1990s has resulted in 14 new agents being licensed as add-on treatment for difficult-to-control adult and pediatric epilepsy, with some becoming available as monotherapy for newly diagnosed patients. Although a large number of antiepileptic drugs are available but their usage become limited due to drug resistance, its toxicity and its interactions with others. It was reported that vigabatrin blocks the GABA transaminase activity and increasing GABA level thus control the seizure; but it has severe retinotoxicity. Similarly, 'Levetiracetam' is another highly effective antiepileptic drug, but it has also some side-effects like increase anxiety, mood change, severe headache etc. (Izumi *et al.,* 2004). Therefore, a new drug with lesser toxicity and highest efficacy is of utmost importance.

In the present day perspectives of neurological disease treatment, the traditional medicine systems have been playing a challenging role in primary health care needs. Medicinal plants are a potential source of new bioactive molecules having remarkable therapeutic effects against the neurological disorders in modern bioassays and many such plants are yet to be scientifically investigated which may possess some potential phytoconstituents (Hegde *et al.,* 2009). Natural products from the traditionally used medicinal plants have contributed significantly in the discovery of new drugs and can be chosen as an alternative source for the discovery of more efficient drugs with better safety and efficacy profiles (Kaushik *et al.,* 2009). Earlier studies have shown the use of natural products/herbal extracts for the prevention and curing of various diseases including neurological disorders. For example, ethanolic extract of *Cynodon dactylon,* methanolic extract of *Bryophyllum pinnatum,* ethanolic extract of *Terminalia chebula,* alcoholic extract from *Punica granatum,* methanolic extract from *Moringa oleifera*, ethanolic extract from *Bacopa monnieri,* ethanolic extract from *Ipomoea aquatica* are extensively used as a brain tonic and uplifting the brain activity. These extracts were used especially as anticonvulsant agent.

There are numerous medicinal plants used against different neurological disorders like epilepsy, convulsion, Parkinson disease, sleeplessness, narcotics, etc. irrespective of its family and plant part utilized. Some bioactive molecules alone or a specific plant extract may be used against these disorders. Common medicinal plants used against different neurological disorders are shown in Table 2.

Table 2: Comprehensive list of natural resources used in different neurological disorders.

Name of the plants	*Family*	*Parts used*	*Used to treat*	*References*
Achillea millefolium L.	Asteraceae	Corymb	Anticonvulsant, antiepileptic	Misra *et al.* (2000)
Alhagi camelorum Fisch.	Fabaceae	Aerial organs	Lumbago	Misra and Kumar (1997)
Amygdalus kotschyi Boiss.	Rosaceae	Seed	Narcotic	Tuli *et al.* (2009)
Anthemis tinctoria L.	Asteraceae	Flowering shoot	Nerve tonic, sedative	Wagner (1985)
Abrus precatorius L.	Fabaceae	Root	Convulsions	Marcy and Douglas (2005)
Acalypha villicaulis Hochst.ex A. Rich.	Euphorbiaceae	Leaf Maceration	Epilepsy	Wagner (1985)
Alchornea cordifolia (Schumach. & Thonn.) Muell.Arg.	Euphorbiaceae	Leaf or leafy stem	Epilepsy	Wagner (1985)
Alstonia boonei. De Wild.	Apocynaceae	Root	Anti-depressant	Misra and Kumar (1997)
Amaranthus viridis L.	Amaranthaceae	Leaf sap	Convulsions, epilepsy	Ragupathi (2017)
Anacardium occidentale L.	Anacardiaceae	Leaf	Anti-depressant	Panjwani (2015)
Andira inermis (Wright) DC.	Fabaceae	Bark	Anti-depressant	Reybellet *et al.* (2015)
Annona senegalensis Pers.	Annonaceae	Root bark	Convulsions, epilepsy	Konate (2012)
Asystasia gangetica (L.)	Acanthaceae	Leaf	Epilepsy decoction	Adetula (2004)
Achyranthes aspera	Amaranthaceae	Seed	Headache of migraine	Balkrishna and Misra (2017)
Acorus calamus	Araceae	Bark	Memory and cures forget fullness, epilepsy, facial paralysis	Balkrishna and Misra (2017)
Adhatoda zeylanica	Acanthaceae	Fruit	Epilepsy disorder	Balkrishna and Misra (2017)
Albizia lebbeck	Mimosaceae	Seed	Cures unconsciousness, psychosis, insanity,anxiety, hysteria	Balkrishna and Misra (2017)

Table 2: (*Contd...*)

Table 2: (*Contd...*)

Name of the plants	*Family*	*Parts used*	*Used to treat*	*References*
Anacyclus pyrethrum	Asteraceae	Flower, root	Hysteria,epilepsy, paralysis,	Balkrishna and Misra (2017)
Allium cepa	Liliaceae	Seed	Beneficial in sleeplessness	Balkrishna and Misra (2017)
Bersama abyssinica Fresen.	Melianthaceae	Root decoction	Epilepsy	Bosch (2008)
Blighia sapida K.D. Koenig.	Sapindaceae	Leaf	Convulsions,	Bosch (2008) epilepsy
Boerhavia diffusa L.	Nyctaginaceae	Aerial parts	Convulsions	Muzila (2006)
Bacopa monnieri	Plantaginaceae	Leaf	Hysteria, epilepsy, memory enhancer	Balkrishna and Misra (2017)
Benincasa hispida	Cucurbitaceae	Leaf	Hysteria, epilepsy	Balkrishna and Misra (2017)
Brassica nigra	Brassicaceae	Seed	Migraine	Balkrishna and Misra (2017)
Cajanus cajan (L.) Millsp.	Fabaceae	Leaf	Epilepsy	Manga *et al.* (2007)
Calycobolus heudelotii (Bak. ex Oliv.) Heine.	Convolvulaceae	Bark	Seizures	Manga *et al.* (2007)
Cassia sieberiana DC.	Fabaceae	Leaf	Convulsions	Misra and Kumar (1997)
Citrus sinensis (L.) Osbeck.	Rutaceae	Leaf, flower, bark, root	Convulsions, epilepsy	Bum (2011)
Cochlospermum tinctorium Perr. ex A.Rich.	Cochlosperma -ceae	Root	Epilepsy	Jansen and Cardon (2005)
Cryptolepis sanguinolenta (Lindl.) Schltr.	Apocynaceae	Leaf	Convulsions, epilepsy	Bum (2011)
Guilandina bonduc	Caesalpiniaceae	Seed, leaf	Headache, epilepsy	Balkrishna and Misra (2017)
Calotropis procera	Asclepiadaceae	Flower, leaf,root	Epilepsy, migraine pain, paralysis	Balkrishna and Misra (2017)
*Cannabis sativa*Linn.	Cannabinaceae	Leaf	Epilepsy, sleeplessness	Balkrishna and Misra (2017)
Cassia occidentalis	Caesalpiniaceae	Whole plant part	Epilepsy and hysteria	Balkrishna and Misra (2017)
Cassia tora	Caesalpiniaceae	Seed	Migraine attack	Balkrishna and Misra (2017)
Celastrus paniculatus	Celastraceae	Seed	Improve memory	Balkrishna and Misra (2017)
Centella asiatica	Apiaceae	Whole plant part	mproves memory power, insomnia, anxiety	Balkrishna and Misra (2017)

Table 2: (*Contd...*)

Table 2: (*Contd...*)

Name of the plants	*Family*	*Parts used*	*Used to treat*	*References*
Citrullus colocynthis	Brassicaceae	Fruit, root	Migraine and ear pain, epilepsy	Balkrishna and Misra (2017)
Citrus aurantifolia	Rutaceae	Seed, fruit	Insanity, anxiety	Balkrishna and Misra (2017)
Clitorea ternatea	Papilionaceae	Seed and root	Migraine pain.	Balkrishna and Misra (2017)
Convolvulus microphyllus	Convolvulaceae	Aerial part	Memory power, strengthens the mind	Balkrishna and Misra (2017)
Coriandrum sativum	Apiaceae	Leaf	Vertigo and headache	Balkrishna and Misra (2017)
Cuscuta reflexa	Cuscutaceae	Leaf	Brain disorders.	Balkrishna and Misra (2017)
Cynodon dactylon	Poaceae	Whole plant part	Madness and epilepsy	Balkrishna and Misra (2017)
Cyperus scariosus	Cyperaceae	Aerial part	Epilepsy	Balkrishna and Misra (2017)
Centaurea cyanus L.	Asteraceae	Corymb	Narcotic	Haidan *et al.* (2016)
Cichorium intybus L.	Asteraceae	Root, Leaf,	Nerves tonic Flower, Seed	Prosper *et al.* (2017)
Coronilla varia L.	Fabaceae	Leaf	Sedative	Marcy (2005)
Cydonia oblonga	Rosaceae	Fruit, Seed	Sedative	Prosper *et al.* (2017)
Datura metel	Solanaceae	Seed	Psychosis	Balkrishna and Misra (2017)
Datura stramonium L.	Solanaceae	Seed	Sedative	Haidan *et al.* (2016)
Daucus carota	Apiaceae	Leaf	Migraine	Balkrishna and Misra (2017)
Daniellia oliveri Hutch. & Dalziel.	Fabaceae	Bark	Epilepsy	Bum (2011) (Rolfe)
Desmodium adscendens (Sw.) DC.	Fabaceae	Leaf	Convulsions	Haidan *et al.* (2016)
Detarium microcarpum Guill. and Perr.	Fabaceae	Bark	Epilepsy	Bum (2011)
Eclipta alba	Asteraceae	Fruit	Migraine	Balkrishna and Misra (2017)
Echium italicum L.	Boraginaceae	Flowering shoot	Anticonvulsant, sedative	Rogawski and Loscher (2004)
Ficus benghalensis	Moraceae	Root bark	Memory power	Balkrishna and Misra (2017)
Ficus religiosa	Moraceae	Branch	Madness	Balkrishna and Misra (2017)
Glycyrrhiza glabra	Papilionaceae	Root	Epilepsy	Balkrishna and Misra (2017)

Table 2: (*Contd...*)

Table 2: (*Contd...*)

Name of the plants	*Family*	*Parts used*	*Used to treat*	*References*
Guiera senegalensis J.F. Gmel.	Combretaceae	Leaf	Depressant	Reybell *et al.* (2015)
Helianthus annuus	Asteraceae	Leaf	Migraine	Balkrishna and Misra (2017)
Hyoscyamus niger	Solanaceae	Seed	Hysteria in women	Balkrishna and Misra (2017)
Hypericum perforatum L.	Asteraceae	Flowering shoot	Headache, sedative	Prosper *et al.* (2017)
Inula oculus-christi L.	Asteraceae	Flowering shoot	Rheumatism, myalgia, bone, pain	Haidan *et al.* (2016)
Indigofera tinctoria L.	Fabaceae	Leaf	Epilepsy	Jansen and Cardon (2005)
Jatropha curcas L.	Euphorbiaceae	Root	Convulsions	Prosper *et al.* (2017)
Jatropha gossypifolia L.	Euphorbiaceae	Leaf	Convulsions	Bum (2011)
Juglans regia	Juglandaceae	Seed	Hysteria	Balkrishna and Misra (2017)
Khaya senegalensis (Desr.)A. Juss.	Meliaceae	Leaf	Anti-depressant	Nikiema and Pasternak (2008)
Landolphia heudelotii A. DC.	Apocynaceae	Root	Mental problems	Reybellet *et al.* (2015)
Lannea velutina A. Rich.	Anacardiaceae	Bark	Epilepsy and insanity	Jansen and Cardon (2005)
Leea guineensis G. Don.	Leeaceae	Leaf	Epilepsy	Manga *et al.* (2007)
Leptoderris brachyptera (Benth.) Dunn.	Fabaceae	Leaf	Seizures	Misra and Kumar (1997)
Lonchocarpus sericeus (Poir.) Kunth ex DC.	Fabaceae	Leaf	Convulsions	Prosper *et al.* (2017)
Moringa oleifera	Moringaceae	Bark, root	Meningitis, epilepsy, hysteria in woman	Balkrishna and Misra (2017)
Mucuna pruriens	Fabaceae	Fruit	Parkinson's disease	Balkrishna and Misra (2017)
Nardostachys jatamansi	Valerianaceae	Leaf	Mental problem	Balkrishna and Misra (2017)
Newbouldia laevis (P. Beauv.) Seeman.	Bignoniaceae	Leaf, stem bark	Convulsions, epilepsy	Ainooson *et al.* (2009)
Nymphaea lotus L.	Nymphaeaceae	Flower	Anti-depressant	Mireille *et al.* (2016)
Ocimum basilicum L.	Lamiaceae	Aerial organs	Sedative	Haidan*et al.* (2016)

Table 2: (*Contd...*)

Table 2: (*Contd...*)

Name of the plants	*Family*	*Parts used*	*Used to treat*	*References*
Papaver somniferum	Papaveraceae	Aerial part	Delirium, sleeplessness, convulsion	Balkrishna and Misra (2017)
Piper longum	Piperaceae	Fruit	Migraine pain	Balkrishna and Misra (2017)
Piper nigrum	Piperaceae	Fruit	Hysteria	Balkrishna and Misra (2017)
Palisota hirsuta (Thunb.) K. Schum.	Commelinaceae	Young stem	Epilepsy	Haidan *et al.* (2016)
Passiflora foetida L.	Passifloraceae	Leaf	Anti-depressant	Prosper *et al.* (2017)
Piper guineense Schum. & Thonn.	Piperaceae	Root	Anti-depressant	Haidan *et al.* (2016)
Prosopis africana (Guill. & Perr.) Taub.	Fabaceae	Leaf	Epilepsy	Bum (2011)
Psidium guajava L.	Myrtaceae	Leaf	Convulsions, epilepsy	Lahon *et al.* (2015); Balkrishna and Misra (2017)
Punica granatum	Punicaceae	Leaf	Insomnia, madness	Balkrishna and Misra (2017)
Papaver rhoeas L.	Papaveraceae	Seed	Narcotic, capsule	Marcy (2005) sedative
Pyrus salicifolia Pall.	Rosaceae	Fruit	Nerve tonic	Haidan *et al.* (2016)
Rauvolfia vomitoria Afzel.	Apocynaceae	Leaf	Convulsions	Olatokunboh *et al.* (2009)
Solanum dulcamara L.	Solanaceae	Stem	Sedative	Prosper *et al.* (2017)
Solanum nigrum L.	Solanaceae	Fruit, Seed	Sedatives, antidepressant	Manga *et al.* (2007)
Sapindus mukorossi	Sapindaceae	Fruit	Migraine pain	Balkrishna and Misra (2017)
Sesbania grandiflora	Fabaceae	Leaf, flower	Epilepsy and migraine	Balkrishna and Misra (2017)
Sida cordifolia	Malvaceae	Leaf	Facial paralysis and anxiety,	Balkrishna and Misra (2017)
Solanum surattense	Solanaceae	Root	Epilepsy	Balkrishna and Misra (2017)
Stachys lavandulifolia	Lamiaceae	Flowering shoot	Narcotic	Misra and Kumar (1997)
Sphaeranthus indicus	Asteraceae	Fruit	Parkinson's Disease	Balkrishna and Misra (2017)
Syzygium aromaticum	Myrtaceae	Fruit	Migraine	Balkrishna and Misra (2017)

Table 2: (*Contd...*)

Table 2: (*Contd...*)

Name of the plants	***Family***	***Parts used***	***Used to treat***	***References***
Terminalia chebula	Combretaceae	Seed	Migraine	Balkrishna and Misra (2017)
Tanacetum parthenium (L.) Schultz.	Asteraceae	Leaf, Flower	Anti-headaches	Haidan *et al.* (2016)
Uvaria chamae P. Beauv.	Annonaceae	Bark	Epilepsy, "bad winds, bad spirits	Reybellet *et al.* (2015)
Vigna subterranea (L.) Verdc.	Fabaceae	Leaf	Epilepsy	Brink *et al.* (2006)
Vitellaria paradoxa C.F. Gaertn.	Sapotaceae	Leaf	Convulsions, epilepsy	Bum, 2014
Valeriana officinalis L.	Valerianaceae	Root, Rhizome	Hypnotic, sedative	Prosper *et al.* (2017)
Vitex negundo	Verbenaceae	Fruit	Mental disorder	Balkrishna and Misra (2017)
Withania somnifera	Solanaceae	Whole plant part	Ischemia	Balkrishna and Misra (2017)
Waltheria indica L.	Sterculiaceae	Aerial	Depressant portion	Hamidu *et al.* (2008)
Xeromphis spinosa	Rubiaceae	Fruit	Migraine headache	Balkrishna and Misra (2017)
Ziziphus mauritiana	Rhamnaceae	Fruit	Epilepsy	Balkrishna and Misra (2017)

3. DRUG DISCOVERY APPROACHES FROM NATURAL RESOURCES TO THE LABORATORY USE

Drug discovery from a medicinal plant involves in-depth exploration, amongst ethnobotanist, ethnopharmacologist, biotechnologist including computational biologist and the animal scientist including medical person. The collection step involves collection and identification of plant species having targeted biological activity which is traditionally used as herbal remedies by the traditional healers. During this step, it must ensure to oblize the country's intellectual property rights (Bakre *et al.,* 1995). Phytochemists or the plant biotechnologists prepare the plant extracts from the selected plant parts and screen the pharmacologically active assays to find out the bioactive assays and further to isolate and characterize the bioactive compound. Molecular biologist and animal biotechnologist plays a key role in drug design and delivery pathway in the cellular environment. Pharmacognosy is the interdisciplinary approach to make a targeted bioactive molecule into competent drug.

Generating a novel drug is a complex problem. Designing of a new drug in terms of its sheer size of the search space of the targeted bioactive molecule is a major challenge for the scientist. The major challenge in drug design is the sheer size of the search space for the novel molecules. Scientists screen the active molecules against the biological target and the modern high-throughput screening principle results in the testing the molecules in the order of 10^6 in the laboratory. But conducting this large number of *in vitro* experiments is exclusively expensive. That is why, it is helpful to have computational biology approach to screen these huge number of source molecules into a small number of entity. Virtual screening is one of the best strategies to screen and select a most efficient drug-like molecule amongst millions of such molecules. Another way of drug development and discovery is the *de-novo* drug design. In this approach, molecules are synthesized according to its required activity towards the desired biological targets. In molecular design approach, molecules are created by computer simulation technique, their drug ability score is counted and filtered for better molecules. Molecules are designed either from predefined groups of atoms or by conducting virtual chemical reactions based on expert coded rules. Thus, the structures of drug-like molecules are generated. However, this approach may sometimes fail in elucidating the structure of the molecule. Molecular docking approach or the machine-learning (ML) approaches help in filtering the undesirable reactive groups (Hartenfeller *et al.*, 2012).

Molecular modelling (MM) is a computational package to presume the efficiency of a drug molecule thus, assisting in drug discovery and development approach. It helps in predicting the ideas of a bioactive molecule *i.e.,* macromolecular 3D conformation, protein-ligand interactions, and its biological behaviour in combination with medicinal chemistry. It is an integral part of explanation and prediction of the functional properties of small drug-like organic molecules. These techniques determine the conformational analysis of the drug target molecules including the virtual screening, docking and molecular dynamics study. Fig. 1 highlights the major steps involved in the process of drug discovery from natural resources to human application.

3.1. Molecular modelling approach for drug discovery

Potential drug development with therapeutic efficiency is a complex and difficult pharmaceutical strategy in the pharma industry in terms of both cost and time. A huge amount of cost and a long period of time are to be devoted in the discovery process. Application of computational approach in the combined chemical and biological efforts in the process of drug discovery, design, development and optimization is of great benefit. *In silico* design is an approach to exploit the hit identification, hit-to-lead selection and to optimize the ADME rules *i.e.,* absorption, distribution, metabolism, excretion

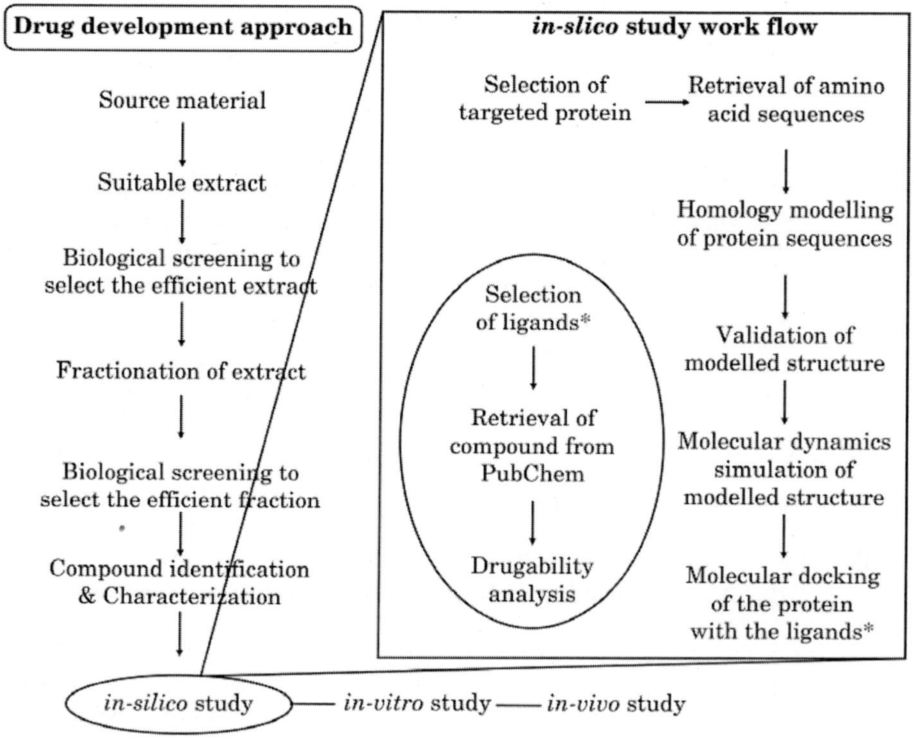

Fig. 1: Flow chart showing different steps of drug discovery.

and toxicity profile of the ligand. Common *in-silico* approach include ligand and structure based drug design, and also the quantitative structure-activity (QSAR) and quantitative structure-property relationships (QSPR).

3.1.1. *Quantitative structure-activity relationship (QSAR)*

It is a computational tool to characterize the topological parameters like hydrogen acceptor, hydrogen donor, electronegativity, logP, molecular weight, molar volume, and molar refractivity of a drug. Hu *et al.* (2006), combined this ANN approach with quantum chemistry and molecular docking principle to design novel Aldose Reductase Inhibitors (ARIs) and also characterized the physicochemical parameters of the molecule including electronegativity and molar volume of the inhibitors. Using these ANN based approach and the topological parameters as input nodes, a novel QSAR model can be constructed to determine the biological activities of new compounds including the neuronal drugs.

3.1.2. *Virtual screening (VS)*

Another computational approach for speeding up the drug discovery approach is the virtual screening to quickly search and identify the compounds with high biological activities from a group of compounds in a database. ANNs-based QSAR models are widely used in the process of virtual screening. Recently, Myint *et al.* (2012) developed a 2D fingerprint-based ANN QSAR (FANN-QSAR) method for virtual screening from huge database of bioactive molecules. They screened and performed a five-fold cross validation of 1699 cannabinoid receptor subtype 2 (CB2) ligands with known activities. A 2D circular topological fingerprint, ECFP6, was chosen as the neural network input. Applying the same principle *i.e.,* the ECFP6-ANN-QSAR model, they predicted GPCR cannabinoid ligand binding affinities of a large number compound database with over 200,000 structurally diverse compounds and two compounds with nanomolar activities were discovered.

3.1.3. *Quantitative structure toxicity relationship (QSTR)*

QSTR predicts the toxicity of bioactive compounds. It defines the mathematical relationship between the chemical's quantitative molecular descriptors and its toxicological activities. QSTR derives the parameters and dataset from the physicochemical properties of the compounds and modelled using computational approach like ANNs. Gao *et al.* (2003) developed an ANN-based ANN-QSTR models for predicting the toxicological effects of substituted benzene and accordingly 78 substituted benzene compounds were validated for its toxicity.

4. PHARMACOKINETIC AND PHARMACODYNAMICS

The computer-aided pharmacodynamical analysis approach offers an exciting alternative to monitor complex interactions between bioactive molecules and the physiological system. Haider *et al.* (2002) established a quantitative computational model for an oral hypoglycemic agent using ANN approach and established a quick and simple method for predicting and identifying significant covariates. Gobburu *et al.* (1996) also applied the ANN tool in drug discovery approach and exhibited its advantages over the conventional model-independent approach.

5. CURRENT TREND IN NEUROLOGICAL DISORDER TREATMENT AND THEIR PROBLEMS

Since the belief, emotion and intuition on the medicinal properties of plants were not supported by the conditions of scientific parameters, they were belittled and replaced by doubt or distrust. With the passage of time, the modern medical methodology sought to break up complicated phenomena and processes into smaller components which had to be dealt with in isolation, often by distinct sub-disciplines, as such largely ignoring the principles of synergy and holism. While in diagnosis, the focus was generally laid on the search for a single illness, to be cured ideally by one remedy, in pharmacology the quest was likewise for one active component to be identified and isolated or synthesized. The development and implementation of the scientific methods and techniques in medicine have brought enormous improvements, especially, in all those cases in which material phenomena, including infection, injury, poisoning, nutrition and hygiene, are major factors in the disease etiology. Of course in public health, modern medicine has substantially contributed to the decrease and eradication of some major epidemic diseases such as typhoid, cholera, bacterial infections, parasitic diseases, smallpox and polio.

In selecting herbal treatments, herbalists may use large base for information because herbs are consumed as vegetables, teas or spices. Therefore, large-scale epidemiological studies become feasible and ethnobotanical studies are further source of information (Anonymous, 1969). It is taken as supporting evidence for its efficacy when indigenous peoples from geographically dispersed areas use closely related herbs for the same treatment (Riddle, 2002).

Most of the plants synthesize substances that are useful to the maintenance of health in humans and other animals. These include aromatic substances, most of which are phenols or their oxygenated derivatives such as phenylpropanoids and lower terpenoids such as mono- and sesquiterpenoids. Many of the herbs and spices used by humans to yield flavor and fragrance are useful medicinal compounds, also (Wagner *et al.*, 1985). These substances help in plant defense mechanisms against different predatory microorganisms, insects, and herbivores (Lai and Roy, 2004; Tapsell *et al.,* 2006). These plants extracts contain a mixture of novel bioactive molecules which can interact with different disease causing molecules thus, signaling in the cellular environment to cure the respective ailment (Abdalla and Ortiz, 2011). Table 3 highlights the major neurological disorders and how they are cured using natural product.

Use of natural product plays a role in preventing a neurological disorder rather than using it as therapy when combined with a healthy life style including a selected dietary habit and a moderate physical activity. These natural products are generally used as some food ingredients. In addition,they contain some bioactive molecules. Designing and development of an effective drug against a neurological disorder is a challenging tough. As mentioned

Table 3: Plant species with their active fraction of extract used in curing different neurological disorders.

Plant species	***Fraction of extract/phyto-chemicals***	***Target molecule in the brain***	***Diseases against which used***	***References***
Arcopus echinatus	Ethanolic extract	$GABA_A$ receptor	Anxiolytic effect of mental disease	Hallam *et al.* (2003)
Artemisia afra	Ethanolic extract	$GABA_A$ receptor	Anxiolytic effect of mental disease	Lo and Liew (2012)
Angelica sinensis	Aqueous	$GABA_A$ receptor	Epilepsy and convulsion	Warner *et al.* (2016)
Ecklonia cava	Polyphenol	$GABA_A$-BZD receptor	Anti-convulsive, sleep-inducing effects, anxiety and insomnia	Dinh *et al.* (2011)
Ephedra sinica	α-tocopherol and ascorbic acid	NMDA, AMPA receptor	BBB disruption, brain edema and brain injury	Hallam *et al.* (2003)
Gentiana macro-phylla	n-Butanol	$GABA_A$ receptor	Epilepsy and convulsion	Warner *et al.* (2016)
Hypericum perfo-ratum	Hexane/dichlo-romethane	Opioid, serotonin, estrogen, histam-ine, neurokinin, and metabotropic glutamate and $GABA_A$ receptor	Anti-depressant effects	Lo and Liew (2012)
Impatiens balsa-mina	Methanolic extract	Opioid receptor	Anti-nociceptive	Lo and Liew (2012)
Lippia alba	Ethanolic extract	$GABA_A$	Epilepsy and convulsion	Lo and Liew (2012)
Melissa officinalis	Volatile compounds such as triterpenoids, phenolic acids, and flavonoid	Acetylcholine-sterase (AChE) inhibition, stimulation of acetylcholine, and $GABA_A$ receptors	Mood, cognition, and memory function	Shakeri *et al.* (2016)
Melissa officinalis	Hexane, acetonitrile	AChE inhibition and cholinergic receptor	Memory enhan-cement, sedative and insomnia	Warner *et al.* (2016)
Mitragyna spe-ciosa	Alkaloid	Monoaminergic and opioid receptors	Mood, recreation and relief of pain	Dinh *et al.* (2011)
Neorautenania mitis	Polyphenol, methanolic extracts	Opioid receptors, NMDA receptor	Brain trauma, brain ischemia, epilepsy and Alzheimer's disease	Dinh *et al.* (2011)

Table 3: (*Contd...*)

Table 3: (*Contd...*)

Plant species	*Fraction of extract/phyto-chemicals*	*Target molecule in the brain*	*Diseases against which used*	*References*
Rhizoma chu-anxiong	Ethanolic extract	$GABA_A$ receptor	Epilepsy and convulsion	Warner *et al.* (2016)
Salvia miltior-rhiza	Aqueous	Benzodiazepine	Anxiety, insomnia, agitation, seizures, muscle spasms, alcohol withdrawal	Shakeri *et al.* (2016)
Scutellaria baicalensis	Methanolic extract	BDZ site in $GABA_A$Receptors	Seizure	Dinh *et al.* (2011)
Storax pili	Oil, flavonoids	GABAA receptor, GABAergic neuromodulation	Epilepsy	Dinh *et al.* (2011)
Tanacetum parth-enium	Ethanolic extract	$GABA_A$ receptor	Epilepsy and prophylactic treatment of migraine	Shakeri *et al.* (2016)
Valeriana adscendens	Methanolic and aqueous	Dopamine D1 receptor	Psychoactive	Shakeri *et al.* (2016)
Valeriana officinalis	Aqueous extract	Ionotropic (iGluR) and metabotropic glutamate receptor NMDA and AMPA receptor binding	Anxiety or insomnia Cognitive and psychomotor effect	Hallam *et al.* (2003)
Ziziphi spinosae	Aqueous	Serotonin 5-HT1A receptors	Panic disorder anxiety and depression	Hallam *et al.* (2003)

earlier in the section 2.1, there are various antiepileptic drugs like vigabatrin, levetiracetam, valproic acid etc. are available in the market. But till date, none of them work in smooth manner. They cause some severe side effects in the physiological systems of the victims. There may be some problems in delivering the drug in the site of action or they may accumulate in the body fluids causing some abnormalities. But when natural products are taken as a food, they can provide additionally the therapeutic value to the body in addition to its normal food value thus, acting as a nutraceutical agent. Moreover, drug from natural product origin are safer than the synthetic drug. Synthetic drugs are made from the cocktails of chemicals which causes an extra harm to the physiology of the organisms than its counterpart natural origin. Hence, in the coming days, the drug molecule derived from the natural product is supposed to be more beneficial having lesser side effects than any other synthetic neuronal drugs.

6. CONCLUSIONS AND FUTURE PERSPECTIVES

Although the theoretical approach to neuronal drug discovery is a very much easy executable but in most times it fails to develop a new and effective drug against a neuronal disorder because of different shortfalls in the drug discovery process. In most cases, either it fails to deliver in the deserved site or it may result in some severe side effects like retinal toxicity, headache, vomiting, mood promotion etc. In the neuronal drug delivery process the blood-brain barrier (BBB) plays a major role to select a drug whether it will be delivered in the required site of action or it will face some physiological traffic in the process.

The most challenging and important step in neuroscience researches and therapy is the selection of a novel technique/strategy for delivering a drug molecule to penetrate the brain barriers. The most applied strategies for drug delivery includes molecular transformation, disruption of the BBB and choosing an alternative route for drug delivery. The methods of molecular transformation involve preparation of lipophilic analogs, development of prodrugs, use of chemical drug delivery systems, application of carrier and receptor mediated drug delivery. But all the methods have some major limitations; like toxic side effects, low efficiency etc. The BBB disruption approach includes osmotic blood-brain barrier disruption and biochemical blood-brain barrier disruption technique. But along with, they also break down the brain's self-defense mechanism and make it vulnerable to damage or infection from all circulating chemicals or toxins. Since these approaches enhance the penetration of drugs to the CNS *via* circulatory system, thus, they will increase the penetration of drugs throughout the entire body resulting in unwanted systemic side effects. Many of the potentially active drug molecules cannot penetrate into the brain environment at therapeutic concentrations. The alternative strategy to enhance the CNS penetration of drug molecules is based on the methodology that does not rely on the cardiovascular system. These strategies circumvent the BBB altogether and do not need drug manipulation to enhance BBB permeability and/or BBBD. Using alternative routes to deliver drugs to the CNS, *e.g.*, intraventricular/intrathecal route and olfactory pathway, is one of these strategies. In spite of a number of modern drugs in the market, but still there is a need to discover and develop new drug molecule because of its common side effects and unsatisfactory mode of work. Drugs from synthetic origin can only for a limited known symptoms of human ailments. Traditional plant drugs still enjoy important status in the modern day drug industries owing to their negligible side effects as well as the synergistic and holistic actions of the combination of a variety of compounds. These traditional plants and plants' extracts, are frequently termed as phytotherapy playing a significant role in human society and civilization exclusively in the healthcare management. Planned and well-designed natural product having the criteria of no side-effects and cost effectiveness may be a better option of use as a neural drug in future.

REFERENCES

Abdalla MS, Ortiz, JG. Selective interactions of *Valeriana officinalis* extracts and valerenic acid with [3H] glutamate binding to rat synaptic membranes. Evidence Based Complementary and Alternative Medicine. 2011: 2011: 1-7.

Adetula OA. *Asystasia gangetica* (L.) T. Anderson. *In:* Grubben, G.J.H. and O.A. Denton (Eds.). PROTA (Plant Resources of Tropical Africa/Resources végétales de l'Afrique tropicale). Recuperado el 18 de Abril de 2011. Disponible en: http://database.prota.org/search.htm, 2004.

Ainooson GK, Woode E, Obiri DD, Koffour GA. Antinociceptive effects of *Newbouldia laevis* (P. Beauv) Stem Bark Extract in a Rat Model. Pharmacognosy Magazine. 2009; 5(17): 49-54.

Anonymous. The Wealth of India. CSIR, New Delhi, India, 1969; Vol. 1-8, pp. 1-384.

Anonymous. WHO Fact sheet no. 134 Traditional Medicine. 2008. http://www.who.int/media centre/factsheets/fs134/en/.

Bakre AG. Quality of life of people with epilepsy: An European study. Epilepsia. 1995; 38: 353–362.

Balkrishna A, Misra LN. Ayurvedic Plants in Brain Disorders: The Herbal Hope. Journal of Traditional Medicine & Clinical Naturopathy. 2017; 6(2): 221.

Barnes J, Ernst E. Traditional herbalists' prescriptions for common clinical conditions: A survey of members of the UK National Institute of Medical Herbalists. Phytotherapy Research. 1998; 12: 369-371.

Bosch CH. *Bersama abyssinica* Fresen. *In:* Schmelzer G.H. and Gurib-Fakim A. (*eds.*). PROTA (Plant Resources of Tropical Africa). 11(1). Medicinal plants 1. PROTA Foundation. Wageningen, Netherlands: Backhuys publishers, 2008, pp. 116.

Brink M, Ramolemana GM, Sibuga KP. *Vigna subterranean* (L) Verdc. *In*: Brink, M. and G. Belay (*eds.*), PROTA I: Cereals and Pulses/ Cereals and Dried Legumes, Wageningen, The Netherlands. 2006, pp. 241-246.

Bum EN, Taiwe GS, Moto FC, Ngoupaye GT, Vougat RR, Sakoue VD, Gwa C, Ayissi ER, Dong C, Rakotonirina A, Rakotonirina SV. Antiepileptic medicinal plants used in traditional medicine to treat epilepsy. *In:* Clinical and genetic aspects of epilepsy 2011. In Tech. doi: 10.5772/18469

Casey MG, Adams J, Sibbritt D. An examination of the prescription and dispensing of medicines by Western herbal therapists: A national survey in Australia. Complementary Therapeutic Medicine, 2007; 15: 13-20.

Dinh LD, Ngyuen LA, Trinh CT, Pham HT. Interaction of various Vietnamese medicinal plant extracts with angiotensin II receptor revealed by fluorescein-labeled ligand receptor binding assays. *In:* Proceedings of the 7th Indochina Conference on Pharmaceutical Sciences and Advancing Pharmacy for ASEAN Community, Bangkok, Thailand, 14–16 December, 2011. P-BB-08.

Ernst E. Herbal medicines: Balancing benefits and risks. Novartis Foundn. Symp. 2007; 282: 154-167.

Gao DW, Wang P, Liang H, Peng YZ. A study on prediction of the bio-toxicity of substituted benzene based on artificial neural network. Journal of Environmental Science and Health. 2003; 38: 571-579.

Ghosh A, Chakraborty K, Mattoo SK. Newer molecules in the treatment of schizophrenia: A clinical update. Indian Journal Pharmacology. 2011; 43(2): 105-112.

Gobburu JV, Chen EP. Artificial neural networks as a novel approach to integrated pharmacokinetic-pharmacodynamic analysis. Journal of Pharmaceutical Science. 1996; 85: 505-510.

Greig N, Lahiri D, Sambamurti K. International Psychogeriatrics, 2002; 14(1): 77-91.

Haidan Y, Qianqian M, Li Y, Guangchun P. The Traditional Medicine and Modern Medicine from Natural Products. Molecules. 2016; 21: 559.

Haider SH, Johnson SB, Fossler MJ, Hussain AS. Modeling the pharmacokinetics and pharmacodynamics of a unique oral hypoglycemic agent using neural networks. Pharmaceutical Research. 2002; 19: 87-91.

Hallam KT, Olver JS, McGrath C, Norman TR. Comparative cognitive and psychomotor effects of single doses of *Valeriana officinalis* and triazolam in healthy volunteers. Human Psychopharmacology. 2003; 18 (8): 619-25.

Hamidu LJ, Ayo AO, Adelaiye AB, Abubakar MS. Sedative and Anticonvulsant Effects of Ethyl Acetate Fraction of *Waltheria indica* in Mice. Journal of Pharmacology and Toxicology. 2008; 3(4): 261-266.

Hartenfeller M, Zettl H, Walter M, Rupp M, Reisen F, Proschak E. DOGS: Reaction-Driven de novo Design of Bioactive Compounds. PLoS Computational Biology. 2012; 8(2): e1002380.

Hegde K, Thakker SP, Joshi AB, Shastry CS, Chandrashekhar KS. Tropical Journal of Pharmaceutical Research. 2009; 8(2): 117.

Hshieh TT, Fong TG, Marcantonio ER, Inouye SK. Cholinergic deficiency hypothesis in delirium: A synthesis of current evidence. The Journals of Gerontology. 2008; 63 (7): 764-72

Hu L, Chen G, Chau RM. A neural networks-based drug discovery approach and its application for designing *Aldose reductase* inhibitors. The Journal of Molecular Graphics and Modelling. 2006; 24: 244-253.

Husain A, Virmani OP, Popli SP, Misra LN, Gupta MM, Srivastava GN, Abraham Z, Singh AK. Dictionary of Indian Medicinal Plants, 1992. CIMAP, Lucknow, India.

Husain A, Virmani OP, Sharma A, Kumar A, Misra LN. Major essential oil bearing plants of India. CIMAP, Lucknow, India, 1988.

Izumi Y, Ishikawa M, Benz AM, Izumi M, Zorumski CF, Thio LL. Acute vigabatrin retinotoxicity in albino rats depends on light but not GABA. Epilepsia. 2004; 45(9): 1043-8.

Jansen PCM, Cardon D. Plant Resources of Tropical Africa 3 (eds). Dyes and tannins. PROTA Foundation, Wageningen, Netherlands/Backhuys Publishers, Leiden, Netherlands/CTA, Wageningen, Netherlands. 2005.

Kariya S, Isozaki S, Masubuchi Y, Suzuki T, Narimatsu S. Possible pharmacokinetic and pharmacodynamic factors affecting Parkinsonism inducement by cinnarizine and flunarizine. Biochemical Pharmacology. 1995; 50(10): 1645-1650

Kaushik D, Khokra SL, Kaushik P, Saneja A, Arora D. Pharmacology online. 2009; 3: 101-106.

Kehne JH. The CRF1 receptor, a novel target for the treatment of depression, anxiety and stress related disorder, CNS Neurological Disorders and Drug Targets. 2007; 6(3): 163-82

Konate A, Sawadogo WR, Dubruc F, Caillard O, Ouedraogo M, Guissou IP. Phytochemical and anticonvulsant properties of *Annona senegalensis* Pers. (Annonaceae), plant used in Burkina folk medicine to treat epilepsy and convulsions, British Journal of Pharmacology and Toxicology. 2012; 3(5): 245-250.

Lahon J, Phukan S, Lahkar M, Sharma U. Anticonvulsant potential of leaves of *Psidium guajava* LINN. In MES and PTZ induced convulsion in experimental animals. International Journal of Pharmaceutical Sciences and Research. 2015; 6(9): 3946.

Lai PK, Roy J. Antimicrobial and chemopreventive properties of herbs and spices. Current Medicinal Chemistry 2004; 11: 1451-1460.

Lo DC, Hughes RE. Neurobiology of Huntington's disease: Applications to drug discovery. Boca Raton (FL): CRC Press/Taylor & Francis, 2011.

Lo KS, Liew KC. Influence of different extraction solvents on lipophilic extractives and *Acacia* hybrid in different wood portions. Asian Journal of Applied Sciences. 2012; 5: 107-116.

Marcy JB, Douglas K. Drug discovery from medicinal plants. Life Sciences. 2005; 78: 431-441.

Bernard SC, Simpson N, Join-Lambert O, Federici C, Laran-Chich MP, Maïssa N, Bouzinba-Ségard H, Morand PC, Chretien F, Taouji S, Chevet E. Pathogenic Neisseria meningitidis utilizes CD147 for vascular colonization. Nature Medicine. 2014; 20(7): 725-31.

Mireille KP, Paul Desire DD, Claude BD, Sandrine MNY, Marguerite M, Chantal NM, Rodrigue N, Agnes OC, Theophile D, Pierre K. Protective effects of *Nymphaea lotus* Linn. (Nymphaeaceae) aqueous extract against chronic unpredictable mild stress induced testicular lipid peroxidation. Asian Journal of Biomedical and Pharmaceutical Sciences. 2016; 6(54): 01-06.

Misra LN, Kumar S. Indian medicinal plants as the potential source of therapeutic agents. *In*: Harvesting Herbs-2000, Nautiyal, A.R. (*ed.*). Bishen Singh Mahendra Pal Singh Press, Dehradun, India, 1997. pp. 13-27.

Misra LN, Siddiqui MS, Singh AK, Shukla YN. Essential oils of *Cymbopogons*: Chemistry, uses and biological activities. *In*: Aromatic Grasses, Kumar, S. (*eds.*). CIMAP, Lucknow, 2000. pp. 315-367.

Mittal D, Ali A, Md S, Baboota S, Sahni JK, Ali J. Insights into direct nose to brain delivery: Current status and future perspective. Drug Delivery. 2013; 21: 75-86.

Muzila M. *Boerhavia diffusa* L. *In:* Schmelzer, GH, Gurib-Fakim A, (*eds.*) Prota 11(1): Medicinal plants/Plantes médicinales 1. [CD-Rom]. PROTA, Wageningen, Netherlands, 2006.

Myint KZ, Wang L, Tong Q, Xie XQ. Molecular fingerprint-based artificial neural networks QSAR for ligand biological activity predictions. Molecular Pharmaceutics. 2012; 9: 2912-2923.

Nadembega P, Boussim JI, Nikiema JB, Poli F. Antognoni F. Medicinal plants in Baskoure, Kourittenga Province, Burkina Faso: An ethnobotanical study. Journal of Ethnopharmacology. 2011; 133: 378-395.

Nikiema A, Pasternak D. *Khaya senegalensis* (Desr.) A. Juss. [Internet] Record from PROTA4U. 2008.

Olatokunboh AO, Kayode YO, Adeola OK. Anticonvulsant activity of *Rauvolfia Vomitoria* (Afzel). African Journal of Pharmacy and Pharmacology. 2009; 3(6): 319-322.

Panjwani D, Purohit V, Siddique HH. Antidepressant like effects of *Anacardium occidentale* L. leaves in the mouse forced swim and tail suspension tests. Pharmacologia. 2015; 6(5): 186-191.

Poli FP, Deste G, Smieskova R, Barlati S, Yung AR, Howes O, Stieglitz RD, Vita A, Guire MP, Borgwardt S. Cognitive Functioning in Prodromal Psychosis: A meta-analysis. Archives of Gynecology and Psychiatry. 2012; 69: 562–571.

Prosper TK, Patrice Z, Samson G, Moussa C, Alin C, Martin K. Medicinal plants used for neuropsychiatric disorders treatment in the Hauts Bassins region of Burkina Faso. Medicines. 2017; 4: 32. doi: 10.3390/medicines4020032

Ragupathi G. Neuropharmocological effects of methanolic extract of leaves of *Amaranthus viridis*. L. in rats and mice. Dissertation submitted to the Tamil Nadu Dr. M.G.R Medical University 2017.

Reybellet P, Quoi de. neuf dans le traitement des psychoses, Current Opinion in Psychiatry, 2015; 1: 1-26.

Riddle JM. History as a tool in identifying new old drugs. Advances in Experimental Medicine and Biology; 2002: 505: 89-94.

Rogawski MA, Loscher W. The neurobiology of antiepileptic drugs. Nature Reviews Neuroscience. 2004; 5: 553-564.

Shakeri A, Sahebkar A, Javadi B. *Melissa officinalis* L. — A review of its traditional uses, phytochemistry and pharmacology, Journal of Ethnopharmacology. 2016; 188: 204-228.

Starling J, Feijo I. Schizophrénie et autres troubles psychotiques à début précoce. IACAPAP E-textb. Child Adolesc. Mental Health. 2012; 4(2): 1–24.

Taiwe GS, Kuete V. Neurotoxicity and neuroprotective effects of African medicinal plants. In toxicological survey of African medicinal plants, Elsevier: London, UK, 2014. pp. 423-444.

Tapsell LC, Hemphill I, Cobiac L, Patch CS, Sullivan DR, Fenech M, Roodenrys S, Keogh JB, Clifton PM, Williams PG, Fazio VA, Inge KE. Health benefits of herbs and spices: The past, the present, the future. The Medical Journal of Australia, 2006; 185(4 Suppl): 4-24.

Tapsoba H, Deschamps JP. Use of medicinal plants for the treatment of oral diseases in Burkina Faso. Journal of Ethnopharmacology. 2006; 104: 68–78.

Tiziana C, Sergio P. Molecular targets for improvement of Parkinson's disease therapy, Brain Disorder Therapy. 2015; 4: 173.

Tuli R, Sangwan RS, Kumar S, Bhattacharya S, Misra LN. *Ashwagandha (Withania somnifera:* A Model Indian Medicinal Plant. CSIR, New Delhi, 2009.

Wagner H, Hikino H, Farnsworth NR. Economic and Medicinal Plant Research. SPCK Publishing, London & Academic Press, London, 1985. pp. 1-4.

Warner ML, Kaufman NC, Grundmann O. The pharmacology and toxicology of kratom: From traditional herb to drug of abuse. The International Journal of Legal Medicine. 2016; 130: 127–138.

Yasamy MT, Maulik PK, Tomlinson M, Lund C, Van OM, Saxena S. Responsible Governance for Mental Health Research in Low Resource Countries. PLoS Medicene. 2011; 8:1-6.

Zerbo P, Compaore M, Meda NTR, Lamien MA, Kiendrebeogo, M. Potential medicinal plants used by traditional healers in western areas of Burkina Faso. World Journal of Pharmacy and Pharmaceutical Sciences. 2013; 2: 6706-6719.

5

Phytochemistry and Pharmacological Properties of a Neglected Tropical Plant *Averrhoa carambola* L. (Star Fruit): A Review

MANJESHWAR SHRINATH BALIGA[1*], GANESH BHANDARI[2], ROMITH PERIERA[2], JAFFY MARY MATHEW[2], PRINCY LOUIS PALATTY[2] AND MALLAPPA KUMARA SWAMY[3,4*]

ABSTRACT

Averrhoa carambola L., (Family: Oxalidaceae) colloquially known as the star fruit tree is one of the most underutilized plant. The fruits of which are like a star shaped and are sweet when ripe, but have a slight hint of astringency. These trees are found growing in the warmer tropical and sub tropical areas of the world. The tree prefers full sun exposure and well draining soil. The tree grows normally to a medium size, and is also used as an ornamental tree for decorative purposes. They also have culinary uses and are used in confectionaries preparation. The bark, leaves and roots have been used extensively as medicinal agent for curing various human ailments in various traditional systems of medicine. In the recent past, studies have shown that many of their ethnomedicinal uses are validated scientifically. In this chapter, phytochemistry and pharmacological properties of star fruit are addressed in detail.

Key words: *Averrhoa carambola*, Star fruit, Phytochemistry, Traditional uses & pharmacology.

[1] Mangalore Institute of Oncology, Pumpwell, Mangalore, Karnataka, India 575002
[2] Father Muller Medical College, Father Muller Road, Mangalore, Karnataka, India 575002
[3] Department of Crop Science, Faculty of Agriculture, Universiti Putra Malaysia, Serdang 43400, Selangor, Malaysia
[4] Department of Biotechnology, East West First Grade College, Bengaluru, Karnataka, 560091, India.
**Corresponding author:* msbaliga@gmail.com; swamy.bio@gmail.com

1. INTRODUCTION

The plant, *Averrhoa carambola* L., commonly known as the starfruit plant is widely distributed throughout the globe, particularly in the tropical nations including Indonesia, Malaysia, Philippines, and India. The plant belonging to the genus, *Averrhoa.* There are about 5 reported species of *Averrhoa*, namely *A. carambola, A. bilimbi, A. leucopetala, A. dolichocarpa,* and *A. microphylla*. Amongst them, *A. carambola* is extensively cultivated in many tropical countries, such as South-east Asia and Malaysia on a large scale (Khoo *et al.,* 2016; Muthu *et al.,* 2016). In addition, people in the United States of America, South Pacific Islands, and Australia likes this fruit, and it is one of their favorite and popular fruit (Ray, 2012). Starfruits are crunchy, fleshly, juicy, but they are somewhat bitter, acidic, and sweeter in the sense of taste. The highly valued part of the plant is its fruits which is known to possess superior antioxidant activity and scavenge free radical ions effectively. Moreover, the fruit improves the health condition of patients suffering from hypoglycemia and hypocholesterolemia (Chau *et al.,* 2004a,b; Shui *et al.,* 2006; Muthu *et al.,* 2016). Starfruits are usually utilized in preparing juices, pickles, and fruit salads. However, the fruit is also eaten raw, and for cleaning of utensils due to the fact that it effectively remove the rust caused by iron oxidation. Starfruits are documented with many bioactive phytocompounds, such as cis-abscisic acid, abscisic acid-s-D glucopyranosyl ester, trans-abscisic acid, abscisic alcohol, abscisic acid-β-D-glucopyranosyl ether, vomifoliol, roseoside, epicatechin, quercetin-3-O-β-D-glucoside, rutin, β-sitosterol, lupeol, anthraquinone glucoside, cyanidin-3-O-β-D-glucoside, cyanidin-3,5-O-β-D-diglucoside, β-amirin, apigenin-6-C-β-L-fucopyranoside, apigenin-6-C-(200-O-α-L-rhamnopyranosyl)-β-L-fucopyranoside and carambolaflavone. Considering these fact, the present chapter is aimed to provide a comprehensive information from the available literatures on the starfruit plant's nutritional, phytochemistry and pharmacological properties. Moreover, the chapter highlights on the toxicological aspects of the starfruit plant.

2. BOTANICAL DESCRIPTIONS, MORPHOLOGY, OCCURRENCE

Averrhoa carambola L. belonging to the family, Oxalidaceae is a plant originally indigenous to Ceylon and the Moluccas (Morton, 1978; Manda *et al.,* 2012; Dasgupta, 2013). However, today the tree is also found growing in warmer tropical countries like Philippines, Indonesia, India, Southeast Asia, Southern China, Taiwan, Australia (Queensland), South Pacific, East Asia, Peru, Colombia, Trinidad, Ecuador, Guyana, Dominican Republic, United States, in South Florida, Hawaii and in tropical west Africa, south Florida, and Hawaii. In colloquial terms the plant is known as 'Kamrakh' or 'Star fruit' tree. The other vernacular names are enlisted in Table 1 (Morton 1978; Manda *et al.*, 2012; Dasgupta 2013).

Table 1: The different vernacular names of *Averrhoa carambola* L.

Local language	***Common Name***
Assamese	Kordoi/Rohdoi
Bengali	Kamranga
Chinese	Gooseberry
English	Star fruit
Filipino	Balimbing, saranate
Gujarati	Kamrakh
Hindi	Kamrakh, karmal
Indonesian	Belimbing
Kannada	Carambola fruit
Malay	Belimbing
Malayalam	Caturappuli
Marathi	Karambal
Sanskrit	Karmaranga
Sinhala	Kamaranga
Tamil	Thambaratham/Tamarattai
Telugu	Ambanamkaya

The fruits of the plant appear to have a star shape and hence, the name Star fruit (Fig. 1). When cut across the middle of the fruit is the most important valued plant part possessing both dietary and medicinal uses (Dasgupta, 2013). This fruit also goes by many other names including: bilimbi, belimbing, Chinese star fruit, five-angled fruit and the star apple. With regard to the fruits, there are two documented types; the tart and sweet varieties. The average length of the fruit is about 10-20 cm with the diameter of about 6-10 cm. The average weight of each fruit will be approximately 150-500 g. An unripe star fruit is preserved in many parts of the Southeast

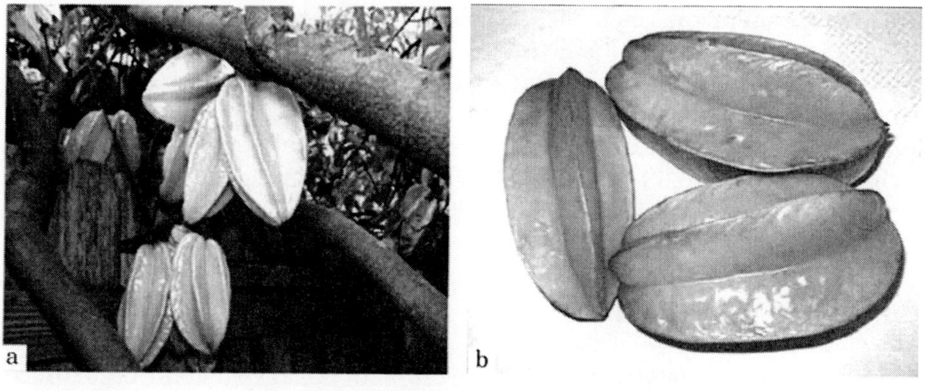

Fig. 1: Picture showing *Averrhoa carambola* L. tree (a) and fruit (b)

Asia, and is used as a traditional remedy for treating several health problems. Morphologically, overripe fruit will be yellowish with brown spots (Dasgupta, 2013).

The fruits have a waxy translucent skin, and appear golden yellow (ripe) to green color skin (unripe). The aroma of the fully ripe fruit is sweet and candy-like, and fruity. The taste is slightly sweet, fruity and mild with a slight hint of astringency, but no obvious oxalic acid flavor (Morton, 1978, Manda *et al.*, 2012, Dasgupta, 2013). Carambolas are the best consumed when ripe, and when they are yellow with a light shade of green. The tart varieties typically have narrowly spaced ribs, while sweet varieties tend to have thick, fleshy ribs. The fruit is harvested mainly during the months of June to August, and a fully grown well-nourished mature tree can produce from 200 to 400 pounds (91 to 180 kg) of fruits each year (Morton, 1978; Manda *et al.*, 2012; Dasgupta, 2013).

2.1. Scientific classification

Kingdom: Plantae
Division: Plantae
Class: Magnoliopsida
Order: Oxalidales
Family: Oxalidaceae
Genus: *Averrhoa*
Species: *carambola*

3. PROXIMATE COMPOSITION OF THE FRUIT

The fruits have been investigated for their nutritional values, and reports indicate that it possess the important water soluble Vitamin C (L-ascorbic acid), carotene, tartaric acid, oxalic acid, α-ketoglutaric acid and citric acid. Dietary intake of 100 g of the fruit is reported to provide, 35.7 g calories, 0.38 g proteins, 9.38 g carbohydrates, 0.80-0.90 g dietary fiber, 0.8 g fat, 4.4-6.0 mg calcium, 0.32-1.65 mg iron, 15.5-21.0 mg phosphorus, and 2.35 mg potassium. The fruits also contain various amino acids like 0.03-0.038 mg of thiamine, 0.019-0.03 mg of riboflavin, 0.294-0.38 mg of niacin, 3 mg of tryptophan, 2 mg of methionine, and 26 mg of lysine (Morton, 1978; Manda *et al.*, 2012; Dasgupta, 2013).

4. PHYTOCHEMISTRY

Phytochemical characterization of starfruit plant has revealed the occurrence of various biologically important chemical compounds. Some of the determined compounds include cis-abscisic acid, abscisic acid-s-D glucopyranosyl ester, trans-abscisic acid, abscisic alcohol, abscisic acid-β-D-glucopyranosyl ether, vomifoliol, roseoside, epicatechin, quercetin-3-O-β-D-glucoside, rutin, β-sitosterol, lupeol, anthraquinone glycosides, proanthocyanidin, cyanidin-3-O-β-D-glucoside, cyanidin-3,5-O-β-D-diglucoside, β-amirin, apigenin-6-C-β-L-fucopyranoside, apigenin-6-C-(200-O-α-L-rhamnopyranosyl)-β-L-fucopyranoside and carambolaflavone (Morton 1978; Manda *et al.*, 2012; Dasgupta 2013). Some of these important phytochemicals are depicted in Fig. 2.

5. TRADITIONAL USES

Star fruit has been used since time immemorial as a dietary agent in various parts of the world. The ripe yellow fruits are generally eaten freshly, and is

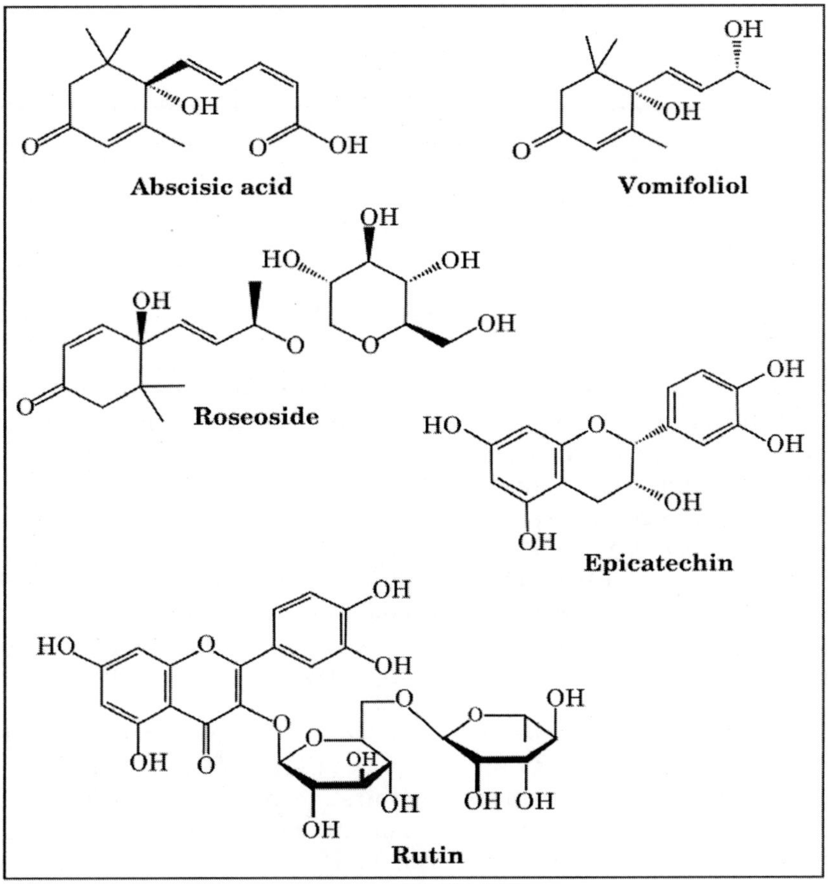

Fig. 2: (*Contd...*)

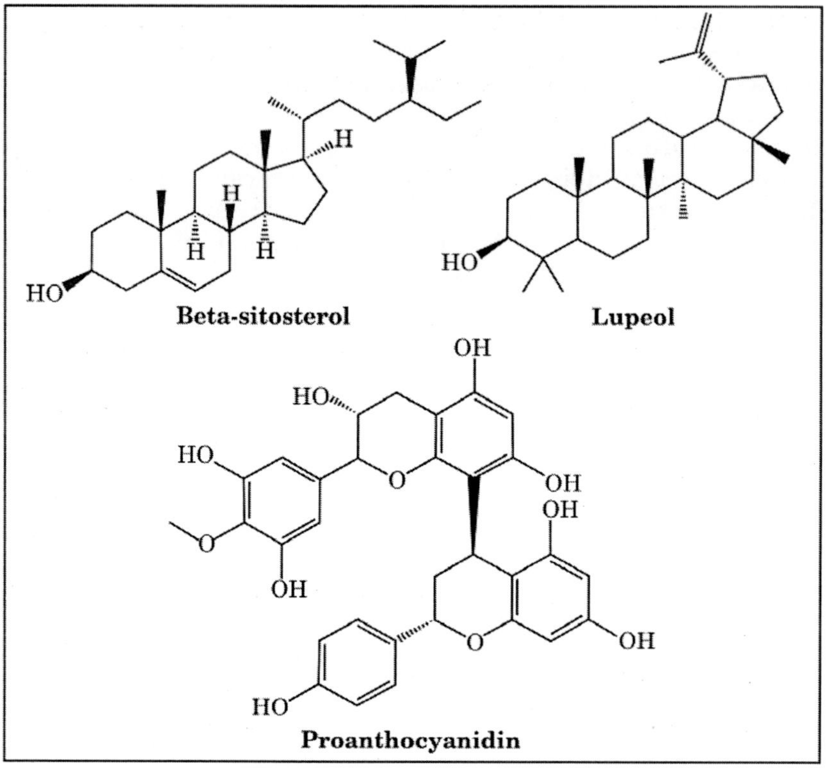

Fig. 2: Some of the major phytochemicals identified from *Averrhoa carambola* L.

highly recommended as diet fruit because of its high fiber and low calorie content. In addition to this, the fruits are also used in making jelly, confectionaries, as a garnishing agent for salads and drinks, and in making pickles. The fruit juice is an excellent appetite stimulant and a diuretic agent. It is also used in treating sore eyes, as anti- diarrheal, febrifugal agent, and expectorants *i.e.,* as mucolytics, a medical preparation that mediate in coughing up of mucus from the bronchial passages and to removes phlegm from the lungs. In the traditional medicine preparations, the ripe fruit is utilized as a good remedy for the treatment of internal piles, and to eliminate intestinal worms (Manda *et al.,* 2012; Dasgupta, 2013).

In Brazil, the carambola is recommended as a diuretic agent for treating kidney and bladder complaints, while in the Chinese *Materia Medica,* they are supposed to be useful in quenching thirst, to increase salivary secretion, and reduce fever. The ripe fruit is considered as a tonic and improves the digestive process when consumed. The fruit is also been used to treat sore eyes, even for nursing mothers as it is commonly believed to stimulate the flow of milk. Its high vitamin C content can help ward off winter colds and flu. It is also used topically on poisonous bites and stings. The fruits are also used to treat of eczemas, sunstroke, diarrhea, vomiting, hemorrhoids, intermittent fever, scabies and general debility (Manda *et al.,* 2012; Dasgupta, 2013).

In addition to the fruits, the leaves are supposed to be useful as anti-pruritic, anti-pyretic, anthelmintic agents, and it is effective in treating scabies, healing fractured bones, to eliminate intestinal worms and as an antidote for various poisoning. The leaf decoction is also used to treat diabetes, hypertension and to act as a stimulator of appetite, anti-scurry agent and antipyretic agent. The tea prepared with the leaves has also been used to treat headaches, vomiting, to mitigate cough and hangovers. A decoction of the leaves and roots either alone or in combination is also believed to help cure ringworm and chickenpox (Manda *et al.*, 2012; Dasgupta, 2013).

6. SCIENTIFICALLY VALIDATED PHARMACOLOGICAL PROPERTIES

In the past decade, there has been a renewed interest in validating the various ethnomedical uses attributed to the plant and fruits of *A. carambola* in specific. Various studies involving both *in vitro* approaches, use of animal cell lines cultures as well as *in vivo* animal models have been carried out by many researchers in the past. They have scientifically validated this plant for several pharmacological properties. In the subsequent sections, findings of these validated properties are addressed in detail.

6.1. Antimicrobial activity

Drug resistance in bacteria is a growing problem, and there is a need for the development effective novel antimicrobial agents. Thus, it has become an important avenue for research. In this regard, several research efforts are required to overcome this problem. A study by Sripanidkulchai *et al.* (2002) has shown that the stem extracts of the plant possess antibacterial activity against *Staphylococcus aureus* and *Klebsiella* sp. The minimal bactericidal concentration (MBC) was observed to be 15.62 mg/ml and 125 mg/ml, respectively for *S. aureus* and *Klebsiella* sp. Subsequent studies have also shown that methanolic extract and its petroleum ether, carbon tetrachloride, chloroform and aqueous soluble fractions of the bark were effective against the growth of Gram-positive bacteria like *Bacillus cereus, B. megaterium, B. subtilis,* and *S. aureus*; the Gram-negative bacteria like *Escherichia coli, Pseudomonas aeruginosa, Salmonella typhi, S. paratyphi*;

and the fungi, *Candida albicans, Aspergillus niger,* and *Saccharomyces cerevisiae* (Masum *et al.,* 2007).

6.2. Anti-inflammatory activities

Innumerable studies have shown that the inflammatory cascade is detrimental to health and that an ideal non-toxic anti-inflammatory agent, possibly from the dietary source is highly desired (Cabrini, 2011). Experimental studies with the crude ethanolic extract of the leaves and its hexane, ethyl acetate, and butanol fractions and two of its isolated flavonoids, when applied to the croton oil-induced ear edema model of inflammation in mice have shown that the topically application of the ethanolic extract was effective in reducing the edema in a concentration-dependent manner. Further various fractions of the ethanolic leaf extract were also effective in reducing the inflammation with the best effect being observed with the ethyl acetate fraction application in the animal model. Mechanistic studies showed that the observed anti-inflammatory activities were mediated partly by the inhibition of the myeloperoxidase activity (Carbini *et al.,* 2011). However, contrary to the extract, the isolated phytochemicals, such as apigenin-6-C-β-l-fucopyranoside and apigenin-6-C-(23-O-α-l-rhamnopyranosyl)-β-l- fucopyranoside were observed to be ineffective in reducing the inflammatory response. Further studies have also shown that the pure compound, 2-Dodecyl-6-Methoxycyclohexa-2,5-Diene-1,4-Dione isolated from the plant was effective against the palmitic acid-induced inflammation and exhibited apoptosis in Min6 Cells, and that the effects were mediated at least in part by inhibiting the TLR4-MyD88-NF-κB signaling pathway (Xie *et al.,* 2016).

6.3. Gastroprotective effects

Gastric ulcers are a common health problem in many individuals, and the imbalance between the acid and pepsin along with weakness of the mucosal barrier is supposed to be a responsible factor for the underlying pathogenesis. Using an animal model studies, researchers shown that the pretreatment with hydroalcoholic extract of the leaves was effective in reducing the ethanol-induced gastric ulcerogenesis. A dose dependent cytoprotective effects was observed when 800 and 1200 mg/kg were tested in laboratory rats (Goncalves *et al.,* 2006).

6.4. Photoprotective effects

Globally, skin cancers are the most common cancer types, and the UV-induced damage is a major contributor for the condition. Recent studies by Ronpirin *et al.* (2016) have shown that the aqueous and the ethanolic extracts of *A. carambola* was effective in reducing the UV-induced apoptotic cells, to induce DNA repair and significantly decrease the percentage of cyclobutane pyrimidine dimers. All these observations are suggestive to the fact that *A. carambola* possess a strong photoprotective effects, and hence it can be used as an ideal skin protective agent.

6.5. Anticancer studies

Cancer is a multi-disease characterized by an uncontrolled growth of abnormal cells with the potential of either localized to one particular tissue or can spread to other parts of the body (metastasis). In recent times, it has become one of the most common cause of death and the number of deaths related to cancer is on a rise throughout the world. Hepatocellular carcinoma, commonly known as liver cancer is one of the more severe forms, and its prevention is a priority (Singh *et al.,* 2010). Animal studies with laboratory mice have shown that prophylactic treatment of the fruit (25 mg/kg bwt/day for 5 consecutive days) was effective in reducing the incidence of hepatocellular carcinoma, and degree of malignancy of the diethylnitrosamine-induced and CCl_4-promoted hepatocarcinogenesis. Administration of fruit resulted in a significant reduction in the tumor incidence, tumor yield, and tumor burden.

Further, the mechanistic studies indicated that when compared to the carcinogen treated control that were fed with the placebo, the cohorts that were administered with the fruit caused a significant reduction in the levels of lipid peroxidation, and concomitantly increased the activities of enzymatic antioxidants (superoxide dismutase, and catalase) and that of the nonenzymatic antioxidant (reduced glutathione), and total proteins (Singh *et al.,* 2010).

Subsequent studies have also shown that 2-Dodecyl-6-methoxycyclohexa-2,5-diene-1,4-dione, a cyclohexanedione found in the roots of *A. carambola* suppressed the growth of breast carcinoma cells, but not normal mammary epithelial cells (Gao *et al.,* 2015). Mechanistic studies revealed that the anticancer activities were mediated by increasing the level of intracellular reactive oxygen species, inhibiting NF-κB signaling pathway, TNF-α production, phosphorylation of NF-κB, p65 and IκBα, as well as TNF-α activated NF-κB p65 nuclear translocation, inducing G1 phase cell cycle arrest, oxidative stress and apoptosis.

6.6. Hypocholesterolaemic and hypolipidemic activity

Hypercholesterolaemia which is characterized by the increase in cholesterol, and hyperlipidemia are an important metabolic conditions that progressively lead to multitude of health issues, especially to the cardiac ailments. Seminal studies by Chau *et al.* (2004a) have shown that the water-insoluble fiber rich fraction isolated from the pomace of the fruit was effective in lowering the serum concentration of triglycerol, liver cholesterol and increased the concentration of total lipids, cholesterol and bile acids in faeces, indicating its usefulness in these conditions.

6.7. Hypotensive effects

Hypertension which in colloquial terms is known as high blood pressure is a medical condition in which the arterial blood pressure is constantly elevated. This may consequentially lead to blood clots in the arteries and may cause cardiac arrest and stroke. Seminal studies by Soncini *et al.* (2011) have shown that the aqueous extract of *A. carambola* was effective in reducing the mean arterial pressure in anesthetized rats. Additionally, *in vitro* studies with thoracic aortic rings isolated and suspended in organ bath showed that when compared to the placebo controls, the extract caused a depression in the E(max) response to phenylephrine without a change in sensibility. Further studies confirmed that the extract inhibited the contractile mechanisms involving extracellular Ca^{2+} influx. Together, all these observations suggest that the aqueous extract possess hypotensive effects, and these effects may be due to the inhibition of Ca^{2+} ions.

6.8. Anti-diabetic effects

Diabetes has become today's leading endocrine dysfunction ailment globally, and is associated with significant morbidities (Shahreen *et al.,* 2011; Xu *et al.,* 2014). Since time immemorial the leaves and roots of *A. carambola* have been used as a antidiabetic agent and studies by Shahreen *et al.* (2011) have shown that the administration of graded doses of methanolic extract of leaves one hour prior to glucose administration was effective in reducing hyperglycemia (Xu *et al.,* 2014). When compared to control animals that were fed with placebo water, the optimum effect was observed at 400 mg extract per kg body weight, the highest dose as it caused a 34.10% reductions in the serum glucose levels (Xu *et al.*, 2014). However the extract was not as effective as the standard antihyperglycemic drug, glibenclamide that caused a 57.3% reduction in serum glucose levels versus control.

Reports also indicate that the aqueous and ethanolic extracts of the roots significantly decreased the serum levels of blood glucose, total cholesterol, triglycerides and free fatty acids, while concomitantly increasing the serum insulin content in the streptozotocin - induced diabetic mice (Xu *et al.,* 2014). Immunohistochemical studies with the pancreatic β cells showed that the administration of root extract caused a significant decrease in the expressions of apoptosis-related regulators like caspase-3, caspase-8, caspase-

9 and modulating the levels of Bax and Bcl-2 protein. These observations clearly indicate that the anti-diabetic effects were mediated by ameliorating the metabolic functions and inhibiting apoptosis in the pancreatic tissue.

With regard to phytochemicals experiments with hyperglygemic rats have also shown that apigenin-6-C-(2"-O-alpha-l-rhamnopyranosyl)-beta-L-fucopyranoside, an important constituent of *A. carambola* was effective in stimulating glucose uptake and to have a dual target of action, as an insulin-secretagogue and an insulin-mimetic agent (Cazarolli *et al.,* 2009). Subsequent studies have also shown that 2-dodecyl-6-methoxycyclohexa-2,5-diene-1,4-dione, isolated from the roots were effective in reducing the advanced glycation end-product-mediated renal injury in type 2 diabetic KKAy mice (Zheng *et al.,* 2013).

Following this experiments have shown that lyoniresinol 3α-O-β-D-glucopyranoside isolated from the extract were effective in mitigating the renal injury in streptozotocin-induced diabetic mice (Wen *et al.,* 2013). Lyoniresinol 3α-O-α-D-glucopyranoside was observed to be devoid of hypoglycemic effects but the diabetes-dependent alterations in the kidney like as glomerular hypertrophy, excessive extracellular matrix amassing, and glomerular and tubular basement membrane thickening were improved after the administration of the phytochemical for 14 consecutive days. Mechanistic studies showed that administering lyoniresinol 3α-O-β-D-glucopyranoside decreased the expression of nuclear factor-κB (NF-κB), caspase-3, -8, -9, and Bcl-associated X protein (Bax).

7. CONCLUSIONS

In the recent past, scientific studies have shown that *A. carambola,* possesses myriad pharmacological benefits like anti-inflammatory, gastroprotective, photoprotective, anticancer, hypotensive and anti-diabetic effects. Starfruit is very nutritious and hence, beneficial for human health. Nevertheless, because of the caramboxin and oxalate contents in the starfruit, it is very toxic to individuals having renal complications. Future studies should be carried out to isolate and purify more phytochemicals from this plant and to evaluate their vital pharmacological properties based on the traditional applications. Further, more research are required to improve our understanding on the mechanism of action responsible for various beneficial effects of *A. carambola* compounds. More advances approaches like genomics, transcriptomics, and metabolomics application in this plant may be very advantageous for us to know about genes, their expression for the biosynthesis of bioactive metabolites. The discovery of novel genes that are involved in the biosynthesis of caramboxin and oxalate could allow us to express them in other plants or heterologous systems. Moreover, it facilitates the genetic manipulation of genes to improve the biosynthetic pathways in a specific way in order to enhance the nutritional quality of fruits.

REFERENCES

Chau CF, Chen CH, Wang YT. Effects of a novel pomace fiber on lipid and cholesterol metabolism in the hamster. Nutrition Research. 2004a, 24(5):337-45.

Cabrini DA, Moresco HH, Imazu P, da Silva CD, Pietrovski EF, Mendes DA, da Silveira Prudente A, Pizzolatti MG, Brighente IM, Otuki MF. Analysis of the Potential Topical Anti-Inflammatory Activity of *Averrhoa carambola* L. in Mice. Evidence Based Complement Alternat Med. 2011, 11:908059. doi: 10.1093/ecam/neq026.

Cazarolli LH, Folador P, Moresco HH, Brighente IM, Pizzolatti MG, Silva FR. Mechanism of action of the stimulatory effect of apigenin-6-C-(2"-O-alpha-l-rhamnopyranosyl)-beta-L-fucopyranoside on 14C-glucose uptake. Chemical and Biological Interaction. 2009, 179(2-3):407-12.

Chau CF, Chen CH, Lin CY Insoluble fiber-rich fractions derived from *Averrhoa carambola*: Hypoglycemic effects determined by *in vitro* methods. LWT-Food Science and Technology, 2004b; 37(3):331-5.

Chau, C., Chen, C. and Lin, C. [-]. Effects of a novel pomace fiber on lipid and cholesterol metabolism in the hamster. Nutrition Research. 2004, 24:337–45.

Dasgupta P., Chakraborty P., Bala N. N. *Averrhoa carambola*: An Updated Review. International Journal of Pharma Research and Review, 2013, 2(7) [-]:54-63

Gao Y, Huang R, Gong Y, Park HS, Wen Q, Almosnid NM, Chippada-Venkata UD, Hosain NA, Vick E, Farone A, Altman E. The antidiabetic compound 2-dodecyl-6-methoxycyclohexa-2,5-diene-1,4-dione, isolated from *Averrhoa carambola* L., demonstrates significant antitumor potential against human breast cancer cells. Oncotarget. 2015, 6: 24304-19.

Goncalves S, Baroni S, Bersani-Amado FA, Melo GAN, Cortez DAG, Bersani-Amado CA, Roberto K. Cuman Preliminary studies on gastric anti-ulcerogenic effects of *Averrhoa carambola* in Rats. Acta Farm. Bonaerense, 2006, 25: 245-7.

Khoo HE, Azlan A, Kong KW, Ismail A. Phytochemicals and medicinal properties of indigenous tropical fruits with potential for commercial development. Evidence-Based Complementary and Alternative Medicine. 2016, 2016:1-20. doi.org/10.1155/2016/7591951

Manda H, Vyas K, Pandya A, Singhal G. A complete review on: *Averrhoa carambola*. World Journal of Pharmacy and Pharmaceutical Sciences, 2012, 1:17-33.

Masum MM, Rahman SM, Begum K, Begum B, Rashid AM. Phytochemical and Biological studies of *Averrhoa carambola*. J. Pharm. Sci. 2007; 6(2): 125-128.

Morton J.F. Fruits of Warm Climates. Flair Books, Miami, FL, 1978, 125–128.

Muthu N, Lee SY, Phua KK, Bhore SJ. Nutritional, Medicinal and Toxicological Attributes of Star-Fruits (*Averrhoa carambola* L.): A Review. Bioinformation. 2016, 12(12):420.

Ray, PK. Breeding Tropical and Subtropical Fruits. Springer Science & Business Media. 2012

Ronpirin C, Pattarachotanant N, Tencomnao T. Protective Effect of *Mangifera indica* Linn., *Cocos nucifera* Linn., and *Averrhoa carambola* Linn. Extracts against Ultraviolet B-Induced Damage in Human Keratinocytes. Evid Based Complement Alternat Med. 2016. doi: 10.1155/2016/1684794.

Shahreen S, Banik J, Hafiz A, Rahman S, Zaman AT, Shoyeb MA, Chowdhury MH, Rahmatullah M. Antihyperglycemic activities of leaves of three edible fruit plants (*Averrhoa carambola*, *Ficus hispida* and *Syzygium samarangense*) of Bangladesh.

African Journal of Traditional, Complementary and Alternative Medicine. 2011, 9(2):287-91.

Shui G, Leong LP. Residue from star fruit as valuable source for functional food ingredients and antioxidant nutraceuticals. Food Chemistry. 2006, 97(2):277-84.

Singh R, Sharma J, Goyal PK. Prophylactic Role of *Averrhoa carambola* (Star Fruit) [-] Extract against Chemically-Induced Hepatocellular Carcinoma in Swiss Albino Mice. Advances in pharmacological sciences. 2014. doi: 10.1155/2014/158936.

Soncini R, Santiago MB, Orlandi L, Moraes GO, Peloso AL, dos Santos MH, Alves-da-Silva G, Paffaro VA Jr, Bento AC, Giusti-Paiva A. Hypotensive effect of aqueous extract of *Averrhoa carambola* L. (Oxalidaceae) in rats: An *in vivo* and *in vitro* approach. Journal of Ethnopharmacology. 2011, 133 (2):353-7.

Sripanidkulchai B, Tattawasart U, Laupattarakasem P, Wongpanich V. Anti-inflammatory and bactericidal properties of elected indigenous medicinal plants used for dysuria. Thailand Journal of Pharmaceutical Science, 2002, 26(1-2):33-38.

Wen Q, Liang T, Qin F, Wei J, He Q, Luo X, Chen X, Zheng N, Huang R. Lyoniresinol 3α-O-β-D-glucopyranoside-mediated hypoglycaemia and its influence on apoptosis-regulatory protein expression in the injured kidneys of streptozotocin-induced mice. PLoS One. 2013, 8(12):e81772.

Xie Q, Zhang S, Chen C, Li J, Wei X, Xu X, Xuan F, Chen N, Pham T, Qin N, He J, Ye F, Huang W, Huang R, Wen Q. Protective effect of 2-dodecyl-6-methoxycyclohexa-2, 5-diene-1, 4-dione, isolated from *Averrhoa carambola* L., against palmitic acid-induced inflammation and apoptosis in min6 cells by inhibiting the TLR4-MyD88-NF-κB signaling pathway. Cell Physiol Biochem. 2016, 39(5):1705-1715.

Xu X, Liang T, Wen Q, Lin X, Tang J, Zuo Q, Tao L, Xuan F, Huang R. Protective effects of total extracts of *Averrhoa carambola* L. (Oxalidaceae) roots on streptozotocin-induced diabetic mice. Cell Physiology and Biochemistrty. 2014, 33(5):1272-82.

Zheng N, Lin X, Wen Q, Kintoko, Zhang S, Huang J, Xu X, Huang R. Effect of 2-dodecyl-6-methoxycyclohexa-2,5-diene-1,4-dione, isolated from *Averrhoa carambola* L. (Oxalidaceae) roots, on advanced glycation end-product-mediated renal injury in type 2 diabetic KKAy mice. Toxicology Letters. 2013, 219(1):77-84.

6

Medicinal Values and Health Benefits of Dalchini (*Cinnamomum zeylanicum* Blume) Essential Oil

ANGANA BORAH[1] AND MOHAN LAL[1*]

ABSTRACT

Cinnamomum zeylanicum Blum, an evergreen tropical plant, belonging to the family, Lauraceae is well-known for its uses in the traditional medicine since ages. It is also known as the 'true cinnamon' or 'Ceylon cinnamon' or 'dalchini'. It is native to Sri Lanka and the south Indian regions. It grows principally in the tropical rainforest region. The inner bark of C. zeylanicum is used as a spice all over the world. Essential oil can be yielded from some parts of the plant, mainly from the leaves and the inner bark. It is seen that the amount of oil extracted from the leaves and barks of cinnamon tree yields about 1.6 and 1.8% and 0.5 to 1% of essential oil, respectively. The major chemical components of the bark oil are cinnamaldehyde, trans-cinnamaldehyde, linalool, and eugenol. In the leaf oil eugenol as the major component while, cinnamyl acetate is the major component of the oils extracted from the fruit and flower. Several studies have confirmed that the essential oils of C. zeylanicum possess antimicrobial, antidiabetic, anti-inflammatory, antioxidant, anti-cancer and wound healing properties. Moreover, the essential oil extracted from its bark and leaves are used as an aromatic compound in flavouring, perfumes, aromatherapy and beverages. Cinnamon is also an imperative constituent in the Ayurvedic medicines against toothache, sore gums, joint pain, etc. This chapter illustrates the significant health benefits of C. zeylanicum and various medicinal properties

[1] Medicinal, Aromatic and Economic Plants Group, Biological Sciences and Technology. Division, CSIR-North East Institute of Science and Technology Jorhat-785006, Assam, India.

**Corresponding author:* mohan@neist.res.in

of its essential oil. The chemical composition of its essential oil and traditional utilization in medicines is also highlighted in this chapter.

Key words: *C. zeylanicum*, Essential oil, Eugenol, Traditional medicine, Therapeutic property, Health benefits.

1. INTRODUCTION

Cinnamomum zeylanicum Blume (commonly known as cinnamon) is a small evergreen tropical plant. It is native to Sri Lanka and the south Indian regions. It belongs to the family, Lauraceae and mainly, it is grown in the tropical forest regions of the world, although nearly 80-90% of its cultivation is from Sri Lanka. It is also known as 'Ceylon cinnamon' (the source of its Latin name, zeylanicum) or 'true cinnamon' or Dalchini (Ranasinghe *et al.*, 2002). Its use in the traditional medicines including Ayurveda is well-known world-wide from ancient ages. The dried inner bark of the plant is used as a spice for centuries all over the world (Ulbricht *et al.*, 2011). It is also used as an aromatic compound due to its fragrance in different perfumes, food products, aromatherapy and medicinal products (Huang *et al.,* 2007). Essential oil is extracted from several parts of this plant (Fig. 1). Various research studies have shown that the essential oil contains various bioactive

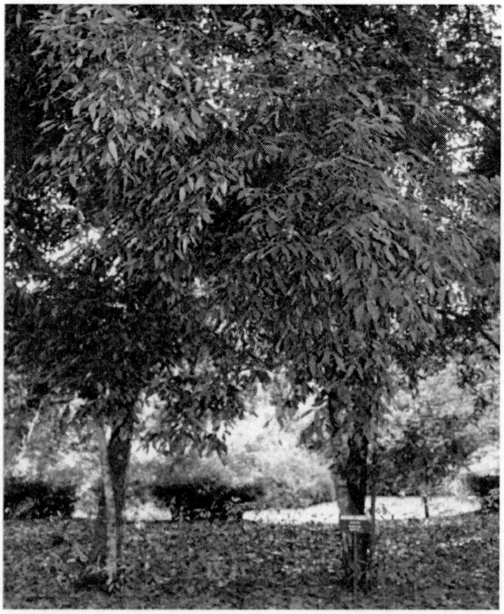

Fig. 1: *Cinnamomum zeylanicum* Blume. tree (Grown at CSIR-NEIST experimental farm, Jorhat, India)

compounds possessing beneficial medicinal effects. These bioactive phytocompounds include alkaloids, steroids, tannins, and phenol compounds, flavonoids, steroids, resins, fatty acids, and gums which can produce a definite physiological action on body (Joshi *et al.,* 2009).

Essential oil can be extracted from various parts of *C. zeylanicum* through hydro-distillation and the volatile compounds could be identified through Gas chromatography coupled with mass spectrophotometry (Wang *et al.,* 2009). The major constituent of the cinnamon bark includes cinnamaldehyde (60–70%) and cinnamyl acetate (8–10%). (Ehlers *et al.,* 1995). While, (E)-Cinnamyl acetate (36.59%) and eugenol are the main constituents of the fruit stalks (Jayaprakasa *et al.,* 2007). Another comparative study conducted by Paranagama *et al.* (2001) on the essential oil of cinnamon (bark, leaf, root and fruit) have also confirmed the occurrence of these chemical constituents in their essential oil. Studies have been confirmed the health benefits rendered by their chemical compounds, which makes *C. zeylanicum* a medicinally important tree to be used by pharmaceutical industry.

The knowledge of *C. zeylanicum* bioactive components and their different pharmacological uses can be beneficial for human kind. In this chapter, we have tried to highlight the major uses of cinnamon. The information will be very useful to the pharmaceutical industries, especially in formulating herbal drugs.

2. PHYTOCHEMISTRY

In plants, various bioactive compounds are present in the essential oil, which renders it their pharmaceutical properties. The essential oil of *C. zeylanicum* has been studied and their different compounds were identified. Many researchers have carried out a study to identify the bioactive components of cinnamon essential oil by using gas chromatography, coupled with mass-spectrometry. They have reported that the major compounds present in the oil are (E)-cinnamaldehyde (68.95%), benzaldehyde (9.94%), trans-α-bergamotene (7.97%), caryophyllene oxide (7.2%) and (E)-cinnamyl acetate (7.44%). Also, the essential oil of bark extracted by supercritical fluid extraction (SCFE) contained several other compounds, such as limonene, copaene, naphthalene, heptane, bicyclo[4.2.0]octa-1,3,5-triene and 2-propenal were observed from supercritical fluid extraction method of oil (Fig. 2) (Jayaprakasha *et al.,* 2000; Unlu *et al.,* 2010; Saleem *et al.*, 2015).

3. TRADITIONAL USES

Since ancient times, cinnamon bark has been used as an aromatic spice all over the world. The part used as a spice is its dried inner bark. Cinnamon

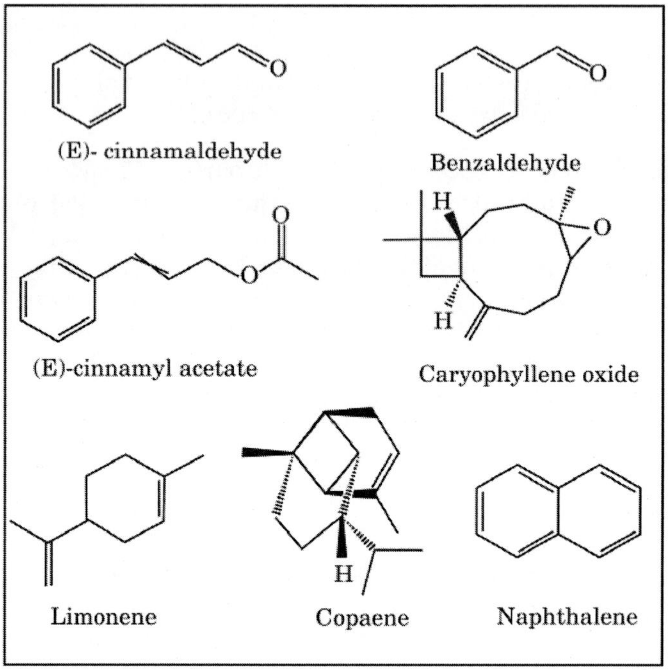

Fig. 2: Chemical structures of major bioactive components in essential oil of *Cinnamomum zeylanicum* Blume.

has an ancient history in the Ayurvedic medicine as well as Chinese medicines. In the Ayurvedic medicine, it is used to treat common cold, cough, diabetes, fever, flatulence, indigestion, sinusitis and sore throat. It is also used for its mouth refreshing activities as it can remove bad breath (Jakhetia *et al.,* 2010). Therefore, it has been used in tooth powders and to treat dental problems. In Chinese medicine, it is used toxins from the body and improving blood circulation. Cinnamon also acts as a blood thinner, which helps in preventing heart attack. Moreover, it is one of the major spice used in every household since ancient time. Its aroma is derived from a compound, cinnamaldehyde (Fig. 2), which is present in its bark essential oil (Ribeiro-Santos *et al.,* 2017). Cinnamon can also be found in Iranian traditional medicines. It is found in their antibacterial and antifungal herbal medicines (Bonjar *et al.,* 2004).

4. MEDICINAL PROPERTIES AND HEALTH BENEFITS

It has been reported that the constituents of the extracted essential oil of the plant renders its medicinal properties (Table 1). The oil is aromatic, and the oil's colour varies from yellow to red-brown, being extracted from leaves and bark respectively. The essential oil is useful for its several health benefits.

Table 1: Pharmaceutical properties of *Cinnamomum zeylanicum* essential oil.

Sl. no.	*Properties*	*References*
1.	Anti-microbial	Goubran and Holmes (1993); Barattha *et al.* (1998); Matan *et al.* (2006); Agastha *et al.* (2009); Joshi *et al.* (2009); Parthasarathy and Thombare (2013); Ranasinghe *et al.* (2013)
2.	Anti-diabetic	Kannappan *et al.* (2006); Babu *et al.* (2007)
3.	Anti-inflammatory	Han and Parker (2017)
4.	Anti-oxidant	Mathew and Abraham (2004); Jayaprakasha *et al.* (2007)
5.	Anti-cancer	Kwon *et al.* (1997), Jeong *et al.* (2003); Lu *et al.* (2010); Varalakshmi *et al.* (2013)
6.	Wound healing ability	Kamath *et al.* (2003); Farahpour and Habibi (2012)

4.1. Antimicrobial activity

Till date, several studies on the antimicrobial properties of *C. zeylanicum* have been reported. Antimicrobials that are of plant origin have benefits over synthetic antimicrobial agents, as they do not have any side-effects (Joshi *et al.,* 2009). A study conducted by Matan *et al.,* (2006) and reported that cinnamon oils can inhibit different bacterial (*Pediococcus halophilus* and *Staphylococcus aureus),* fungal (*Aspergillus flavus, Mucor plumbeus, Penicillium roqueforti,* and *Eurotium sp.*), and yeast species (*Candida lipolytica, Pichia membranifaciens, Debaryomyces hansenii,* and *Zygosaccharomyces rouxii*). Studies conducted by Joshi *et al.* (2009), have also reported that, cinnamon oil can inhibit *Bacillus thuringiensis, Bacillus cereus* and *Bacillus subtilis*. Cinnamon oil is also a good alternative to few of the fungicides. It has been shown that it can inhibit the growth of *Monilia, Botrytis* and *Mucor* sps. (Goubran and Holmes, 1993). The essential oil can also inhibit several food-poisoning/spoiling organisms like *Clostridium perfringens, E. coli, Klebsiella pneumonia, Pseudomonas aeruginosa, S. aureus, S. faecalis and Yersinia enterocolitica.* (Baratta *et al.,* 1998; Agasthya *et al.,* 2009).

Another study conducted on the antimicrobial effect of *Azadirachta indica, Syzygium aromaticum* and *Cinnamomum zeylanicum* against oral microflora, has found that *C. zeylanicum* aqueous extract was the most effective compared to the other two (Parthasarathy and Thombare, 2013). Likewise, Agastha *et al.* (2009) has reported the antimicrobial property of cinnamon extract against *Brucella melitensis.* Moreover, it also has the inhibitory effect against anthracnose and crown rot pathogens that infect banana plants

(Ranasinghe *et al.,* 2013). Thus, *C. zeylanicum* could be used as a natural antimicrobial agent and can be used as an alternate therapeutic agent.

4.2. Antidiabetic

Diabetes mellitus is a major source of epidemics all over the world. According to the latest global estimate from the International Diabetes Federation (IDF 2016), there were 415 million people with diabetes mellitus and that by 2040 the number will be 642 million. Diseased person shows decrease in the insulin level of blood. There are several studies on the prevention and cure of diabetes.

It has been demonstrated that when a person consumes cinnamaldehyde (20 mg/kg bw), his total cholesterol and triglyceride levels decreases and simultaneously plasma insulin, hepatic glycogen, and high-density lipoprotein-cholesterol levels in the blood increases (Babu *et al.*, 2007). *C. zeylanicum* can also expressively improve metabolic derangements, which are related to insulin resistance as stated by Kannappan *et al.* (2006).

4.3. Anti-inflammatory

Studies on *C. zeylanicum* and its essential oil have indicated their anti-inflammatory properties. The cinnamon bark essential oil contains various flavonoids that give it their anti-inflammatory property. A previous study was conducted on a mimicked disease micro-environment of inflamed human skin cells using dermal fibroblast cell system, HDF3CGF. It was found that cinnamon bark oil can pointedly inhibit the production of several protein biomarkers which are involved in inflammation and tissue re-modelling of human cells. Moreover, the study also observed that the essential oil has anti proliferative activity against the inflamed skin cells used (Han and Parker, 2017). So, in this way, the essential oil can be used in the production of different drugs.

4.4. Antioxidant

Phenolic compounds present in cinnamon have antioxidant ability. Cinnamon bark extracts possess 2,2-Diphenyl-1-picrylhydrazyl (DPHH) free-radical scavenging activity and can be regarded as potent antioxidant agent (Mathew and Abraham, 2004). Also, the antioxidant activity of the dried fruit extracts has been reported (Jayaprakasha *et al.,* 2007). They have determined the antioxidant property of cinnamon oil using β carotene-linoleate model. The ability of the essential oil to reduce beta-carotene-linoleic acid co-oxidation enzymatically induced by 1,1-diphenyl-2-picrylhydrazyl determined their comprehensive antioxidant ability.

4.5. Anti-cancer

Studies on cinnamon extracts have been done and it has been noted that they also have anti-cancer properties. It was reported that cinnamon extract can inhibit the angiogenesis of cancer by preventing vascular endothelial growth factor subtype 2 (VEGFR2). This study confirmed that cinnamon can be used in the prevention of cancer (Lu *et al.,* 2010). Another study also confirmed that, cinnamaldehydes (present in cinnamon essential oil) have the ability to inhibit angiogenesis (Kwon *et al.*, 1997). Jeong *et al.,* 2003 reported that CB403, which is derived from cinnamaldehyde can inhibit tumour growth. Their study shows the ability of CB403 against tumour and cancer growth inhibitory proteins.

Another study was carried out by Varalakshmi *et al.* (2013) reported that the anticancer activity of cinnamon bark using MTT assay. The assay was performed on Human hepatocellular carcinoma cells (HepG-2 cell line) and it was found that the cinnamon extract was toxic to more than 50% of HepG2 cells. In the present era, cancer has large impact on human beings. Further studies and research can lead to the use of cinnamon essential oil in drugs developed against cancer as it has the potential.

4.6. Wound-healing property

Previous studies using the ethanolic extract of cinnamon has reported that it also possesses wound-healing properties. Drugs developed from plant extracts have faster healing effect than the synthetic ones. A study was conducted on incision wound of Wistar rats, (Kamath *et al.*, 2003). They have found that when the rats were fed with cinnamon extract, the wound-breaking strength was boosted noticeably.

Another study conducted by Farahpour and Habibi (2012), confirmed that the cinnamon extract accelerates the wound-healing process, when the rats were induced by excision wound. The oral administration of cinnamon extract recovers the wound-site, which ultimately acts as a good curative. This activity of cinnamon is rendered by the presence of cinnamaldehyde and eugenol compounds in the essential oils.

5. CONCLUSIONS AND FUTURE PROSPECTS

This present chapter emphasizes on the various medicinal and therapeutic uses of the cinnamon essential oil. The oil is usually extracted from the bark and leaves of the plant and sometimes from the fruits and stalks. The major provider of cinnamon oil to all parts of the world is Sri Lanka. From the various research analyses, it is clear that the major components of the essential oil is cinnamaldehyde and eugenol, which gives the plant its various therapeutic properties.

It is reported to demonstrate anti-microbial, antidiabetic, anti-inflammatory, anti-oxidant and would healing ability. So, we can conclude that *C. zeylanicum* Blume is a major tree of utmost pharmacological importance and various advances have been made in pharmacology of the active constituents of its essential oil. A clear knowledge of its chemical constituents and their medicinal values is advantageous for human beings and the society. It could indicate the possibility of the potential use of cinnamon in natural remedies against treatment and prevention of various major diseases like cancer and its ultimate use as a source of alternate therapy. Thus, cinnamon is highly beneficial and can be used as a vital therapeutic agent.

REFERENCES

Agasthya AS, Jayapal N, Naveenkumar E, Goud NR, Vijayanand J, Hemapriya J. *In vitro* study of antimicrobial activity of the South Indian spices against enteric pathogens. Asian Journal of Microbiology, Biotechnology and Environmental Science. 2009; 11: 173–180.

Babu S, P., Prabuseenivasan, S., Ignacimuthu, S. Cinnamaldehyde: A potential antidiabetic agent. Phytomedicine. 2007; 14(1): 15–22.

Baratta MT, Dorman HJD, Deans SG, Figueiredo AC, Barroso JG, Ruberto G. Antimicrobial and antioxidant properties of some commercial essential oils. Flavour Fragrance Journal. 1998; 13: 235–244.

Bonjar GHS, Aghighi S, Nik AK. Antibacterial and antifungal survey in plants used in indigenous herbal-medicine of south-east regions of Iran. Journal of Biological Sciences. 2004; 4(3): 405-412.

Ehlers D, Hilmer S, Bartholomae S. HPLC analysis of supercritical Co2 cinnamon and cassia extracts in comparison with cinnamon and cassia oils. European Food Research and Technology. 1995; 200: 282–288.

Farahpour MR, Habibi M. Evaluation of the wound healing activity of an ethanolic extract of Ceylon cinnamon in mice. Veterinarni Medicina. 2012; 57(1): 53–57

Goubran FH, Holmes RJ. The development of alternative fungicides from essential oils victoria, Australia: Institute for Horticultural Development, Knoxfield, Department of Agriculture. 1993.

Han X, Parker TL. Anti-inflammatory activity of cinnamon (*Cinnamomum zeylanicum*) bark essential oil in a human skin disease model. Phytotherapy Research. 2017; 31(7): 1034-1038.

Huang TC, Fu HY, Ho C, Tan D, Huang Y, Pan M. Induction of apoptosis by cinnamaldehyde from indigenous cinnamon *Cinnamomum osmophloeum* Kaneh through reactive oxygen species production, glutathione depletion, and caspase activation in human leukemia K562 cells, Food Chemistry. 2007; 103(2): 434–443.

IDF (International Diabetes Federation) Diabetes Atlas 7th edition. 2016. http://www.diabetesatlas.org

Jakhetia V, Patel R,Khatri P, Pahuja N, Garg S, Pandey A, Sharma S. Cinnamon: A pharmacological review. Journal of Advanced Scientific Research. 2010, 1(2): 19–12.

Jayaprakasha GK, Jagan Mohan Rao L, Sakariah KK. Chemical composition of the flower oil of *Cinnamomum zeylanicum* Blume. Journal of Agricultural and Food Chemistry. 2000; 48(9): 4294-5.

Jayaprakasha GK, Rao JML and Sakarriah KK. Volatile Constituents from *Cinnamomum zeylanicum* Fruit Stalks and Their Antioxidant Activities. Journal of Agriculture and Food Chemistry. 2007; 51(15): 4344-8.

Jeong, HW, Han DC, Son KH, Han MY, Lim JS, Ha JH, Lee CW, Kim HM, Kim HC, Kwon BM. Antitumor effect of the cinnamaldehyde derivative CB403 through the arrest of cell cycle progression in the G2/M phase. Biochemical Pharmacology. 2003; 65(8): 1343–1350.

Joshi B, Lekhak S, Sharma A. Antibacterial Property of Different Medicinal Plants: *Ocimum sanctum, Cinnamomum zeylanicum, Xanthoxylum armatum* and *Origanum majorana,* Kathmandu University Journal of Science, Engineering and Technology. 2009; 5(1): 143-150.

Kamath JV, Rana AC, Chowdhury AR. Prohealing effect of *Cinnamomum zeylanicum* bark. Phototherapy Research. 2003; 17(8): 970-972.

Kannappan S, Jayaraman T, Rajasekar P, Ravichandran MK, Anuradha CV. Cinnamon bark extract improves glucose metabolism and lipid profile in the fructose-fed rat. Singapore Medical Journal. 2006; 47(10): 858–863.

Kwon BM, Lee SH, Cho YK, Bok SH, So SH, Youn MR, Chang SI. Synthesis and biological activity of cinnamaldehydes as angiogenesis inhibitors. Bioorganic and Medicinal Chemistry Letters.1997; 7(19): 2473-2476.

Lu J, Zhang K, Nam S, Anderson RR, Jove R, and Wen W. Novel angiogenesis inhibitory activity in cinnamon extract blocks VEGFR2 kinase and downstream signalling. Carcinogenesis. 2010; 31(3): 481–488.

Matan N, Rimkeeree H, Mawson AJ, Chompreeda P, Haruthaithanasan V, Parker M. Antimicrobial activity of cinnamon and clove oils under modified atmosphere conditions. International Journal of Food Microbiology. 2009; 107(2): 180–185.

Mathew S, Abraham TE. Studies on the antioxidant activities of cinnamon (*Cinnamomum verum)* bark extracts, through various *in vitro* models. Food Chemistry. 2004; 94:520–528.

Paranagama PA, Wimalasena S, Jayatilake GS, Jayawardena AL, Senanayake UM, Mubarak AM. A comparison of essential oil constituents of bark, leaf, root and fruit of cinnamon (*Cinnamomum zeylanicum* Blum) grown in Sri Lanka. Journal of the Natural Science Foundation of Sri Lanka. 2001; 29(3&4): 147-153.

Parthasarathy H, Thombare S. Evaluation of antimicrobial activity of *Azadirachta indica, Syzygium aromaticum* and *Cinnamomum zeylanicum* against oral microflora, Asian Journal of Experimental Sciences. 2013; 27(2): 13–16.

Ranasinghe L, Jayawardena B, Abeywickrama K. Fungicidal activity of essential oils of *Cinnamomum zeylanicum* (L.) and *Syzygium aromaticum* (L.) Merr et L.M. Perry against crown rot and anthracnose pathogens isolated from banana. Letters in Applied Microbiology. 2002; 35(3): 208–211.

Ranasinghe P, Pigera S, Premakumara GAS, Galappaththy P, Constantine GR, Katulanda P. Medicinal properties of 'true' cinnamon (*Cinnamomum zeylanicum*): A systematic review. BMC Complementary and Alternative Medicine. 2013; 13:275.

Ribeiro-Santos R, Andrade M, Madella D, Martinazzo AP, Moura LD, de Melo NR, Sanches-Silva A. Revisiting an ancient spice with medicinal purposes: Cinnamon. Trends in Food Science and Technology. 2017; 62: 154-169.

Saleem M, Bhatti HN, Jilani MI, Hanif MA. Bioanalytical evaluation of *Cinnamomum zeylanicum* essential oil. Natural Product Research. 2015; 29(19):1857-1859.

Ulbricht C, Seamon E, Windsor RC, Armbruester N, Bryan JK, Costa D, Giese N, Gruenwald J, Iovin R, Isaac R, Grimes Serrano JM. An Evidence-Based Systematic Review of Cinnamon (*Cinnamomum* spp.) by the Natural Standard Research Collaboration, Journal of Dietary Supplements. 2011; 8(4): 378–454.

Unlu M, Ergene E, Unlu GV, Zeytinoglu HS, Vural N. Composition, antimicrobial activity and *in vitro* cytotoxicity of essential oil from *Cinnamomum zeylanicum* Blume (Lauraceae). Food Chemistry and Toxicology. 2010; 48(11): 3274-80.

Varalakshmi B, Vijaya AA, Karpagam T, Suguna Bai J, Manikandan R. *In vitro* antimicrobial and anticancer activity of *Cinnamomum zeylanicum* Linn bark ex-tracts. International Journal of Pharmacy and Pharmaceutical Sciences. 2013; 6(1): 12-18.

Wang R., Wang R. and Yang B. Extraction of essential oils from five cinnamon leaves and identification of their volatile compound compositions. Innovative Food Science & Emerging Technologies. 2009; 10(2): 289-292.

7

Botany, Chemistry and Pharmacological Aspects of Safed Musli (*Chlorophytum borivilianum* Santapau & Fernandez)

Bhaskar Protim Mahanta[1], Saikat Haldar[1] and Mohan Lal[1]*

ABSTRACT

The trend of using products which are found in their natural habitat or grown in a natural process is increasing. This is as a result of increasing awareness among related consumers. The modern market has a higher quantum of demand for such products. Chlorophytum borivilianum is one of such eminent traditionally used herb of India which is a member of Liliaceae family. Because of its high value of medicinal property it is designated as 'white gold' in Indian system of medicine. In Ayurveda, C. borivilianum occupies a good position in the 'Vajikaran Rasayana' group in support of its rejuvenation capacity, aphrodisiac and efficiency in reducing sexual disorders. It helps in curing physical illness and weakness; it also cures arthritis, diabetes; acts as an aphrodisiac agent and revitalizer, as general sex tonic, remedy for rheumatism and joint pains, as antimicrobial, anti-inflammatory, antitumor agent and it also helps in increasing body immunity and also useful for diarrhoea, dysentery leucorrhoea, gonorrhoea etc. The roots of C. borivilianum are rich in many phytochemical components that include steroidal and triterpenoidal saponins, sapogenins and fructons which act in many therapeutic purpose and hence widely used. The report were also found that the plant is a rich source of over 25 alkaloids, fibers, steroids, carbohydrate, proteins, vitamins, saponins, potassium, magnesium,

[1] Medicinal, Aromatic and Economic Plants Group, Biological Sciences and Technology Division, CSIR-North East Institute of Science and Technology Jorhat-785006, Assam, India.

**Corresponding author*: mohan@neist.res.in

calcium, fructose, glucose, mannose, galactose, xylose etc. Thus, the present chapter is an attempt to provide an overview of this medicinal plant i.e., Safed musli and focuses mainly on its botany, chemistry and pharmacological aspects.

Key words: *Chlorophytum borivilianum*, Safed musli, Aphrodisiac agent, Tuber extraction, Phytochemistry, Saponin.

---

1. INTRODUCTION

As stated, 'Prevention is better than cure' and with the arising awareness of people regarding one's health, the prevailing food and medicinal habits, a desperate preference for the nutritional organic food and herbal preventives against diseases is seen almost everywhere across the sections of people. Production and marketing of such items is an upcoming strategy of modern trade also. Remedial plants and herbs were discovered and used in conventional medicine practices since pre-historic times. The use of plants for herbal remedies can be traced back to over 5000 years. The Vedas are considered to be the earliest reliable resource of information about the herbal medicine, and more specifically Yajurveda has been depicted as the main source of such information (Thakur *et al.*, 2009). Experiences from far and near past reveal that the use of chemical drugs or allopathic medicines have various side effects on the human body. Moreover, they actually are unable to cure most of the diseases; in fact they just subside the symptoms of the diseases and suppress the disease as long as their doses are taken as directed by the physicians. So, it is observed that, it is better to prevent rather than curing any disease. Medicinal plants play vital roles in disease prevention. Their promotion and use fit into all existing prevention strategies. As a normative basis for the maintenance of good health, the use of medicinal plants and herbs in most of the countries has been widely observed. Due to its high reliability, the extraction and development of several drugs and chemotherapeutics from such remedial plants as well as from conventional used rural herbal remedies are now in the modern trend (Kumar *et al.*, 2004). Besides low cost personal health care, the demand for these plants is also increasing due to their utility as secondary metabolites (Swamy and Sinniah, 2015; Swamy and Sinniah, 2016; Swamy *et al.*, 2016; Swamy *et al.*, 2017).

Here, in this chapter the topic of discussion is emphasized on the chemistry and pharmacological aspects of *Chlorophytum borivilianum* (Safed musli), which is a member of Liliaceae family and is one of the well-known therapeutically used medicines in the Ayurvedic, Unani, Homeopathic and Allopathic systems of medicine (Nakasha *et al.*, 2016). With respect to its great medicinal property, Indian system of medicine considered Safed musli as 'White Gold' or 'divya aushad' (Kirtikar, 1975; Nakasha *et al.*, 2016; Nakasha *et al.*, 2017a,b). Safed musli has a wide diversity of medicinal properties and is mainly grown-up in the thick, tropical moist and dry deciduous forest of India. Out of the 256 species found in different tropical and sub-tropical regions of the world, 17 species were reported to have discovered in India (Sharma, 2017; Nakasha *et al.*, 2016; Nakasha *et al.*, 2017a,b). The medicinal uses of these herbs differ from each other but due to the lack of desirable information, they together known as Safed musli. The roots of Safed musli contain phytochemical components which include steroidal and triterpenoidal saponins, sapogenins and fructans that act as therapeutic agents and hence widely used.

The productivity of Safed musli is quite low, as compared to its market demand. The pursuit of bridging the production and demand of this high valued medicinal plant, it encounters certain adulteration with closely resembling medicinal inferior species, during the process. The studies on these plants reported lack of substantial evidences and they don't stand the list of critical assessments. Hence, to meet the increasing demand of the root there is an urgent need to understand the current scenario of its cultivation and new medicinal properties. Thus, the present chapter is undertaken to provide valuable information on the importance of this plant and to focus mainly on botanical, chemical and pharmacological aspects of the traditional use of Safed musli and to explore it worldwide.

2. BOTANICAL DESCRIPTION OF *CHLOROPHYTUM BORIVILIANUM*

Safed musli is an herbaceous plant found mainly in tropical wet forests of India. It consists of firm stem disc from where the whorl of leaves originates. The appearance of the leaves is ovate, linear and sessile in nature with a length and breadth of 10-40 cm and 0.6-0.4 cm respectively. The flora is found to be pedicellate with joints, white, small, tasteless, bracteates and Zygomorphic. The perianth of the flower with six tepals are designed in two heteromorphous series consisting of three tepals in each and the androecium of six stamens are designed opposite to the tepals. The Stamen is present quite away from the stigma and is shorter as compared to that of the Pistil. Anthers of the flower are found to be longer than its filament. Bracts are linear, papery and purplish with 1.0-10.5 cm longs, pedicle, whitish and 6-10 mm long.

The plant bears green and yellow coloured fruits which length and breadth are almost equal in size. The fruit is said to be capsule producing 3-12 seeds inside which are black coloured, endospermic and angular in shape and small in size. Modification on the fibrous roots of the plant is made turn it into fleshy roots, considering it to be economically important (Fig. 1). Its

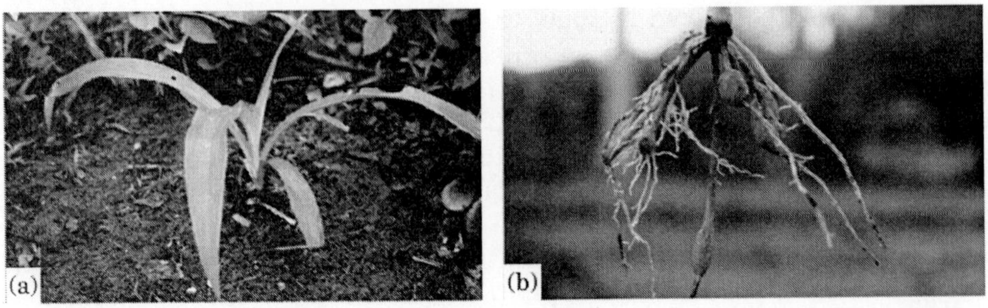

Fig. 1: (a) *Chlorophytum borivilianum* plant; (b) *Chlorophytum borivilianum* plant tubers (Taken from the Experimental Farm at CSIR-NEIST, Jorhat, India)

tuber roots are plump and cylindrical with a number of about 5-20 originating from the stem disc. It has 6-13 radicals spirally imbricate and slightly narrowed at the base and spread in horizontal way with smooth surfaces, wavy margins and parallel venation.

3. PHYTOCHEMISTRY

Safed musli is characterized and identified for the occurrence of a wide variety of phytochemical constituents in its plant organs, mainly in roots. The constituents present in this herb mainly include alkaloids, saponins, phenolic acids, and flavonoids (Visavadiya *et al.*, 2007; Nakasha *et al.*, 2017a,b). A report has been found that the roots of this herb consist of Carbohydrates of 42%, fibre of 3-4%, protein of 8-9% and saponins of 2-17% (Thakur *et al.*, 2009). In addition to all these, triterpenoids, gallotannins, steroid, magnesium, vitamins, calcium, potassium and also some rare elements *viz* Cu, Zn, P, resins along with some other phyto constituents such as large quantity of simple sugars like fructose, glucose, galactose, mannose, sucrose and xylose were discovered to have present in the plant (Jamal, 2005; Thakur and Dixit, 2005; Singh *et al.*, 2012). Besides, the study also suggested that the plant contains phenolics, proteins and Mucilage (Thakur and Dixit, 2005). Saponins are considered to be chief medicinal compounds present in the roots of Safed musli. According to research study, saponins are formed by the admixture of sapogenins along with sugar moiety and are proved to be highly responsible for medicinal properties. They are also easily soluble in water. Although, complete investigation was yet to be found on the species of *Chlorophytum,* but in recent years several sapogenins, saponins, spirostane glycosides and furostane came to light (Kaushik, 2005). The inulin type 2-1 linked fructans first reported by Kothari and Singh (2004) along with the extracts was indicated to be significantly important as antidiabetic activity in streptozotocin induced diabetic animals (Kothari and Singh, 2004). Moreover, after investigating the species of *Chlorophytum*, it can be suggested that out of all the species available, *Chlorophytum borivilianum* has the highest saponin content and is capable of producing maximum root powder.

3.1. Saponins of *Chlorophytum borivilianum*

A wide range of herbs from the genus *Chlorophytum* are known for their therapeutic potential. Saponins are rich in many therapeutic potential. They are proved to be different from other glycosides due to their surface active properties (Tyler *et al.*, 1981). The saponins present in *Chlorophytum borivilianum* are steroidal spirostane and steroidal furostane (Fig. 2) which were of much interest for their structural variety and therapeutic capacity (Bruneton, 1995). The chief secondary metabolites of this plant are saponins along with stigmasterol and hecogenins, where stigmasterol contributes the aphrodisiac action of the herb while the later helps in producing anabolic hormones. These secondary metabolites are together considered to be responsible for antioxidant, aphrodisiac, anti-cancer activities and for immune booster (Kumar *et al.*, 2011). Many researchers have made qualitative analysis of saponins in order to standardize both saponins as well as sapogenins by analysing High Performance Thin Layer Chromatography (HPTLC) and High Performance Liquid Chromatography (HPLC) (Govindarajan *et al.*, 2005a; Narasimhan *et al.*, 2006).

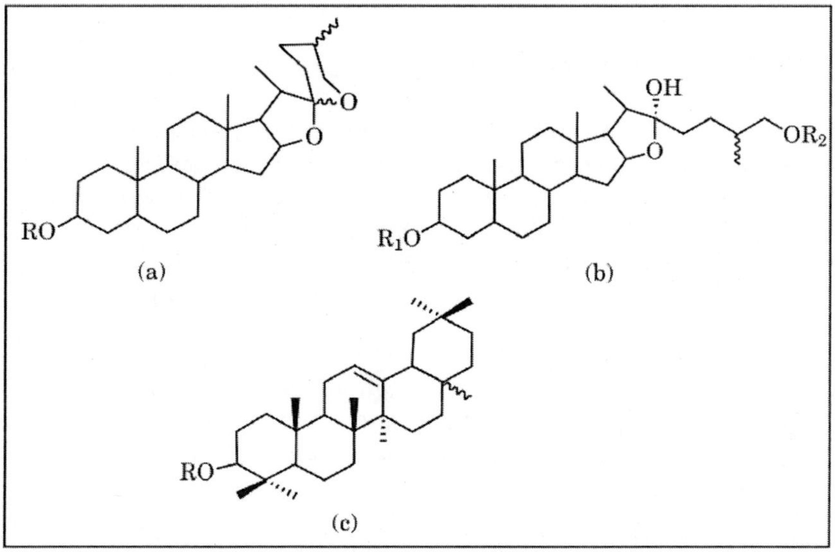

Fig. 2: (a) Steroidal spirostane, (b) Steroidal furostane, (c) Triterpenoid saponins, R = Sugar moiety.

Though only a few studies made by the researchers on systematic isolation of saponin till date. Later, researchers have successfully reported 20 steroidal saponins by working on butanol (n-BuOH) layer of ethanol extract of the roots of Safed musli (Acharya *et al.* (2008a) and Acharya *et al.*, 2009). Also it has been reported with 4 new insecticidal and cytotoxic furostane kind of saponins for the first time by Acharya *et al.* (2007). Further, Acharya *et al.*, (2008a) investigated n-BuOH layer of ethanolic extract of *C. borivilianum* roots which led to the isolation of six new steroidal saponins out of which two were considered to be furostanol and another four were spirostanol steroid type saponins. In the same year, Acharya *et al.* (2008b) made another study where he successfully obtained four new furastanol steroid saponins, borivillianoside A, B, C and D. They found glucose, galactose, and rhamnose are present as sugar moieties in borivillianoside A and B, while borivillianoside C and D was found to contain glucose, galactose, and xylose. Another study conducted by Acharya *et al.* (2009) identified another four new spirostane-type saponins, borivillianoside E, F, G and H from ethanol extract of the roots of *C. borivilianum.* Likewise, a novel furostanol saponin named chlorophytoside-I was successfully isolated by Deore and Khadabadi (2010) from methanolic extract of *Chlorophytum borivilianum* roots. Although there is lack of investigation and many chemical compounds, saponins are the mainly isolated from butanol fraction of ethanolic extract, however still there exist enough scope for further investigation on various extracts and other remaining parts of the plant *viz.*, leaves and flowers.

4. MEDICINAL ASPECTS OF *CHLOROPHYTUM BORIVILIANUM*

C. borivilianum is an established herbal plant with medicinal importance, occurs very rarely in tropical and sub-tropical regions of India. The plant is well recognized for therapeutical medicine and there is evidence of using this herb in Unani, Ayurvedic, Homeopathic and Allopathic medicinal system. It is also called as divine herb in Atharvaveda for its medicinal qualities. Its roots are mainly used in therapeutic application such as immunomodulatory, aphrodisiac, antidiabetic and adaptogenic (Nakasha *et al.*, 2016). It is curative for natal and post-natal problems and increases lactation in feeding mothers. It is a general sex tonic, used in diarrhoea, dysentery, gonorrhoea, leucorrhoea etc. It is designated as alternative 'Viagra' due to the presence of spermatogenic property. Its roots are indicated by pharmacological studies as antiviral (Siddiqui, 2005), anticancer (Jamal, 2005), antioxidant (Govindarajan *et al.*, 2005a; Govindarajan *et al.*, 2005b; Kenjale *et al.*, 2007; Sreevidya *et al.*, 2006), antidiabetic (Panda *et al.*, 2007; Mujeeb *et al.*, 2009), antistress (Gopalkrishna and Patil, 2006; Deore and Khadabadi, 2009b), aphrodisiac (Thakur and Dixit, 2007; Thakur and Dixit, 2006), antimicrobial (Deore and Khadabadi, 2007), hypolipidemic (Visavadiya and Narasimhacharya, 2007), hypochloremic (Deore and Khadabadi, 2009a), anti-inflammatory (Deore and Khadabadi, 2008), immunomodulatory activities (Thakur *et al.*, 2007). The chief constituents of this medicinal plant are steroidal saponins, polysaccharides, fructans and fructo-oligosaccharides, stigmasterol, Beta sitosterol, hecogenin and mucilage. Hence, all these components of *C. borivilianum* act as therapeutic agents in various therapeutic applications.

4.1. Immunomodulatory activity

Scientific literature has mentioned repeatedly about the immunomodulatory activity present in plant drugs. The term 'Immunomodulation' represents a change, a strengthening of suppression, of the indicators of cellular and humoral immunity and non-specific defence factors. Its aspect is to act as pharmacological agent under numerous dose and time regimes and to reveals an immunomodulating effects. Immunostimulating and immunosuppression are biologically active substances of immunomodulatory actions and both these agents considered to have their own standing and can search for better agents by exerting these activities, which has begun to receive much attention throughout the world (Smirnov and Suskova, 1989). Moreover, immonumodulatory activity was evaluated by ethanolic extract of the tubers of *C. borivilianum* and sapogenins. This provides more remarkable activity towards the ethanolic extract and proved to be more patent as compared to that of sapogenin fraction of the herb.

4.2. Aphrodisiac activity

In Greek the word 'Aphrodisiac' denotes goddess of love. Aphrodisiac is defined as a substance that enhance the sexual wish and useful for the treatment of sexual dysfunction (Triveni, 1977). Its study was 1st conducted on animals and has become the most leading supporting scientific evidence for using the herb as aphrodisiac agent. The aphrodisiac activity of the herb was first tested on albino rats with roots ethanolic extract and sapogenin extract with the doses of 200 mg/kg and 100 mg/kg body weight respectively and was found that the treated animal showed anomalous sexual behaviour as well as their reproductive organs also gained weight. Hence, from the findings of the study it certifies the use of this herb as strong sexual stimulant.

4.3. Antidiabetic activity

Diabetes, a disease emerged as a most serious threatening to human health in this modern world. According to recent study, among the developing nations of the world, India merged as the leading country in this respect with a population of over 1 billion. *C. borivilianum* plant is famous for anti-diabetic activity from past days. In recent years, studies have been performed on this herb for antidiabetic property against streptozotin induced diabetes and provide ample evidences for the potency of the herb (Mujeeb *et al.*, 2009). From a different study, it was found that the attendance of fructans in the herb reduces the chances of diabetes by normalizing glucose level of blood.

4.4. Effectiveness against lipid metabolism

The tuber crush of *C. borivilianum* is very effective and controls the hyperlipidemic/hypercholesterolemic conditions that occur mostly in male albino rats (Visavadiya and Narasimhacharya, 2007). In an experiment on hypercholesterolemic rats, two doses of root powder *i.e.,* 0.75 and 1.5 g root powder/ rat per day was chosen for execution for four weeks and was found that high density lipoprotein cholesterol level increased and the plasma along with hepatic lipid profiles decreased. Interestingly in control normocholestremic animals no noteworthy evident variation has been found in lipid profiles. Therefore, to ameliorate the lipid metabolism in hypercholesterolemic animals the *C. borivilianum* herb is very effective. Later, Sreevidya *et al.* (2006) stated that due to the presence of fructans in the herb, it may be regarded as one of the most leading factor for proper management of hypercholesterolemic.

4.5. Antiulcer activity

The alcoholic extract of Safed musli shows ulcer healing property. Gastric ulceration which is induced by cold stress was selected as a model for the assessment of this property. The ulcer index was reduced ($p<0.001$) by evaluating the alcoholic extract at the dosage of 200 mg/kg in comparison to that of control group (Singh *et al.*, 2012).

4.6. Analgesic activity

Analgesic, better acknowledged as painkiller or pain reliever belongs to the assorted group of drugs which reduces or eliminates pain. This kind of drugs acts in various ways in the central nervous system which include paracetamol, the non-steroidal anti-inflammatory drugs (NSAIDS) like salicylates. It also acts as narcotic drugs like morphine as well as synthetic drugs that have narcotic properties like tramadol etc.

The effectiveness of methanolic extracts of *Chlorophytum borivilianum* used in treating pain has been reported by Panda *et al.* (2007), where the study was mainly focused on the utilization of the traditional demand of the herb against rheumatoid arthritis. Thus, the present investigation suggests that the herb has analgesic activity used as an ointment to relieve pain.

4.7. Anti-tumour and anti-mutagenic activity

The roots of Safed musli consist of cytotoxic steroidal glycoside Saponin chloromaloside-A and Spirostanolpentaglycosides, which embraces beta-D-apiofuranose that responsible for anti-cancer property (Kumar *et al.*, 2010). The aqueous extract of the tuber roots of *C. borivilianum* having anti-tumour and anti-mutagenic property have established when reported that skin papillomagenesis studies helps to determine significantly ($P<0.001$) the decreasing of cumulative number of Papilloma (Mimaki *et al.*, 1996). Moreover, tumour incidence, the size of tumour along with tumour weight also increases in noteworthy way ($P<0.01$) at usual latent period when the extracts of the roots of the herb was possessed by animals. Its dose level was 800mg/kg body weight/day orally in double distilled water which was done during the beginning stages of carcinogenesis. It was moreover observed that the chromosomal aberration frequency along with micronuclei was decreased in treated animals in a significant way than that of carcinogen controls (Sharma *et al.*, 2017). Thus, from the present study it can be suggested that *C. borivilianum* has Anti-tumour property, anti-mutagenic as well as chemomodulatory effects (Khanam *et al.*, 2013).

4.8. Anthelmintic activity

Saponin extract of Safed musli proved to have contained anthelmintic property. The result was found as it is checked on *Pheretima posthuma* and also *Ascaridia galli* by using methanolic extract along with crude saponin and purified saponin extract. It also uses Piperazine as model drug and distilled water as control. Parameters were measured by using time required for paralysis and that of time required for death of the worm (Deore and Khadabadi, 2010; Singh *et al.*, 2012). Although anthelmintic activity on selected worms could be found from all extracts but the extract of purified saponin has proved to be more vigorous in contrast to others (Deore and khadabadi, 2010).

4.9. Antimicrobial activity

Four pathogenic fungi and eight bacteria were investigated next to the antimicrobial capability of *C. borivilianum* with micro-broth dilution assay. The extract with least concentration that can inhibit all kind of microbial propagation by the treatment of p-lodonitrotetrazolium violet was treated as minimum concentration of inhibition. The extract of water of the herb proved to have antimicrobial activity which ranges from 75-1200 mg/ml (Singh *et al.*, 2012; Sharma *et al.*, 2017).

4.10. Larvicidal activity

The saponin extracts of Safed musli was reported to have larvicidal properties which was being examined for the mosquito species such as *Anopheles stephensi*, *Aedes aegypti* and *Culex quinquefasciatus* on the basis of LC_{50} and EC_{50} values. Among all the extracts having larvicidal activity, the purified saponin fraction showed highest effectiveness. Besides larvicidal activity *C. borivilianum* extract also reported to have antiviral activity which shows a potent antiviral activity BHV-1 virus (Goel *et al.*, 2011). Antibacterial property of *C. borivilianum* was investigated by using different extract of the herb against 4 bacteria, *Staphylococcus aureus*, *E. coli*, *Pseudomonas aeruginosa* and *Bacillus subtilis* by using cup diffusion method and was found that acetic acid extract shows antibacterial activity against all these 4 bacteria in the order of sensitivity as *Staphylococcus aureus, Pseudomonas aeruginosa, E. coli* and *Bacillus subtilis* (Sundarum *et al.*, 2011).

5. CONCLUSIONS

In the approach to conclude the above discussion, the various studies found many utilities of Safed musli (*C. borivilianum*) roots, though these studies don't validate its efficiency as antipyretic, anti-diarrhoea, anti-dysentery, anti-ageing, anti-obesity and gynaecological disorders, as claimed in the traditional system. The medicinal properties and their uses for treatment need more scientific research approach to achieve precision in the process of using it for medicinal purposes considering their possible side effects or toxicities. Certain international products of *C. borivilianum* like GAP, GMP, and GSP should also be implemented with HACCP approach.

Moreover, the illegal movement of forest products to meet the increasing market demand should be checked and regulated through strict implementation of existing laws (Indian Forest Act, 1927). There still exist a huge gap of insufficient knowledge and awareness among people, which is to be filled up with proper orientation and approach of scientific research in order to gain universal acceptance as a plant with usable medicinal values.

REFERENCES

Acharya D, Mitaine-Offer AC, Kaushik N, Miyamoto T, Lacaille-Dubois MA. Furostanol glycosides from the roots of *Chlorophytum borivilianum*. Planta Medica. 2007; 73(09): 430.

Acharya D, Mitainea-Offer AC, Kaushik N, Miyamoto T, Paululat T, Lacailleâ, Dubois MA. Furostane-Type Steroidal Saponins from the Roots of *Chlorophytum borivilianum*. Helvetica Chimica Acta. 2008a; 91(12): 2262-9.

Acharya D, Mitaine-Offer AC, Kaushik N, Miyamoto T, Paululat T, Lacaille-Dubois MA. Steroidal saponins from the roots of *Chlorophytum borivilianum*. Planta Medica. 2008b; 74(09): PB23.

Acharya D, Mitaine-Offer AC, Kaushik N, Miyamoto T, Paululat T, Mirjolet JF, Duchamp O, Lacaille-Dubois MA. Cytotoxic spirostane-type saponins from the roots of *Chlorophytum borivilianum*. Journal of Natural Products. 2009; 72(1): 177-81.

Bruneton J. Pharmacognosy, phytochemistry, medicinal plants: Lavoisier publishing; 1995.

Deore SL, Khadabadi SS. *In vitro* antimicrobial studies of *Chlorophytum borivilianum* (liliaceae) root extracts. Asian Journal of Microbiology Biotechnology and environmental Science. 2007; 9(4): 807.

Deore SL, Khadabadi SS. Antiinflammatory and antioxidant activity of *Chlorophytum borivilianum* root extracts. Asian Journal of Chemistry. 2008; 20(2): 983.

Deore SL, Khadabadi SS. A study of hypocholesteremic effects of *Chlorophytum borivilianum* tubers in rats. Pharmacology Online. 2009a; 1: 398-403.

Deore SL, Khadabadi SS. Screening of antistress properties of *Chlorophytum borivilianum* tuber. Pharmacology Online. 2009b; 1: 320-8.

Deore SL, Khadabadi SS. Isolation and characterization of phytoconstituents from *Chlorophytum borivilianum*. Pharmacognosy Research. 2010; 2(6): 343.

Goel A, Singh R, Dash S, Gupta D, Pillai A, Yadav SK, *et al.* Antiviral activity of few selected indigenous plants against Bovine Herpes Virus-1. Journal of Immunology and Immunopathology. 2011; 13(1): 30-37.

Gopalkrishna B, Patil SH. Preliminary phytochemical investigation and *in-vitro* Anti-stress activity of Safed musli, *Chlorophytum borivilianum*. Indian Drugs. 2006; 43(11): 878-880.

Govindarajan R, Sreevidya N, Vijayakumar M, Thakur M, Dixit VK, Mehrotra S, *et al. In vitro* antioxidant activity of ethanolic extract of *Chlorophytum borivilianum*. Natural product sciences. 2005a; 11(3): 165-169.

Govindarajan R, Vijayakumar M, Pushpangadan P. Antioxidant approach to disease management and the role of Rasayana herbs of Ayurveda. Journal of ethnopharmacology. 2005b; 99(2): 165-178.

Jamal MA (*ed*). Effects of Safed musli on cell kinetics and apoptosis in human breast cancer cell lines. International conference on promotion and development of botanicals with international coordination exploring quality, safety, efficacy and regulation organized by School of natural product study, Jadavpur University, Kolkata, India; 2005.

Kaushik N. Saponins of *Chlorophytum* species. Phytochemistry Reviews. 2005; 4(2-3): 191-196.

Kenjale RD, Shah RK, Sathaye SS. Anti-stress and anti-oxidant effects of roots of *Chlorophytum borivilianum* (Santa Pau and Fernandes). Indian Journal of Experimental Biology. 2007; 45(11): 974.

Khanam Z, Singh O, Singh R, Bhat IU. Safed musli (*Chlorophytum borivilianum*): A review of its botany, ethnopharmacology and phytochemistry. Journal of Ethnopharmacology. 2013; 150(2): 421-441.

Kirtikar KR. Liliaceae: Chlorophytum. Indian medicinal plants. 1975.

Kothari SK, Singh K. Safed musli (*Chlorophytum borivilianum*) revisited. Journal of Medicinal and Aromatic Plant Sciences. 2004; 26: 60-63.

Kumar A, Nandi SK, Chandra B, Pal M. Conservation of some Idmalayan Medicinal Plants Using Biotechnological Approaches. Indian Forester. 2004; 130(2): 187-199.

Kumar M, Meena P, Verma S, Kumar M and Kumar A. Anti-tumour, anti-mutagenic and chemomodulatory potential of *Chlorophytum borivilianum*. Asian Pacific Journal of Cancer Prevention. 2010; 11(2): 327- 334.

Kumar KA, Chitra V, Krishna VL, Soujanya J. Evaluation of immunomodulatory effect of hydroalcoholic root extract of *Chlorophytum arundinaeceum* Baker in mice. International Journal of Pharmacy and Pharmaceutical Sciences. 2011; 3: 355-359.

Mimaki Y, Kammoto T and Sashida Y. Steroidal Saponins from the underground parts of *Chlorophytum* and their inhibitory activity on tumor promoter-induced phospholipids metabolism of HeLa cells. Phytochemistry. 1996; 41: 1405-10.

Mujeeb M, Khan SA, Ali M, Mall A, Ahmad A. Antidiabetic activity of the aqueous extract of *Chlorophytum borivilianum* L. in streptozotocin induced-hyperglycemic rats: A preliminary study. Journal of Pharmacy Research. 2009; 2(1):51-53.

Nakasha JJ, Sinniah UR, Kemat N, Mallappa KS. Induction, subculture cycle, and regeneration of callus in safed musli (*Chlorophytum borivilianum*) using different types of phytohormones. Pharmacognosy Magazine. 2016; (Suppl 4):S460-464.

Nakasha JJ, Sinniah UR, Shaharuddin NA, Hassan SA, Subramaniam S, Swamy MK. Establishment of an efficient *in vitro* regeneration and Agrobacterium rhizogenes-mediated genetic transformation protocol for Safed musli (*Chlorophytum borivilianum* Santapau & RR Fern.). *In vitro* Cellular and Developmental Biology-Plant. 2017a; 53(6): 571-578.

Nakasha JJ, Sinniah UR, Puteh AB, Kumara Swamy M. Influence of tuber weight and cutting on growth and yield of safed musli (*Chlorophytum borivilianum*). Archives of Agronomy and Soil Science. 2017b; 63(5): 619-625.

Narasimhan S, Govindarajan R, Madhavan V, Thakur M, Dixit VK, Mehrotra S, *et al*. Action of (2â†' 1) fructo-oligopolysaccharide fraction of *Chlorophytum borivilianum* against streptozotocin-induced oxidative stress. Planta Medica. 2006; 72(15): 1421-1424.

Panda SK, Si SC, Bhatnagar SP. Studies on hypoglycaemic and analgesic activities of *Chlorophytum borivilianum* Sant and Ferz. Journal of Natural Remedies. 2007; 7(1): 31-36.

Sharma P. *Chlorophytum borivilianum* (Safed musli): A Vital Herbal Drug. International Journal of Pharmaceutical and Medicinal Research. 2017; 5(1): 401-411.

Siddiqui YM (*ed*). Potent antiviral effect of Safed musli on poliovirus replication. International conference on promotion and development of botanicals with international co-ordination exploring quality, safety, efficacy and regulation organized by School of natural product study, Jadavpur University, Kolkata, India; 2005.

Singh D, Pokhriyal B, Joshi YM, Kadam V. Phytopharmacological aspects of *Chlorophytum borivilianum* (safed musli): A review. Int J Res Pharm Chem. 2012; 2(3): 853-859.

Smirnov LD, Suskova VS. Modulation of an immune-response of antioxidants. Khimiko Farmatsevticheskii Zhurnal. 1989; 23(7): 773-784.

Sreevidya N, Govindarajan R, Vijayakumar M, Thakur M, Dixit VK, Mehrotra S, Madhusudan KP. Action of fructo-oligo polysaccharide fraction of *Chlorophytum borivilianum* against streptozotocin induced oxidative stress. Planta Medica. 2006; 72(15): 1421-1424.

Sundarum S, Dwivedi P, Purwar S. Antibacterial activity of crud extract of *Chlorophytum borivillianum* to bacterial pathogens. Research Journal of Medicinal Plant. 2011; 1:1-5.

Swamy MK, Sinniah UR. A comprehensive review on the phytochemical constituents and pharmacological activities of Pogostemon cablin Benth.: An aromatic medicinal plant of industrial importance. Molecules. 2015; 20(5): 8521-8547.

Swamy MK, Sinniah UR. Patchouli (*Pogostemon cablin* Benth.): Botany, agrotechnology and biotechnological aspects. Industrial Crops and Products. 2016; 87: 161-176.

Swamy MK, Arumugam G, Kaur R, Ghasemzadeh A, Yusoff MM, Sinniah UR. GC-MS based metabolite profiling, antioxidant and antimicrobial properties of different solvent extracts of Malaysian *Plectranthus amboinicus* leaves. Evidence-Based Complementary and Alternative Medicine. 2017; 2017: 1-10.

Swamy MK, Akhtar MS, Sinniah UR. Antimicrobial properties of plant essential oils against human pathogens and their mode of action: An updated review. Evidence-Based Complementary and Alternative Medicine. 2016; 2016: 1-21.

Thakur GS, Bag M, Sanodiya BS, Debnath M, Zacharia A, Bhadauriya P, *et al. Chlorophytum borivilianum*: A white gold for biopharmaceuticals and nutraceuticals. Current Pharmaceutical Biotechnology. 2009; 10(7): 650-666.

Thakur M, Bhargava S, Dixit VK. Immunomodulatory activity of *Chlorophytum borivilianum* Sant. F. Evidence-Based Complementary and Alternative Medicine. 2007; 4(4): 419-423.

Thakur M, Dixit VK. Effect of *Chlorophytum borivilianum* on androgenic and sexual behavior of male rats. Indian Drugs-Bombay-. 2006; 43(4): 300.

Thakur M, Dixit VK. Effect of some vajikaran herbs on pendiculation activities and *in vitro* sperm count in male. Sexuality and Disability. 2007; 25(4): 203-207.

Thakur M, Dixit VK. Fructan; The polymer with unexplored potential. Indian Pharmacist. 2005; 4(42): 7-12.

Triveni A. Rasendrasarasangrah: Vajikaranadhikar. Nutan Press, Rajkot; 1977.

Tyler VE, Brady LR, Robbers JE. Pharmacognosy, 8th eds. Lea and Febiger, Philadelphia. 1981: 157-158.

Visavadiya NP, Narasimhacharya A. Ameliorative effect of *Chlorophytum borivilianum* root on lipid metabolism in hyperlipaemic rats. Clinical and Experimental Pharmacology and Physiology. 2007; 34(3): 244-249.

Visavadiya NP, Soni B, Dalwadi N, Madamwar D. *Chlorophytum borivilianum* as potential terminator of free radicals in various *in vitro* oxidation systems. Drug and Chemical Toxicology.2010; 33(2): 173-82.

8

Botany, Chemistry and Pharmaceutical Significance of *Terminalia chebula* Retz. – A Traditionally Important Medicinal Plants of India

Twahira Begum[1] and Mohan Lal[1]*

ABSTRACT

Terminalia chebula Retz. is a significant traditional medicinal plant, natively found in the South East Asia, and has a wide distribution throughout India, Sri Lanka, Myanmar, Bangladesh, Malaysia, Nepal, Cambodia, Laos, Indonesia, Pakistan, Vietnam and Thailand. T. chebula is a deciduous tree of medium to large-size, and fruits occur from January to April. As per the reports of World Health Organization, about 80% people of the world depend on various traditionally valuable medicinal plants for their primary medication. The fruit of T. chebula is majorly used for various treatments against human diseases. The fruit is drupe, faintly 5-angular, glabrous and is yellowish-gray, when ripe. The various medicinal properties of T. chebula can be attributed to phytoconstituents of the fruit. In T. chebula, tannins, which are mostly in hydrolysable form are responsible for the pharmacological activities of T. chebula. Besides, it contains phenolics, such as chebulinic acid, anthraquinones and ellagic acid. Also, minor constituents of polyphenols have been found in T. chebula. The fruit of T. chebula has antibacterial, antifungal and antiprotozoal properties. It is being used since a long time for the control of diabetes and gastrointestinal motility. The cryoprotective effect against oxidative damage induced by UV light has been exhibited by the fruit extracts. Other biological properties include

[1] Medicinal Aromatic and Economic Plants Group, Biological Science and Technology Division, CSIR-North East Institute of Science and Technology, Jorhat, Assam, India
**Corresponding author:* mohan@neist.res.in

antimutagenic, anticarcinogenic, radioprotective, chemopreventive activities, immune modulatory activity, and high antioxidant activities have been documented. In addition, fruits possess anti-inflammatory activity. Thus, T. chebula has immense importance in the Ayurveda and is significantly gaining importance in the modern medicine era.

Key words: *Terminalia chebula*, Phytochemistry, Pharmacological, Traditional knowledge.

1. INTRODUCTION

Medicinal plants are an indispensable part of human life throughout the ancient time. *Terminalia chebula* Retz. is a significant medicinal plant, which has been in use traditionally since many years. It has been used in various treatment purposes in the Ayurveda, Unani and other household remedies, since a long time back. As per the reports of World Health Organization about, 80% people of the world depend on the traditionally valuable medicinal plants for their primary medication (WHO 1993; Swamy and Sinniah, 2015; Swamy and Sinniah, 2016; Swamy *et al*. 2016; Arumugam *et al*., 2016; Swamy *et al*., 2017). The fruit of *T. chebula* has a great medicinal value, and the Tibetans consider it as "the king of medicine" (Klika *et al*., 2004).

T. chebula, belonging to the family, Combretaceae of order Myrtales, class Magnoliopsida and division Magnoliophyta, is an important traditional medicinal plant, native to the South East Asia, and has a wide distribution throughout India, Sri Lanka, Myanmar, Bangladesh, Malaysia, Nepal, Cambodia, Laos, Indonesia, Pakistan, Vietnam and Thailand (Chattopadhyay and Bhattacharyya, 2007; Germplasm Resources Information Network, 2016). In India, *T. chebula* is found throughout the country, especially in areas of light rainfall and deciduous forests (Naik *et al*., 2004). *T. chebula* is commonly known as 'black myrobalan' in English. It is a medium to large-sized deciduous tree and fruiting from January to April. The fruit is drupe, faintly 5-angular, glabrous and yellowish-grey when ripe (The Ayurvedic pharmacopoeia of India, 2001). Various medicinal properties of *T. chebula* has been claimed to be due to the phytochemical constituents present in fruits. The fruit has been used in the formulations of a powdered drug, "triphala" meaning three nuts (*T. chebula*, *T. bellirica* and *Emblica officinalis*). It has great medicinal values, and is consumed in India since a long time back. In *T. chebula,* one of the major phytochemical constituents is the tannins, of which mostly belong to the hydrolysable form, and they are the major compounds responsible for various pharmacological activities. Besides, it contains phenolics, such as chebulinic acid, anthraquinones, ellagic acid, and other minor chemical constituents. Thus, it exhibits various pharmacological properties allowing one to explore in the traditional form of primary health treatments. Although, the traditional uses and nutritive values of the fruit are high, but many of their pharmacological uses are unknown to the common people, hence their pharmacological benefits needs to be published for the common people to be able to ripe the benefits of the fruits for natural treatments as compared to using other unnatural sources of medicines for treatments. Thus, *T. chebula* is a significant medicinal plant having immense valuable properties that can be further explored for use in the Ayurvedic medicine development.

This chapter highlights on the botanical, phytochemical and pharmacological significances of *T. chebula*. This comprehensive updated data will be beneficial to readers interested in plant bioactive compounds and their pharmacological investigations to discover novel drugs.

2. BOTANY

T. chebula is a deciduous tree of medium to large-sized, attaining a height of about 30-50 meters with wide spread branches (Fig. 1a,b). Leaves are ovate, elliptical and alternate or opposite. They have white to yellow colored monoecious flowers, borne in short panicles or terminal spikes. The flowers have a strong unpleasant smell. The fruit of *T. chebula* is drupe, glabrous and 1-2 inches in size. It is faintly five-angular on the outside. The fruit is greenish when unripe and turns yellowish on ripening (Fig. 1b). *T. chebula* fruiting starts from January and ends in the month of April (The Ayurvedic pharmacopoeia of India, 2001; Chattopadhyay and Bhattacharyya, 2007). According to Hooker as mentioned in his Flora of British India, apart from the *T. chebula* six other varieties of *T. chebula* has been mentioned (Hooker 1854; Ratha and Joshi, 2013). The varieties as mentioned by Hooker are:

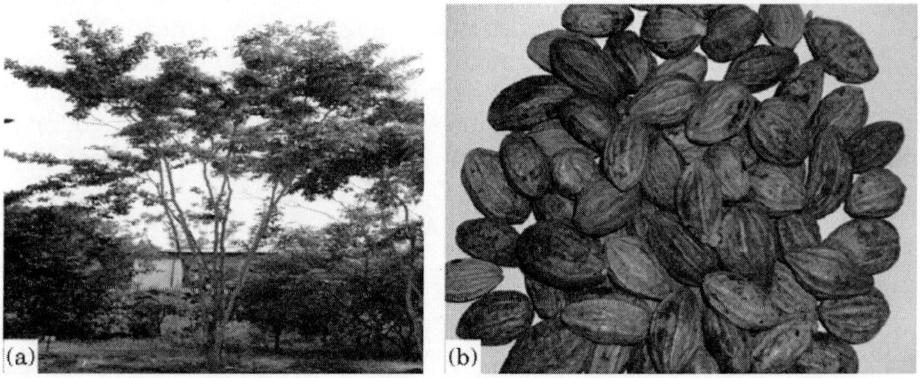

Fig. 1: Fruiting tree of *Terminalia chebula* (a); and dried fruits of *Terminalia chebula* (b)

1. *T. chebula* Retz. (var. chebula proper): The fruits of this variety are 1 to 1.5 inch in size, glabrous and five-ribbed.
2. *T. chebula* (var. typical): The fruits of this variety have young ovary and are shaggy without calyx teeth.
3. *T. chebula* (var. citrina): The fruits of this variety glabrous, ovate fruit, with round base and have young ovary.
4. *T. chebula* (var.): The fruits of this variety are much smaller than the other varieties.
5. *T. chebula* (var. tomentella Kurz): The fruits of this variety are glabrous, ovoid, hardly 1 inch in diameter and has young ovary.
6. *T. chebula* (var. gangetica Roxb.): The fruits of this variety have brown silky hairs covering the twigs. It is similar to that of chebula.
7. *T. chebula* (var. parviflora Thwaitos Enum): The fruit of this variety have more prominent five ribs on the outer side.

3. CHEMISTRY

The various medicinal properties of *T. chebula* can be attributed to the phytoconstituents present in the fruits (Table 1). One of the major phytochemical constituents of *T. chebula* is the tannins, which are mainly believed to be responsible for several pharmacological activities of *T. chebula* (Juang *et al.*, 2004; Han *et al.*, 2006). As per the report, it has been recorded that along with a geographical variation, the tannin content varies (Kumar 2006; Kumar *et al.*, 2009). Various components of hydrolysable tannins have been reported from the fruit of *T. chebula viz.* chebulegic acid, gallic acid, punicalagin, ellagic acid, chebulanin, neochebulinic acid, chebulinic acid, casuarinin, terchebulin, 1,2,3,4,6-penta-O-galloylβ-D-glucose, 1,6-di-o-galloyl-D-glucose, corilagin, 3,4,6-tri-o-glloyl-D-glucose, chebulic acid (Juang *et al.*, 2004; Chattopadhyay and Bhattacharyya, 2007). *T. chebula* fruits are reported to contain phenolic compounds including anthraquinones and ellagic, chebulinic acid, and other polyphenols (Williamson, 2002). The main active constituent present in *T. chebula* is chebulinic acid (Bag *et al.*, 2013; Jami *et al.*, 2014). In addition, it also contains some nutritive valued compounds, such as Vitamin C, amino acid, minerals and protein (Mahesh *et al.*, 2007).

4. PHARMACOLOGICAL SIGNIFICANCE

T. chebula has been used since ancient time as its use has been mentioned by Charaka (the principal contributors to Ayurveda) in preparations, such as Javaghna, Arsoghan, Kustaghna, Kasaghan and Prajasthapana. Besides, *T. chebula* has been used by Vagbhata in Parushakadi and in Amalakyadi, Triphala and Parusakdi by Sushruta, an ancient Indian physician (Sharma *et al.* 2005).

Table 1: Pharmaceutical properties of *Terminalia chebula* seeds.

Sl. no.	*Pharmacological properties*	*References*
1.	Anti-diabetic	Sabu and Kuttan (2002); Senthil Kumar and Subramanian (2008); Kannan *et al*. (2012)
2.	Antimutagenic	Grover and Bala (1992); Naik *et al*. (2004)
3.	Anticarcinogenic	Saleem *et al*. (2002)
4.	Radioprotective	Jagetia *et al*. (2002); Suguna *et al*. (2002); Gandhi and Nair (2005); Gupta *et al*. (2010)
5.	Immune modulator	Hamada *et al*. (1997); Dwivedi *et al*. (2008)
6.	Antioxidant	Klika *et al*. (2004); Naik *et al*. (2004); Okuda *et al*. (2005); Reddy *et al*. (2009); Chang and Lin (2010); Hazra *et al*. (2010)
7.	Anti-inflammatory	Sabina and Rasool (2008); Reddy *et al*. (2009)
8.	Antibacterial	Malekzadeh *et al*. (2001); Khan and Jain (2009); Khan (2009); Aneja and Joshi, (2009); Kumar *et al*. (2011)
9.	Antifungal	Dutta *et al*. (1998); Mehmood *et al*. (1999); Vonshak *et al*. (2003); Shinde *et al*. (2011)
10.	Antiprotozoal	Bagavan *et al*. (2011)
11.	Antiviral	Mekkaway *et al*. (1995); Ma *et al*. (2010)
12.	Astringent	Thomas *et al*. (2000)
13.	Cellular aging	Nam *et al*. (2004a); Na *et al*. (2004b); Manosroi *et al*. (2010)
14.	Melanin inhibition	Jin *et al*. (2006)

4.1. Antidiabetic activity

The methanolic extract of *T. chebula* in combination with *T. bellerica* and *Emblica officinalis*, is used commonly, since a long time back, and is named as 'Triphala', was reported to have antidiabetic potential as it was able to scavenge hydroxyl and peroxide radicals and inhibit lipid peroxide formation in the diabetic rats. Moreover, blood sugar level was observed to be lowered in the normal and alloxan-induced diabetic rats within 4 hrs of oral administration of methanolic extracts of *T. chebula* (75% concentration) (Sabu and Kuttan, 2002). Moreover, as per the report, the fruits and seeds of *T. chebula* have shown a dose dependent reduction in blood glucose level in streptozotocin-induced diabetic rats both in short term and long term study (Senthilkumar and Subramanian, 2008; Kannan *et al*., 2012).

4.2. Antimutagenic activity

In *Salmonella typhimurium,* the antimutagenic activity of *T. chebula* has been demonstrated along with the hydrolysable tannins present in it (Grover and Bala, 1992). The inhibition of strand breaks formation in plasmids induced by gamma radiation in pBR322 DNA has been shown by the aqueous extract of *T. chebula* (Naik *et al*., 2004).

4.3. Anticarcinogenic activity

The phenolics present in *T. chebula* has been found to have an inhibitory effect on the growth of malignant cells. Most of the inhibitory effects on the cancerous cells were found to be by the phenolics, such as ellagic acid, tannic acid and chebulinic acids present in *T. chebula*. It has been reported that 70% methanolic extracts of *T. chebula* was found to be effective in inhibiting cell proliferation, decreasing cell potency, and induction of cell death in a dose-dependent manner in several malignant cell lines, such as human prostate cancer cell line, breast cancer cell line in human and mouse, human osteosarcoma cell line and a non-tumorigenic, immortalized human prostate cell line (Saleem *et al.*, 2002).

4.4. Radioprotective activity

A radio protective activity of *T. chebula* has been demonstrated in mice. It possesses capacity to reduce the damage caused to the DNA due to radiation (Gandhi and Nair, 2005; Gupta *et al.*, 2010). It has been studied that it does so by scavenging free radicals of the radiations (Jagetia *et al.*, 2002). It is also being reported by Suguna *et al.* (2002) that the effect of irradiation on mice under *T. chebula* treatment showed a reduction in peroxidation of membrane lipids in the liver of the mice as well as a reduced level of DNA damage induced by the irradiation, as per the assay results obtained by using a single cell gel electrophoresis (Suguna *et al.*, 2002).

4.5. Immune modulator activity

In the experimental amoebic liver abscess in golden hamsters, the crude extract of *T. chebula* were found to have induced stimulated cell-mediated immune response (Dwivedi *et al.*, 2008). The immunosuppressive effect of chebulagic acid and gallic acid, which are active phytoconstituents of *T.* chebula were evaluated on cytotoxic T lymphocyte (CTL) mediated cytotoxicity. Experimental results showed that the chebulagic and gallic acid blocked the CTL - mediated cytotoxicity and inhibited the killing activity of CTL+CD8 clone at IC_{50} values of 30 and 50 µM, respectively (Hamada *et al.* 1997).

4.6. High antioxidant activity

The leaves, fruits and bark of *T. chebula* have been found to possess high phenol contents as verified by high performance liquid chromatography (HPLC) analysis. The antioxidant properties of *T. chebula* has been reported to be due to its high phenolic contents. Aqueous extract of *T. chebula* was found to be good scavengers of DPPH radicals. They also have shown to have inhibited xanthine/xanthine oxidase activity (Naik *et al.*, 2004; Chang and Lin, 2010). In an experiment the antioxidant enzymes present in the microsomes and mitochondria of rat liver were protected from the reactive oxygen species produced by gamma radiation by the extracts of *T. chebula* (Naik *et al.*, 2004). Chebulagic and chebulinic acid present in *T. chebula* were also found to have antioxidant activity (Klika *et al.*, 2004; Okuda *et al.*, 2005; Reddy *et al.*, 2009). It has been found that 70% methanolic extracts of 'Triphala' (combination of *T. chebula, T. belerica* and *Emblica officinalis*) can be used as a good source of natural antioxidant (Hazra *et al.*, 2010).

4.7. Anti-inflammatory activity

Chebulagic acid present in the fruit of *T. chebula* has been reported to be responsible for the anti-inflammatory effect (Reddy *et al.*, 2009). The anti-inflammatory effect against inflammation in mice induced by monosodium urate crystal was found to be effective by extract of *T. chebula* in formulation as 'Triphala'. It also has shown significance results in gouty arthritis (Sabina and Rasool, 2008).

4.8. Antibacterial activity

The solvent extracts of *T. chebula* have been shown to have an antibacterial activity against both Gram-negative and Gram-positive human pathogenic bacteria (Malckzadeh *et al.*, 2001; Khan and Jain, 2009; Khan, 2009). The extracts of *T. chebula* were tested against two dental caries causing bacteria and the extract was able to inhibit their growth. Thus, it can be effective alternative medication against dental caries causing bacteria (Aneja and Joshi, 2009). It has been reported that 15% aqueous and methanolic extract of *T. chebula* seeds were able to inhibit the growth of *E. coli* and *S. aureus* with 12 mm and 13 mm of zone of inhibition, respectively (Kumar *et al.*, 2011). The aqueous extract of *T. chebula* seeds were tested against *Helicobacter pylori* by agar diffusion method. It showed a minimum inhibitory concentration of 125 mg/L and minimum bactericidal activity of 150 mg/L (Malekzadeh *et al.*, 2001).

4.9. Antifungal activity

The aqueous extract of *T. chebula* seeds has been reported to have antifungal activity against yeast (*Candida albicans*) and a number of dermatophytes (*Epidermophyton, Trichophyton rubrum, Floccosum* and *Microsporum gypseum*) (Dutta *et al.*, 1998; Mehmood *et al.*, 1999; Vonshak *et al.*, 2003). The extracts of *T. chebula* were tested using paper disc method against five pathogenic fungi (*Aspergillus niger, Aspergillus flavus, Helminthosporium tetramera, Alternaria alternata* and *Alternaria brassicicola*) and were found to be effective against them as compared to Carbendazim (Shinde *et al.*, 2011).

4.10. Antiprotozoal activity

T. chebula is known to possess antiprotozoan activity. There is only a single report on the antiplasmodial activity against *Plasmodium falciparum,* which was reported when used with the acetone extracts of *T. chebula* seeds (Bagavan *et al.*, 2011).

4.11. Antiviral activity

The acetone extract of *T. chebula* seeds were evaluated against swine influenza a virus, and it showed antiviral properties (Ma *et al.*, 2010). The inhibitory effect has been shown by the solvent extract of *T. chebula* seeds on the human immunodeficiency virus-1 reverse transcriptase (Mekkaway *et al.*, 1995).

4.12. Astringent activity

The extract of *T. chebula* seeds is used in the allopathy medicine system, and mainly used as an astringent (Thomas *et al.*, 2000).

4.13. Cellular aging activity

T. chebula seed extract has been found to exhibit a significant cellular aging inhibitory effect (Nam *et al.*, 2004). The galls of *T. chebula* has been in use for medicinal plant recipes since from a long time traditionally for increasing the longevity. Thus, it can be used and developed further for making anti-aging products (Manosroi *et al.*, 2010). The extract of *T. chebula* was found to be effective against the inhibition of the age-dependent shortening of telomeric DNA length and oxidative stress (Na *et al.*, 2004).

4.14. Melanin inhibition activity

The methanolic extracts of *T. chebula* at 100 ppm or more than 90% exhibit a melanin inhibitory effect. The extracts of *T. chebula* can be thus used as a good source of de-pigmenting agent as compared to other de-pigmenting agents like kojic acid which have been found to be carcinogenic (Jin *et al.*, 2006).

5. CONCLUSIONS

The plant *T. chebula* is a valuable medicinal plant that has immense importance in Ayurveda system of medicine. Due to its various pharmaceutical uses it is significantly gaining importance in modern era of medicine. In Indian kitchen the fruits are used as pickle, dried or sweets. The plants have unique properties due to various types of phytoconstituents present in the fruit having different types of healing activities in human disease. The fruits can be used as an agent to overcome the drug resistance. Although the plant and its fruit has been in use since ancient times but nowadays the ancient knowledge of various uses of the plant has decreased and the common people needs to know the various uses of the plants so that they can use the plant for treatments in various ailments rather than opting for the allopathy or other medications. In the modern era of medicine people believes more on natural medicine. In this context *T. chebula* could be a source of alternate medicine to the common man. This plant can also pave the way for new drug designing and can be a very valuable natural medicine for the mankind.

REFERENCES

Aneja KR, Joshi R. Evaluation of antimicrobial properties of fruit extracts of *Terminalia chebula* against dental caries pathogens. Jundishapur Journal of Microbiology. 2009, 2(3), 105-111.

Arumugam G, Swamy MK, Sinniah UR. *Plectranthus amboinicus* (Lour.) Spreng: Botanical, phytochemical, pharmacological and nutritional significance. Molecules. 2016, 30;21(4):369.

Bagavan A, Rahuman AA, Kamaraj C, Kaushik KN, Mohankrishnan D, Sahal D. Antiplasmodial activity of botanical extracts against *Plasmodium falciparum*. Paracitology Research 2011, 108(5), 1099-11

Bag A, Bhattacharya KS, Pal N, Chattopadhyay R. Anti-inflammatory, anti-lipid peroxidative, antioxidant and membrane stabilizing activity of hydroalcoholic extract of *Terminalia chebula* fruits. Pharmaceutical Biology. 2013, 5(12), 1515-20

Hazra *et al*. Comparative study of the antioxidant and reactive oxygen species scavenging properties in the extracts of the fruits of *Terminalia chebula, Terminalia belerica* and *Emblica officinalis*, BMC Complementary and Alternative Medicine. 2010, 10:20. 10.1186/1472-6882-10-20

Chang LC, Lin SC. Development of antioxidant activity and pattern recognition of *Terminalia chebula* Retz. extracts and its fermented products. Hung Kuang Journal 2010, 61, 115-129

Chattopadhyay RR, Bhattacharyya SK. Plant Review *Terminalia chebula*. Pharmacognosy Review 2007, 23, 145-150

Dwivedi S, Dwivedi A, Kapadia R, Kaul S. Anthelmintic activity of alcoholic and aqueous extracts of fruits of *Terminalia chebula* Retz. Ethnobotany Leaflets. 2008, 12, 741-743

Dutta KB, Rahman I, Das KT. Antifungal activity of Indian plant extracts. Mycoses. 1988, 41(11-12), 535-36

Gandhi N M, Nair CK. Radiation protection by *Terminalia chebula*: Some mechanistic aspects. Molecular and Cellualar Biochemistry. 2005, 277 (1-2), 43-8.

Germplasm Resources Information Network (GRIN). Agricultural Research Service (ARS), United States Department of Agriculture (USDA). "*Terminalia chebula* Retz". 2016, Retrieved on 6 Aug 2017.

Grover SI, Bala S. Antimutagenic activity of *Terminalia chebula* (myroblan) in *Salmonella typhimurium*. Indian Journal of Experimental Biology. 1992, 30(4), 339-341

Gupta A, Mishra KA, Bansal P, Singh R, Kumar S, Gupta V, Phytochemistry and pharmacological activities of Haritaki- A review. J Pharm Res. 2010, 3(2), 417

Hamada, S., T. Kataoka, J.T. Wo, A. Yamada and T. Yoshida *et al*. Immunosuppressive effects of gallic acid and chebulagic acid on CTL-mediated cytotoxicity. Biol. Pharma Bulletin. 1997, 20: 1017-1019

Han Q, Song J, Wong L, Xu H, Preparative isolation of hydrolysable tannins chebulagic acid and chebulinic acid from *Terminalia chebula* by high-speed counter-current chromatography. Journal of Separation Science. 2006, 29, 1653-165

Hooker DJ, Flora of British India. Part 2. London: Oxford. 1845, 443-9

Jagetia CG, Baliga SM, Malagi JK, Sethukumar Kamath M. The evaluation of the radioprotective effect of Triphala (An Ayurvedic rejuvenating drug) in the mice exposed to gamma-radiation. Phytomedicine. 2002, 9(2), 99-108

Jami SI, Sultana Z, Ali E, Begum M, Haque M. Evaluation of analgesic and anti-inflammatory activities on ethanolic extract of *Terminalia chebula* fruits in experimental animal models. American Journal of Plant Sciences. 2014, 5 (1), 63-9

Jin Yin-Z, Li Guan G-Hua, Ahn So-Young, Row Kyung-Ho, Kim Eun-Ki. Extraction and purification of Depigmenting agent from Chinese plants. Chemistry Research Chinese. 2006, 22(2), 162-167

Juang JL, Sheu JS, Lin CT. Determination of hydrolysable tannins in the fruit of *Terminalia chebula* Retz. by high performance liquid chromatography and capillary electrophoresis. Journal of Separation Science. 2004, 27 (9), 718-724

Kannan RV, Rajasekar SG, Rajesh P, Balasubramanian V, Solomon K E, Nivas D, Chandru S. Anti-diabetic activity on ethanolic extracts of fruits of *Terminalia chebula* Retz. Alloxan induced diabetic rats. American Journal of Drug Discovery and Development. 2012, 2, 135-142

Khan HK. The effect of regular intake of *Terminalia chebula* on oxidative stress in mice originated from *Salmonella typhimurium*. EurAsian Journal of BioScience. 2009, 3, 113-121

Khan HK, Jain KS. Regular intake of *Terminalia chebula* can reduce the risk of getting typhoid fever. Advanced Biotechnology. 2009, 8(9), 1015

Klika KD, Saleem A, Sinkkonen J, Kähkönen M, Loponen J, Tähtinen P, Pihlaja K. The structural and conformational analyses and antioxidant of Chebulinic acid and its thrice-hydrolyzed derivative, 2,4,- chebuloyl-ßd- glucopyranoside, isolated from the fruit of *Terminalia chebula*. ARKIVOC. 2004, 7, 83-105

Klika KD, Saleem A, Sinkkonen J, Kähkönen M, Loponen J, Tähtinen P, Pihlaja K. The Structural and Conformational analyses and antioxidant of Chebulinic acid and its thrice-hydrolyzed derivative, 2,4,- chebuloyl-ßd- glucopyranoside, isolated from the fruit of *Terminalia chebula*. ARKIVOC. 2004, 7, 83-105

Kumar A, Lakshman K, Jayaveera K, Satish K, Tripathi MS. Estimation of rutin and quercitin in *Terminalia chebula* by HPLC. International Journal of Aesthetic Medicine. 2009, 2(1), 3

Kumar JK. Effect of geographical variation on content of tannic acid, gallic acid, chebulinic acid and ethyl gallate in *Terminalia chebula* fruits. Natural Products. 2006, 2(3), 170-175

Ma H, Diao Y, Zhao D, Li K, Kang T. A new alternative to treat swine influenza A virus infection: Extracts from *Terminalia chebula* Retz. African Journal of Microbiology Research. 2010, 4(6), 497-9

Mahesh R, Ramesh T, Nagulendran RK, Velayan S, Hazeena VB (2007). Effect of *Terminalia chebula* on monoamine oxidase and antioxidant enzyme activities in aged rat brain. Pharmacognosy Magazine 2007, 3, 12-16

Malckzadeh F , Eshanifar H, Shahamat N, Levin M, Colwell RR. Antibacterial activity of black myrobalan (*Terminalia chebula* Retz.) against *Helicobacter pylori*. International Journal of Antimicrobial Agent. 2001, 18(1), 85-88

Manosroi A, Jantrawut P, Akihisa T, Manosroi W, Manosroi J. *In vitro* anti-aging activities of *Terminalia chebula* gall extract. Pharmaceutical Biology. 2010, 48, 469- 481

Mehmood Z, Ahmad I, Mohammad F, Ahmad S. Indian medicinal plants: A potential source for anticandidal drugs. Pharmaceutical Biology. 1999, 37(3), 237-42

Mekkaway SE, Meselhy MR, Kusumoto IT, Kadota S, Hattori M, Namba T. Inhibitory Effects of egyptian folk medicines on human immunodeficiency virus (HIV) reverse transcriptase. Chemical and Pharmaceutical Bulletin. 1995, 43(4), 641-48

Naik HG, Priyadarsini IK, Naik BD, Gangabhagirathi R, Mohan H. Studies on the aqueous extract of *Terminalia chebula* as a potent antioxidant and a probable radioprotector. Phytomedicine. 2004, 11(6), 530-538

Na MK, Bae KH, Kang SS, Min BS, Yoo JK, Kamiryo Y, Snoo YI, Yokoo S, Miwa N. Cytoprotective effect on oxidative stress and inhibitory effect on cellular aging of *Terminalia chebula* fruit. Phytotherapy Research. 2004, 18(9), 737-41

Nam M, Bae K, Kang SS, Min SB, Yoo KJ, Kamiryo Y, Yokoo S, Miwa. Cytoprotective Effect on oxidative stress and inhibitory effect on cellular aging of *Terminalia chebula* fruit. Phytotherapy Research. 2004, 18(9), 737-41

Okuda T. Systematics and health effects of chemically distinct tannins in medicinal plants. Phytochemistry. 2005, 66(17), 2012-31

Ratha KK, Joshi CG. Haritaki (Chebulic myrobalan) and its varieties. Ayu. 2013, 34(3), 331-4

Reddy BD, Reddy MCT, Jyotsna G, Sharan S, Priya N0, Laxmipathi V, Pallu R. Chebulagic acid, a COX-LOX dual inhibitor isolated from the fruits of *Terminalia chebula* Retz. Induces apoptosis in COLO-205 cell line. Journal of Ethnopharmacology. 2009, 124(3), 506-12

Sabu, MC and Kuttan R. Anti-diabetic activity of medicinal plants and its relationship with their antioxidant property. Journal of Ethnopharmacology. 2002, 81, 155-160

Sachin Kumar, Hotam Singh Choudhary, Chandrabhan Seniya. *In vitro* antibacterial study of aqueous and methanolic extracts of some selected medicinal plants. Journal of Chemical and Pharmaceutical Research. 2011, 3(4), 854-860

Senthilkumar PG, Subramanian PS, Biochemical studies on the effect of *Terminalia chebula* on the levels of glycoproteins in streptozotocin-induced experimental diabetes in rats. Journal of Applied Biomedicine. 2008, 6, 105-115

Sabina PE, Rasool M. An *in-vivo* and *in-vitro* potential of Indian Ayurvedic herbal formulation Triphala on experimental gouty arthritis in mice. Vascular Pharmacology. 2008, 48(1), 14-20

Saleem A, Husheem M, Harkonen P, Pihlaja K. Inhibition of cancer cell growth by crude extract and phenolics of *Terminalia chebula* fruit. Journal of Ethnopharmacology. 2002, 81, 327-336

Sharma CP, Yelne BM, Dennis JT, Joshi A. Database on medicinal plants in Ayurveda. Vol. 2. Reprint 2005. New Delhi: Documentation and Publication Division, CCRAS. 2005, p.29

Shinde SL, More SM, Junne SB, Wadje SS. Tha antifungal activity of five *Terminalia* species checked by paper disc method. International Journal of Pharmaceutical Research and Development. 2011, 3(2): 36-39

Suguna L, Singh S, Sivakumar P, Sampath P, Chandrakasan G. Influence of *Terminalia chebula* on dermal wound healing in rats. Phytotherapy Research. 2002, 16, 227-231

Swamy MK, Sinniah UR. A comprehensive review on the phytochemical constituents and pharmacological activities of *Pogostemon cablin* Benth.: An aromatic medicinal plant of industrial importance. Molecules. 2015, 12;20(5):8521-47.

Swamy MK, Sinniah UR. Patchouli (*Pogostemon cablin* Benth.): Botany, agrotechnology and biotechnological aspects. Industrial Crops and Products. 2016, 87:161-76.

Swamy MK, Arumugam G, Kaur R, Ghasemzadeh A, Yusoff MM, Sinniah UR. GC-MS based metabolite profiling, antioxidant and antimicrobial properties of different solvent extracts of Malaysian *Plectranthus amboinicus* leaves. Evidence-Based Complementary and Alternative Medicine. 2017;1517683.

Swamy MK, Akhtar MS, Sinniah UR. Antimicrobial properties of plant essential oils against human pathogens and their mode of action: An updated review. Evidence-Based Complementary and Alternative Medicine. 2016;3012462.

The Ayurvedic pharmacopoeia of India. New Delhi: Government of India, Ministry of Health and Family Welfare Department of Indian System of Medicine & Homeopathy. 2001, p-47, 143.

Thomas J, Joy PP, Mathew G, Skaria S, Duethi PB, Joseph ST. Agronomic Practices for aromatic and medicinal plant, Directorate of arecanut and spices Development of India, Calicut, Kerela, India. 2000, p-124-128

Vonshak, A., O. Barazani, P. Sathiyamoorthy, R. Shalev, D. Vardy and A. Golan-Goldhirsh. Screening South Indian medicinal plants for antifungal activity against cutaneous pathogens. Phytotherapy Research. 2003, 17, 1123-1125

Williamson NE. Major herbs of Ayurveda. Edinburgh, Churchill Livingstone. 2002, p. 299.

9

Lantana camara Linn.: Ethnobotany, Phyto-chemistry and Pharmacological Importance

MALLAPPA KUMARA SWAMY[1,2*], GREETHA ARUMUGAM[2], RADHAKRISHNAN NARAYANASWAMY[3], GUDEPALYA RENUKAIAH RUDRAMURTHY[2], VASUDEVAN RAMACHANDRAN[4], BOREGOWDA PURUSHOTHAM[2] AND UMA RANI SINNIAH[1]

ABSTRACT

Lantana camara Linn. *is an aromatic shrub and has the ability to grow under any climatic conditions. Due to its several medicinal values, it is highly valued in the modern medicinal field. The traditional and folk healers in south Asia have essentially used L. camara to relieve various human ailments, such as dermatological, gastrointestinal disorders, tetanus, malaria, cancers, bilious fever, malaria, whooping cough, tetanus, eczema, cancers, asthma, bronchitis, ulcer, itches, cuts, cold, headache, hypertension and rheumatic fever for many centuries. Recently, researchers have scientifically validated its therapeutic potentials. Studies involving phytochemistry evaluation have revealed the occurrence of several bioactive compounds from the different parts of L. camara. The major classes of chemical compounds belongs to terpenoids, phenolics, phenylethanoid glycosides, flavonoids, iridoid glycosides, furanonaphthoquinones, and*

[1] Department of Crop Science, Faculty of Agriculture, Universiti Putra Malaysia, 43400 Serdang, Selangor, Malaysia
[2] Department of Biotechnology, East West First Grade College, Bengaluru- 560091, India
[3] Bio Incubator and Lab, Vel Tech Technology Incubator, Vel Tech Rangarajan Dr. Sagunthala R & D Institute of Science and Technology, Chennai, India
[4] Malaysian Research Institute on Ageing, Universiti Putra Malaysia, Serdang, Malaysia
**Corresponding author:* swamy.bio@gmail.com

steroids. Various biological properties exhibited by this plant are related to its chemical composition. This chapter compiled the knowledge on the distribution, botanical characteristics, phytochemistry and medicinal properties of L. camara.

***Key words*:** Red sage, Phytoconstituents, Pharmacological activity, Medicine, herbs.

---

1. INTRODUCTION

Lantana camara Linn. is commonly known as wild or red sage and it is an evergreen aromatic shrub that belongs to Verbenaceae family. It is a perennial plant, which can grow up to 3 m tall and form dense thickets in a variety of environmental conditions (Sharma, 1981). Since from the 16th century, *L. camara* has been planted as an ornamental plant, attributed to its vibrant flower colours ranging from yellow-orange to pink-violet and white (Bouda *et al.,* 2001; Yadav and Tripathi, 2003; Munsif *et al.,* 2007). Due to an extensive selective breeding approaches throughout the 17th and 18th centuries for its use as an ornamental plant, there are many different *L. camara* cultivars have been found. It is well established, and expanding in many regions of the world, often as a result of clearing of forest for timber or agriculture. Easy hybridization and high ecological tolerance gives the possibly of some 650 varieties of *L. camara* in over 60 countries worldwide (Howard, 1969). Hence, *L. camara* is considered as one of the most noxious weeds (Pereira *et al.,* 2003; Mello *et al.,* 2005). However, it is also listed as one of the most important medicinal plants of the world (Sharma *et al.,* 2000; Barros *et al.,* 2016). There is a growing interest in the pharmacological evaluation of *L. camara,* used for various traditional system of folk medicine and recent scientific studies have emphasized the possible usage in modern medicine too (Kalita *et al.,* 2012; Barros *et al.,* 2016; Ngwewondo *et al.,* 2018). By knowing the value of this plant, this chapter further enhance the comprehensive report on botanical characteristics, distribution, phytochemistry and medicinal properties of *L. camara* and its future prospects for the further scientific exploration and development.

2. DISTRIBUTION

L. camara is native to South America, Central America or southern North America, with a few species occurring naturally in Africa and Asia (Munir, 1996). In its native, this species is poorly investigated, where it is not usually considered to be a serious pest therefore the original native range is still remains unclear. In the West Indies, it is found in dry thickets, and is also documented to be present in the Galapagos Islands of Ecuador (Cruz *et al.,* 1986). *L. camara* was brought in by the Dutch explorers into the Netherlands from Brazil in the late 1600s and later it was introduced to Europe, Great Britain and North America (Ghisalberti, 2000). Later, it moved into Hawaii as a garden flower, and further spread to the islands of the Pacific, Australia and southern Asian countries. Currently *L. camara* has become widespread in Australia, India and South Africa, infesting millions of hectares of land (Bhagwat *et al.,* 2012). In Australia, *Lantana* is mainly found along the east coast from Cape York to southern New South Wales with small infestations Northern Territory and northern Western Australia (Parsons *et al.,* 2001). Whereas in India, it is occurred along the west coast from the north near Jammu to the south near Trichmur, and in the central region near Jabalpur (Thakur *et al.,* 1992) and the list goes on. Presently, *Lantana* is naturalized in approximately 60 countries or island groups between 35°N and 35°S (Day *et al.,* 2003). Distribution of *L. camara* is expending continuously and considered as a major threat to natural ecosystem especially at deforestation area for timber or agriculture.

3. BOTANICAL DESCRIPTION

L. camara is a low erect or sub-scandent vigorous shrub with triangular/quadrangular stem, occasional stout recurved pickles and a strong odour of black currents. This plant can grow up to 1 to 3 metres and it can spread to 2.5 metre in width (Sanjeeb *et al.,* 2012). The posture may be sub-erect, scrambling, or occasionally clambering (ascending into shrubs or low trees, clinging to points of contact by means of prickles, branches, and leaves). Frequently, multiple stems arise from the ground level. The green leaves of *L. camara* are 3-8 cm long by 3-6 cm wide. Shapes of the leaves are ovate or ovate oblong, acute or sub-acute, crenate serrate, rugose above, scabrid on both sides (Sanjeeb *et al.,* 2012). Leaves are covered with rough hairs and have a strong odour when crushed (Rosacia *et al.,* 2004). Shallow root system of *L. camara* forms a dense mat growing mainly within 10-30 cm of the soil. It gives out a new fresh shoots even after repeated cuttings (Sastri *et al.,* 1962).

L. camara has a small tubular shaped flowers with four petals and are arranged in clusters called umbels. Flowers are found at the terminal ends of the stems. Flowers come in many different colours including red, yellow, white, pink and orange which differ depends on the location in the inflorescences itself, and changes as according to age and maturity of the flower (Ram and Mathur, 1984). The calyx is small, corolla tube slender, the limb spreading 6 to 7 mm wide and divided in to unequal lobes. The stamen has two pairs, and ovary has two celled and two ovules. Inflorescences are produced in pairs in the axils of opposite leaves. Inflorescences are compact, dome shaped 2-3 cm across and contain 20-40 sessile flowers. The flowers have fruity smell with a pepper undertone. After pollination the colour of flowers changes (typically from yellow to orangish, pinkish, or reddish) and believed to be a signal to pollinators as well as being sexually viable, thus increasing pollination efficiency (Weiss, 1990).

The fruit of *L. camara* is a berry-like drupe which turns from green to dark purple when mature. The fruit is in round shape, fleshy, 2 seeded drupe, about 5 mm wide, green turning purple then blue-black. Each plant produces up to 12,000 fruits (Priyanka and Joshi, 2013) which are then eaten by birds and other animals to spread the seeds over large distances, facilitating propagation of *L. camara.* Shallow root system and the vibrant colours of flowers allows *L. camara* to propagate *via* both vegetative (asexual) and seed reproduction (asexual) manner.

4. TAXONOMY

The genus *Lantana* consists between 40 and 150 (Gujral and Vasudevan, 1983; Mabberley, 1997) plant species. Most are native to South America, Central America or southern North America, with a few species occurring naturally in Africa and Asia (Munir, 1996). Species under this genus has history of taxonomic uncertainty (Howard, 1969; Stirton, 1977) due to its free-hybridising nature (Sanders, 1989).

L. camara is considered a highly variable species by ecologists around the world. It is widely cultivated for over 300 years giving rise to hundreds of cultivars and hybrids (Howard, 1969) mostly belonging to the *L. camara* complex (Stirton, 1979). In the early days, cultivars were distinguished morphologically through variation in flowers (size, shape and colour), leaves (size, colour and hairiness) and stem thorniness. Since, *L. camara* is an obnoxious weed it was also classified physiologically by the growth rates, tolerance to adverse conditions and toxicity to livestock. Presently, with current biotechnological advances it is being identified by the chromosome number and DNA content (Stirton, 1979; Gujral and Vasudevan, 1983; Scott *et al.,* 1997; Pierre Binggeli, 1999). From this approximately, 650 variety names identified worldwide with many misspellings and synonyms as the detailed botanical descriptions are unavailable (Howard, 1969), highlighting the vast diversity within this complex species (Day *et al.,* 2003). Subsequently, this gave rise to numerous common names around the world and a few are listed in Table 1.

Table 1: Common vernacular names of *L. camara* Linn. (according to the respective region where it is naturalized or cultivated).

Sl. no.	*Region*	*Vernacular names*
1.	Caribbean	White-sage
2.	China	Ma-ying Tan
3.	Indonesia	Kembang telek, Tembelekan, Saliara
4.	Malaysia	Bunga pagar, Bunga tahi ayam, Jebat harimau.
5.	South Africa	Tickberry, Wild lantana, Yellow sage
6.	Spain	Coronitas, Cinco negritosm
7.	Thailand	Kaam kung, Khee kae, Yeesyun
8.	Vietnam	Thomoi
9.	Philippines	Bahug-bahug, sapinit
10.	Portugal	Cambará
11.	Mauritius	Vieille fille
12.	Puerto Rico	Cariaquillo
13.	France	Corbeille d'or, Galabert, Lantanier; Mille fleurs
14.	Assam	Guphul
15.	Brazil	Camara, Camara de espinho
16.	Cambodia	Ach mann
17.	Hawaii	Lakana, Lanakana, Mikinolia hihi
18.	India	Nagaairi, Phullaki, Putus, Tantbi
19.	Japan	Shichihenge
20.	French Polynesia	Tatara moa
21.	Germany	Wandelroschen
22.	Guinea	Boulé kogno, Kogno porto
23.	Venezuela	Cariaquillo, Cariaquito
24.	Sri Lanka	Ganda-pana, Garda-pana
25.	Fiji	Kauboica

5. PHYTOCHEMISTRY

5.1. Occurrence and chemodiversity aspects

The investigations towards obtaining new therapeutically active phytocompounds in *L. camara* species have resulted in several chemocompounds belonging to different chemical families. The phytochemical studies carried out on the *L. camara* species were mainly aimed to elucidate the chemo-profiles of its essential oil obtained from its leaves. Later, various non-volatile compounds were also detected from different parts of the species including stem, flower, and root. The major classes of chemical compounds belongs to terpenoids, phenolics, phenylethanoid glycosides, flavonoids, iridoid glycosides, furano naphthoquinones, and steroids. Various biological properties exhibited by this plant are related to its chemical composition (Sousa *et al.*, 2009; Sousa *et al.*, 2010; Costa *et al.*, 2010; Sousa *et al.*, 2011; Sousa *et al.*, 2012; Medeiros *et al.*, 2012).

The essential oils from *L. camara* are usually obtained by using steam distillation technique using. The yield of essential oils from leaf and flower are ranged between 0.01 and 0.7% (Ghisalberti, 2000; Sousa and Costa, 2012). However, the highest yield is obtained from the leaves. Studies have witnessed that, the varied levels of essential oils and their composition are depends on the samples collected from the different origins. There was a significant variations in the chemical profiles identified from different varieties of *L. camara* species (Ganjewala *et al.,* 2009; Bhakta and Ganjewala, 2009; Swamy *et al.,* 2015). In addition, phytochemicals varied depending on the habitat, environmental factors and growth stages. In some studies, the chromatographic profile of essential oil of *L. camara* evidenced the existence of chemical differences (Sousa *et al.,* 2009; Sousa *et al.,* 2010; Medeiros *et al.,* 2012). Their results indicated the existence of a significant variations in the essential oils yield and chemical composition observed from *L. camara* stems and leaves collected at different seasons in Brazil. The highest yield was noticed when the leaves were collected during the rainy season (Medeiros *et al.,* 2012). The yield of essential oils from leaves were collected during the month of June and September was found to be 0.35% and 0.28% (w/w), respectively. The essential oil yield from stems were collected during June was found to be 0.21% (w/w) while, 0.13% (w/w) yield was recorded during the month, September. Similarly, Ganjewala *et al.* (2009) reported variations in the biochemical composition of the flowers and leaves have 4 varieties (yellow, lavender, red, and white flowers) of *L. camara* plants growing in India. Likewise, Sousa *et al.* (2010) reported different chemotypes of *L. camara* growing in northeastern parts of Brazil. Their study shown a significant differences in the yield and chemical composition with respect to different harvest times. According to them, the best yield can be obtained when leaves were collected at 7:00 pm (0.09% w/v) when compared to morning time before 1:00 pm which results in relatively a lesser yield of only (0.01% w/v).

Mostly, the essential oil appear pale yellow to yellow liquid with a strong terpene-like or basil like, fatty, leathery, and sweaty fragrance (Ghisalberti, 2000). The presence of more than 49 phytochemicals accounts to about 93.3 % of the essential oil. The chief constituents of essential oils are the caryophyllene (34.79 %), geranyl acetate (22.12 %), terpinyl acetate (5.84 %), bornyl acetate (4.13 %), and D-limonene (2.27 %). The occurrence of non-volatile compounds such as flavonoids, steroids, glycosides, etc, were also determined from the different parts of *L. camara* (Begum *et al.,* 2000; Sharma and Sharma, 2006; Naz and Bano, 2013; Swamy *et al.,* 2015). Some of the other constituents of *L. camara* include lantadene A, lantadene B, lantadene C, 22β-angeloyloxy-3β-hydroxyolean-12-en-28-oic acid, oleanonic acid, camarilic acid, camaric acid, ursolic acid, lantacin, α-amyrin, betulinic acid, theveside, geniposide, β-sitosterol, cholesterol, stigmasterol, etc (Ahmed *et al.,* 1972a, 1972b; Goyal and Kumar, 1984; Pan *et al.,* 1992; Misra *et al.,*

1997; Begum *et al.,* 2000; Sharma and Sharma, 2006; Verma and Verma, 2006; Begum *et al.,* 2008b; Julião *et al.* 2009; Ganjewala *et al.,* 2009; Bhakta and Ganjewala, 2009; Sousa and Costa, 2012; Julião *et al.,* 2010; Naz and Bano, 2013; Swamy and Sinniah, 2015; Swamy *et al.,* 2015). The following section presents the summary of these different classes of phytocompounds, their presence in different parts of *L. camara* species harboring in different habitats. Also, various analytical methods employed for the chemical identification are briefly mentioned in the following section.

5.2. Major volatile and non-volatile compounds

The essential oil of *L. camara* include only traces of monoterpene constituents. Among the major identified constituents in the oils include the sesquiterpenes, b-caryophyllene, E and Z-caryophyllene, caryophyllene oxide, isocaryophillene, caryophyllene epoxide, bicyclogermacrene and germacrene D (Sousa and Costa, 2012). Triterpenes include lantadene A, lantadene B, lantadene C, lantadene D, 22b-angeloyloxy-3b-hydroxyolean-12-en-28-oic acid, 3b-hydroxyolean-12-en-28-oic acid, 22b-hydroxyoleanonic acid, oleanonic acid, oleanolic acid, oleanolic acid acetate, 22b-hydroxy-3-oxoolean-12-en-28-oic acid, 22b-dimethylacryloyloxy-24-hydroxy-3-oxo-olean-12-en-28-oic acid, 22b-O-angeloyl-oleanoic acid, 22b-O-senecioyl oleanolic acid, hederagenin, hydroxy-3-oxoolean-12-en-28-oic acid, 21,22b-epoxy-3b-hydroxyolean-12-en-28-oic methyl ester, camarin, lantanone, camaric acid, lantanolic acid, lantanilic acid, camarilic acid, camarinin, arsanilic acid, camaradienone, pomonic acid, ursolic acid, ursolic acid, lantoic acid, camariolic acid, betulonic acid, lantabetulic acid, euphane lactone B, and lantic acid (Sousa and Costa, 2012). Flavonoids, such as lantanoside, linaroside, 3-methoxy-quercetin, 3-methoxy-3, 7-dimethoxy-quercetin, 3,7,4'-trimethoxy-quercetin, pectolinarigenin and pectolinarin are very commonly observed. Likewise, *L. camara* also possess phenylethanoid glycosides, such as calceolarioside E, isonuomioside A, isoverbascoside, derhamnosyl verbascoside, verbascoside, and martynoside. Furanonaphthoquinones, namely 6-methoxydiodantunezone, 6-methoxy-8-hydroxy-diodantunezone, 7-methoxydiodantunezone, 7-methoxy-5-hydroxyisodiodantunezone, 7-methoxy-8-hydroxy-diodantunezone, 6-methoxy-7-hydroxy-diodantunezone, 8-hydroxy-13-(methyldimethyl-hydroxy)-diodantunezone, 5-hydroxy-13-(methyldimethyl-hydroxy)-diodantunezone, diodantunezone and isodiodantunezone are observed from the *L. camara* roots. Similarly, the presence of iridoid glycosides are reported from the roots, leaves and stems of *L. camara* by many authors. The major iridoid glycosides include geniposide, theviridoside, theveside, 8-epiloganin, lamiridoside, and shanzhiside methyl ester. Some steroids, namely b-sitosterol, b-sitosterol-3-O-b-D-glucopiranoside, b-sitosterole, b-sitosterol-3-O-b-D-D-glicoside, b-sitosterol acetate, stigmasterol acetate, stigmasterol, 3b-hydroxystigmast-

5-en-7-one, and campesterol are being observed in the *L. camara* leaves, flowers, and stems (Sousa and Costa, 2012). Some of the major *L. camara* phytocompounds chemical structures are represented in Fig. 1.

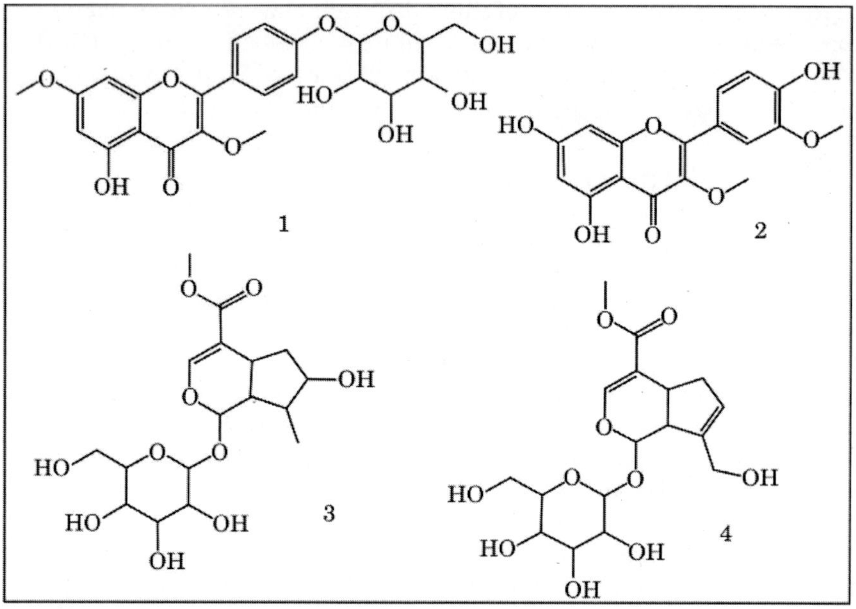

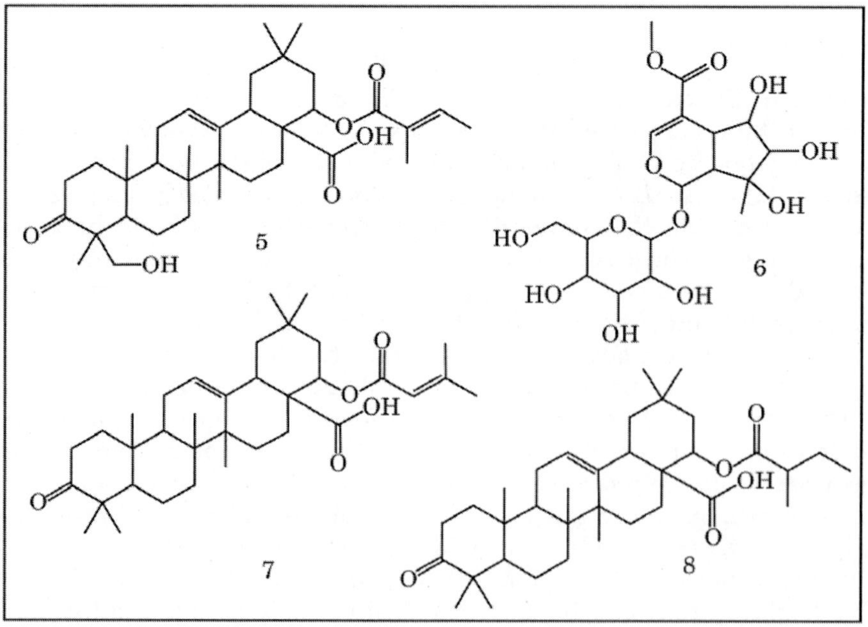

Fig. 1: (*Contd...*)

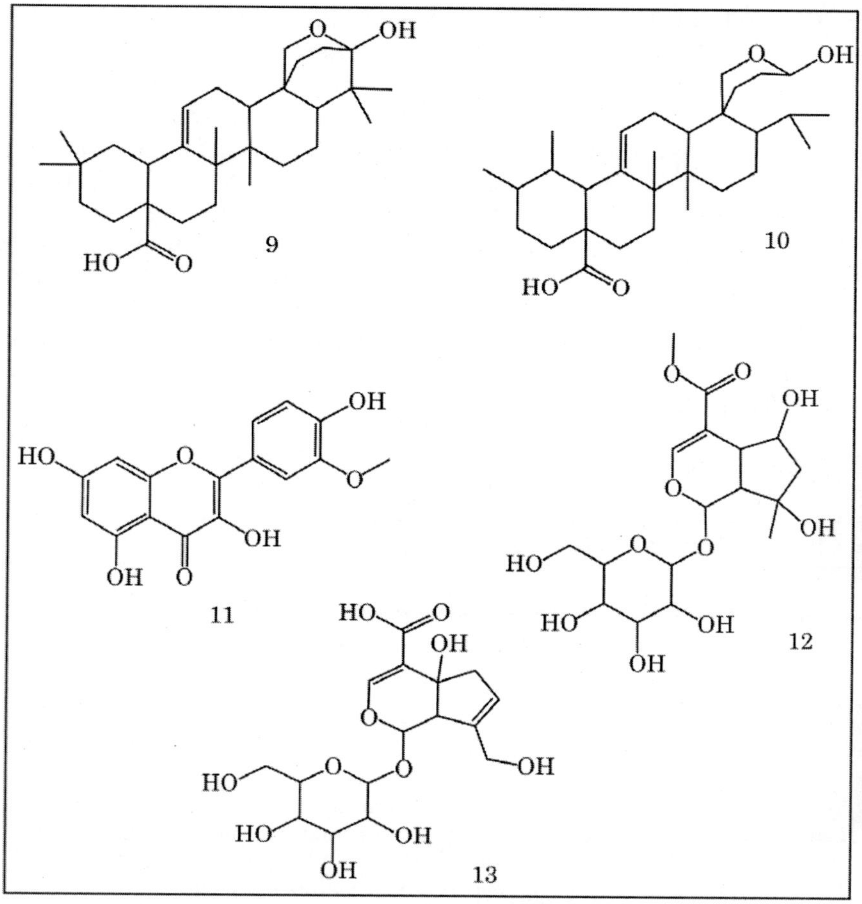

Fig. 1: Chemical structures of *Lantana camara* phytocompounds; 1) Camaroside; 2) 3,3´-Dimethoxy quercetin; 3) Epiloganin; 4) Geniposide; 5) Icterogenin; 6) Lamiridoside; 7) Lantadene B; 8)Lantadene C; 9) Lantanolic acid; 10) Lantic acid; 11) 3-Methoxy quercetin; 12) Shanzhiside methyl ester and 13) Theveside.

6. PHARMACOLOGICAL IMPORTANCE OF *LANTANA CAMARA*

L. camara in its native range is used as a source of medicinal cures, *i.e.,* in Ecuador the leaves are eaten to treat stomach disorders (Ellison and Evans, 1996). Lantana oil is sometimes used for the treatment of skin itches, as an antiseptic for wounds, and externally for leprosy and scabies (Ghisalberti 2000). *Lantana* species extracts are used in folk medicine to treat of cancers, chicken pox, measles, asthma, ulcers, swellings, eczema, tumors, high blood pressure, bilious fevers, catarrhal infections, tetanus, rheumatism, malaria and atoxy of abdominal viscera (Kirtikar and Basu, 1981; Ghisalberti, 2000;

Day *et al.,* 2003). In the recent years, extract of *L. camara* is being studied by the researchers for its potency to act as an anti-microbial, anti-ulcerogenic, hemolytic, anti-hyperglycemic, anti-cancer, anti-inflammatory, anti-diabetic, wound healing, anti-motility and larvicidal treatments. Some compounds are actively being identified as potential drug, *i.e.*, verbascoside, which possesses antimicrobial, immunosuppressive and antitumor activities (Mahato *et al.,* 1994; Day *et al.,* 2003) and lantanoside, linaroside and camarinic acid have been isolated and are being investigated as potential nematicides (Begum *et al.,* 2000; Day *et al.,* 2003). The biological activities of *L. camara* have been discussed in detail in the following sections. Some of the patents obtained from *L. camara* plant and its bioactive constituents for various cosmetic and pharmaceutical applications are detailed in Table 2.

Table 2: List of patents obtained from the *Lantana camara* plant.

Sl. no	*Patent- Country*	*Year*	*Important claim*	*References*
1.	United States (US) Patent	1997	*L. camara* leaves along with potato peel has been claimed as cosmetic agent for treating both skin and hair.	Salinas (1997)
2.	Worldwide (WO) Patent	1998	*L. camara* has been claimed as antithrombin agent.	Francis *et al.* (1998)
3.	Indian Patent (IN)	2009	Botanical formulation containing *L. camara* has been claimed as mosquito control agent.	Virendra Kumar *et al.* (2009)
4.	Indian Patent (IN)	2009	An active compound (oleanolic acid) isolated from *L. camara* roots has been claimed as novel process for obtaining this active compound of interest, which also possesses hepatoprotective activity.	Srivastava *et al.* (2009)
5.	United States (US) Patent	2012	*L. camara* along with other plant extracts has been claimed as skin care agent for treating itching/dry skin.	Florence *et al.* (2012)
6.	Indian Patent (IN)	2013	An active compound (cownaran) isolated from *L. camara* leaves has been claimed as insecticidal agent against stored grain insects.	Rajashekar and Bakthava-tsalm (2013)
7.	Indian Patent (IN)	2014	An active compound (ursolic acid stearoyl glucoside) isolated from *L. camara* leaves has been claimed as cardioprotective agent.	Imran Kazmi *et al.* (2014)

6.1. Enzyme inhibitory activities of *Lantana camara*

6.1.1. *Acetylcholinesterase inhibitory activity*

Acetylcholinesterase (AchE) is an enzyme which catalyzes the breakdown of acetylcholine (substrate) into acetate and choline and has been used as target for managing neurodegenerative disorders. *L. camara* has been reported to inhibit the AchE activity, in dose response manner with inhibition concentration at 50% (IC_{50} value) 47 and 56 µg/ml (root and leaf extract) respectively (Nour *et al.,* 2014).

6.1.2. *Alpha amylase inhibitory activity*

Alpha amylase hydrolyzes carbohydrates (starch) by acting on 1, 4-α linkages. Inhibition of alpha amylase is a prominent target in the management of type 2 diabetes mellitus. *L. camara* leaf extract has been reported to inhibit the alpha amylase activity with IC_{50} value >150 µg/ml (Swamy and Sinniah, 2015).

6.1.3. *Carboxylesterase inhibitory activity*

Carboxylesterases (CES) are group of enzymes belongs to serine hydrolases family, which catalyze the hydrolysis of, amides, carbamates, esters and thioesters. Two human carboxylesterases (hCE1 and hCE2) plays a vital role in drug metabolism. *L. camara* extract has been reported to inhibit the porcine liver CES activity with IC_{50} value <100 µg/ml (Bangou *et al.,* 2011).

6.1.4. *5-lipoxygenase (5-LOX) inhibitory activity*

Lipoxygenases (LOX) are a large monomeric protein family containing dioxygenases that catalyze the polyunsaturated fatty acid (PUFA) as a substrate to yield hydroperoxides. The biological properties of human LOXs had been widely studied due to their involvement in several diseases. The 5-LOX pathway is the source of potent pro-inflammatory mediators. Leukotrienes (LTs) are one such important mediators of allergic asthma produced through 5-LOX pathway. *L. camara* essential oil has been reported to inhibit the 5-LOX activity, with an IC_{50} value 81.5 µg/ml (Benites *et al.,* 2009).

6.1.5. *Glutathione- S-transferase inhibitory activity*

Glutathione- S-transferases (GSTs) are a family of detoxification (phase II) enzymes that plays a major role in protecting the macromolecules from reactive electrophiles. *L. camara* extract has been reported to inhibit the GST activity, 21.83% inhibition at 100 µg/ml level (Bangou *et al.,* 2011).

6.1.6. *Xanthine oxidase inhibitory activity*

Xanthine oxidase (XO) is the key regulatory enzyme in purine (nucleic acid) metabolism which catalyzes the oxidation of hypoxanthine to xanthine and then to uric acid. Hyperuricemia is a metabolic disorder characterized by elevated level of serum uric acid. *L. camara* extract has been reported to inhibit the XO activity, 20.76% inhibition at 100 µg/ml level (Bangou *et al.,* 2011).

6.2. Antimicrobial activity

Several previous reports have described the antibacterial activity of *L. camara* (Kalita *et al.,* 2012). Among those Barreto and co-workers (2010) had reported a good antibacterial activity of *L. camara* (leaves and roots) extracts especially against *Proteus vulgaris* (ATCC 13135) with a minimum inhibitory concentration (MIC) value of 128 and 64 µg/ml respectively. Similarly Dabur and co-workers (2007) had reported a good antibacterial activity of *L. camara* (aqueous) extracts especially against *Staphylococcus aureus* (MTCCB737) with a MIC value of 37.5 µg/ml level. Interestingly, Verma and co-workers (1997) reported that pentacyclic triterpenoids are isolated from *L. camara* has shown an antibacterial activity. Similarly, Saleh and co-workers (1999) had reported that lantic acid (active compound isolated from *L. camara*) has exhibited a board spectrum antibacterial activity against both gram-positive (*Bacillus cereus*) and gram-negative (*Escherichia coli*) organism. The ethanolic leaf extract of *L. camara* was shown to exhibit antibacterial activity against multi-drug resistant (MDR) strains *Pseudomonas aeruginosa* and *E. coli* (Ec 27) with a MIC of 8 µg/ml and 16 µg/ml, respectively (Barreto *et al.,* 2010). Likewise, *L. camara* leaf crude extracts effectively inhibited 3 MDR Gram-positive bacteria (*Streptococcus pyogenes*, methicillin-resistant *Staphylococcus aureus*, and vancomycin-resistant *Enterococcus faecalis* (Dubey and Padhy, 2013). Swamy *et al.* (2015) showed inhibitory activity of *L. camara* leaf extract against bacterial pathogens, such as *E. coli, Klebsiella pneumoniae*, *Bacillus subtilis, Micrococcus luteus,* and *Staphylococcus aureus*. Methanol extract had the highest inhibition activity against all the tested microbes. More recently, terpene-rich leaf extract of *L. camara* was shown to inhibit the growth of mycobacteria (Patil and Kumbhar, 2018; Zamora *et al.,* 2018). *L. camara* leaf extract was effective in inhibiting the growth of fungal pathogens, *Aspergillus flavus*, *Aspergillus niger* and *Colletotrichum falcatum* (Fayaz *et al.,* 2017; Sreeramulu *et al.,* 2017).

6.3. Anti-hyperglycemic/hypoglycemic activity

L. camara (leaves and fruits) extracts have been reported to have anti-hyperglycemic (Ganesh *et al.,* 2010) and hypoglycemic (Venkatachalam *et al.,* 2011) activities in the experimental rat model. Moreover, Ursolic acid, a stearoyl glucoside (active compound isolated from *L. camara*) has been reported to possess hypoglycemic activity in the experimental rat model (Kazmi *et al.,* 2012).

6.4. Anti-inflammatory activity

L. camara (alcoholic and aqueous) extracts have been reported to exhibit anti-inflammatory activity in the experimental rat paw edema model (Forestieri *et al.,* 1996; Shylaja *et al.,* 2008 and Gidwani *et al.,* 2009). The leaf and bark extracts of *L. camara* was documented to possess anti-inflammatory activity by Bairagi *et al.* (2017). According to them, the methanolic leaf extract at 100 mg/kg exhibited a significant anti-inflammatory activity.

6.5. Anti-thrombotic activity

O'Neill and co-workers (1998) reported that tans lactone containing triterpenes (5, 5-trans-fused cyclic lactone euohane triterpenes) isolated from *L. camara* (leaves) shown to inhibit the human alpha-thrombin in dose response manner with inhibition concentration at 50% (IC_{50} value) 18-130 nM.

6.6. Anti-ulcerogenic activity

L. camara (alcoholic) extract has been reported to exhibit anti-ulcer activity in the experimental rat (aspirin/ethanol and cold restraint induced ulcer) models (Thamotharan *et al.,* 2010).

6.7. Anti-filarial activity

Oleanonic acid and oleanolic acid isolated from hexane and chloroform fractions of *L. camara* (stem) extract shown to exerted filaricidal activity (Misra *et al.,* 2006) against human lymphatic parasite (*Brugia malayi*).

6.8. Anti-pyretic activity

L. camara (ethanolic and ethyl acetate) extracts have been reported to exhibit anti pyretic activity in the experimental rabbit model (Jain *et al.,* 2011).

The methanolic leaf and bark extracts at 200 mg/kg exhibit more significant analgesic activity (Bairagi *et al.,* 2017).

6.9. Anti-urolithiatic activity

Urolithiasis is the process of forming urinary calculi, these calculi are formed anywhere in the urinary system. *L. camara* (ethanolic leaves) extracts has been reported to exhibit antiurolithiatic activity against ethylene glycol and ammonium chloride induced urolithiatic (rat) model (Mayee and Thosar, 2011). *L. camara* (ethanolic root) extract and oleanolic acid (isolated from roots of *L. camara*) have been reported to exhibit anti urolithiatic activity against zinc disc implantation induced urolithiatic (rat) model (Vyas and Argal, 2013).

6.10. Nematicidal activity

Lantanillic acid, camaric acid and oleanolic acid (three bioactive compounds isolated from the aerial parts of *L. camara* methanolic extract) have been reported to exhibit nematicidal activity against *Meloidogyne incognita* (Qamar *et al.,* 2005). Similarly, *L. camara* (fresh green leaves) extract has been reported to exhibit nematicidal activity against *M. incognita* (Ahmad *et al.,* 2010). Recently, oleanolic acid (isolated from the aerial parts of *L. camara* extract) has been reported to exhibit nematicidal activity against *M. incognita* at 0.0625% (Begum *et al.,* 2015).

6.11. Wound healing activity

L. camara extract has been reported to have wound healing activity in different wound models such as burn wound (Nayak *et al.,* 2008), excision wound (Dash *et al.,* 2001; Nayak *et al.,* 2009) and diabetic wound model (Mekala *et al.,* 2014) respectively.

6.12. Anti-mutagenic activity

The 22 beta-acetoxylantic acid and 22 beta-dimethylacryloxylantanolic acid (two bioactive triterpenes isolated from *L. camara* extract) have been reported to exhibit anti mutagenic activity against mitomycin-C induced mice model (Barre *et al.,* 1997).

6.13. Anti-proliferative activity

Lantadene A (triterpenoid isolated from *L. camara* leaves extract) has been reported to exhibit anti proliferative activity against human leukemia (HL

60) cell line (Sharma *et al.,* 2007). Similarly, *L. camara* (leaves) extract has been reported to exhibit anti proliferative activity against laryngeal cancer (HEp-2) and lung cancer (NCI-H292) cell lines respectively (Gomes de Melo *et al.,* 2010).

6.14. Antioxidant activity

L. camara (leaves) extract has been reported to exhibit 1, 1-diphenyl-2-picrylhydrazyl (DPPH) radical scavenging activity with inhibition concentration at 50% (IC_{50} value) 27.54 µg/ml (Bhakta and Ganjewala, 2009; Asadu *et al.,* 2015). Similarly, *L. camara* (leaves) extract has been shown to have hydroxyl and superoxide radical scavenging activity with IC_{50} value of 22.18 and 27.94 µg/ml respectively (Asadu *et al.,* 2015). In other report *L. camara* (root-bark) methanolic extract has been shown to have nitric oxide radical scavenging activity with IC_{50} value 145.3 µg/ml (Basu and Hazra, 2006). The methanol solvent extract of *L. camara* was shown to have the highest DPPH radical scavenging activity with IC_{50} value of 165 µg/ml (Swamy *et al.,* 2015). The aerial parts of *L. camara* has shown the capability of scavenging DPPH, nitric oxide, and hydrogen peroxide radicals (Sam *et al.,* 2018).

6.15. Anti-arthritic activity

L. camara (ethanolic leaves) extract has been reported to exhibit anti arthritic activity in acute rat model (Gundamaraju *et al.,* 2012). The methanolic flower extract of *L. camara* was shown to have anti-arthritic activity (Vennila and Kayalvizhi, 2016).

6.16. Anti-fertility activity

L. camara (hydroalcoholic leaves) extract has been reported to exhibit anti fertility activity in the experimental female rat model (Mello *et al.,* 2005).

7. OTHER USES

7.1. Ornamental

The hemispherical clusters of small, bright-colored flowers, of *L. camara* plants are major attraction and frequently used in landscaping as ground cover or border shrubs. In some countries, it is planted as a hedge to contain or keep out livestock (Bradley, 1988; Ghisalberti, 2000). These hardy plants easily adapt to adverse condition, drought-tolerant and require minimal maintenance. The flower attracts butterflies and humming birds during pollination, providing a lovely side to admire. In butterfly gardens *L. camara* is used as a staple plant. In Florida, they are popular hanging baskets. Many cultivars of this species are grown as ornamentals and us hedges in Kenya, Tanzania and Uganda.

7.2. Animal feed, fodder, forage

A number of minor uses of *L. camara* include using the seeds as a source of food for lambs. However, care should be taken as *L. camara* is known to cause acute toxicity to livestock *i.e.,* cattle, sheep and guinea pigs (Sharma *et al.,* 1988).

7.3. Biofuels

L. camara are also used as firewood and mulch in some parts of the world. (Sharma *et al.,* 1988; Sharma, 1989, Day *et al.,* 2003). Lantana twigs and stems serve as fuel for cooking and heating in many developing countries (Sharma *et al.,* 1988). Often *Lantana* straw is mixed with animal dung for biogas production. In 2013, Sunthar and Sharma reported *L. camara* leaf litter that has been spiked with cow dung may be a potential source for vermicompost production for sustainable agriculture.

7.4. Ecology

In some areas, *L. camara* provide shelter and vital winter food for many native birds. A number of endangered bird species utilise the thickets when their natural habitat is unavailable. In Australia, the vulnerable black-breasted buttonquail, *Turnix melanogaster*, feeds and roosts in lantana thickets adjacent to its more favoured habitat, vine forest (Smith *et al.,* 1998; Day *et al.,* 2003). Buttonquails prefers intact vine forest and *L. camara* provides temporary refuge for them between forest remnants (Smith *et al.,* 1998; Day *et al.,* 2003). In central Kenya, the endangered Hinde's babbler, *Turdoides hindei*, has become dependent on lantana thickets. When the natural riverine thickets have been almost completely cleared, the survival of *T. hindei* became highly dependent on the retention of lantana infestations (Njoroge *et al.,* 1998).

7.5. Environmental protection

L. camara is considered as a good ground cover preventing erosion. At some mountainous areas like Tanzania and India the presence of *L. camara* used as ground cover to prevent soil erosion, *L. camara* is used as a live fence in certain parts of Eastern Africa (Howes, 1946). In Ethiopia the establishment of *Lantana* fence to protect crops from domestic animals was taken up by local villagers in the 1990s. However, this quickly led to the loss of rough grazing land through the rapid spread of this plant (Binggeli and Desissa, 2002).

7.6. Food and beverage

In many regions *L. camara* is considered as an important honey source for nectar collecting bees (Fichtl and Admasu Adi, 1994). Their numerous flowers and vibrant colours also attract many bird species and is a major nectar source of butterflies and moths. Fruits of *L. camara* are eaten raw in Pakistan and India once it get ripened. Ripen *L. camara* fruits can be used as flavouring and to make jams, jellies, pies, and cordials. In India the leaves of the plant are boiled for tea for its aromatic, minty taste and the decoction is a remedy against cough (Saxena *et al.,* 2012). On the contrary, children have died from ingesting ripen fruits in Canada, and caused acute toxicity in adults at Hawaii and Florida. Recent reports suggested that, the different varieties of *L. camara* are highly toxic based on the region it's naturalized in therefore care should be taken when the fruits are used in food or food substances.

7.7. As Materials

Apart from that, essential oils from the flowers and leaves may have some value to the perfume industry as beneficial drugs (Ahmad *et al.,* 1962). The fruits can be used to produce a light purple dye. The stems of *L. camara,* if upon treatment by the sulphate process, can be used to produce pulp for paper suitable for writing and printing (Gujral and Vasudevan, 1983; Day *et al.,* 2003). Nevertheless, it is hard to harvest, so is likely to be uneconomical. In Taiping, Malaysia toothbrushes are made from the *Lantana* stems. The roots of *L. camara* contain a substance that may possibly be used for rubber manufacture (Gujral and Vasudevan, 1983). The leaf extracts have strong insecticidal activity whereby storing potatoes with *L. camara* leaves almost eliminates damage by the potato tuber moth *Phthorimaea operculella* (Lal 1987).

8. CONCLUSIONS

In conclusion, although *L. camara* is a weed, it possess several medicinal properties. It has been widely used in various folk and traditional healing systems. From this chapter, it is very clear that *L. camara* possessing many bioactive phytocompounds, such as to terpenoids, phenolics, phenylethanoid glycosides, flavonoids, iridoid glycosides, furanonaphthoquinones, steroids, etc., are attributed to function in treating several human health problems. The plant crude extract or its isolated specific compounds have been scientifically proven to cure a number of human diseases, such as ulcer, inflammations, microbial infections, cancer, insect attack, skin itches, leprosy, etc. However, further research works are necessary to investigate to understand the molecular mechanisms of actions of *L. camara* phytocompounds having medicinal properties. Thus, *L. camara* is considered as one of the major ethnomedicinal plant in the present time, and scientific explorations are required to further to identify its unknown bioactive compounds and other medicinal properties. It can be represented as one the potent medicinal herb for the future drug development.

REFERENCES

Ahmad F, Rather MA, Siddiqui MA. Nematicidal activity of leaf extracts from *Lantana camara* L. against *Meloidogyne incognita* (kofoid and white) chitwood and its use to manage roots infection of *Solanum melongena* L. Brazilian Archives of Biology and Technology. 2010; 53(3):543-8.

Asadu CL, Anosike CA, Uzoegwu PN, Abonyi O, Ezugwu AL, Uroko RI. *In vitro* antioxidant activity of methanol extract of *Lantana camara* leaves. Global Veterinaria. 2015; 14(4):595-602.

Bairagi SM, Pathan IB, Nitin NE. Analgesic and anti-inflammatory activity of crude leaf and bark extract of *Lantana Camara*. Marmara Pharmaceutical Journal. 2017; 21(4):810-7.

Barre JT, Bowden BF, Coll JC, De Jesus J, Victoria E, Janairo GC, Ragasa CY. A bioactive triterpene from *Lantana camara*. Phytochemistry. 1997; 45(2):321-4.

Barreto FS, Sousa EO, Campos AR, Costa JG, Rodrigues FF. Antibacterial activity of *Lantana camara* Linn and *Lantana montevidensis* brig extracts from Cariri-Ceará, Brazil. Journal of young pharmacists: JYP. 2010; 2(1):42.

Barros LM, Duarte AE, Morais-Braga MF, Waczuk EP, Vega C, Leite NF, de Menezes IR, Coutinho HD, Rocha JB, Kamdem JP. Chemical characterization and trypanocidal, leishmanicidal and cytotoxicity potential of *Lantana camara* L. (Verbenaceae) essential oil. Molecules. 2016; 21(2):209.

Basu S, Hazra B. Evaluation of nitric oxide scavenging activity, *in vitro* and *ex vivo*, of selected medicinal plants traditionally used in inflammatory diseases. Phytotherapy Research. 2006; 20(10):896-900.

Begum S, Ayub A, Shaheen Siddiqui B, Fayyaz S, Kazi F. Nematicidal triterpenoids from *Lantana camara*. Chemistry and Biodiversity. 2015; 12(9):1435-42.

Begum S, Wahab A, Siddiqui BS, Qamar F. Nematicidal constituents of the aerial parts of *Lantana camara*. Journal of Natural Products. 2000; 63(6):765-7.

Benites J, Moiteiro C, Miguel G, Rojo L, Lopez J, Venancio F, Ramalho L, Feio S, Dandlen S, Casanova H, Torres I. Composition and biological activity of the essential oil of Peruvian *Lantana camara*. Journal of the Chilean Chemical Society. 2009; 54(4):379-84.

Bhagwat SA, Breman E, Thekaekara T, Thornton TF, Willis KJ. A battle lost? Report on two centuries of invasion and management of *Lantana camara* L. in Australia, India and South Africa. PloS One. 2012; 7(3):e32407.

Bhakta D, Ganjewala D. Effect of leaf positions on total phenolics, flavonoids and proanthocyanidins content and antioxidant activities in *Lantana camara* (L). Journal of Scientific Research. 2009; 1(2):363-9.

Binggeli P. Verbenaceae, *Lantana camara*, fankatavinakoho, fotatra, mandadrieko, rajejeka, radredreka, ramity. The Natural History of Madagascar. University of Chicago Press, Chicago. 2003, pp. 415-7.

Bouda H, Tapondjou LA, Fontem DA, Gumedzoe MY. Effect of essential oils from leaves of *Ageratum conyzoides*, *Lantana camara* and *Chromolaena odorata* on the mortality of *Sitophilus zeamais* (Coleoptera, Curculionidae). Journal of Stored Products Research. 2001; 37(2):103-9.

Bradley PN. Survey of woody biomass on farms in Western Kenya. Ambio. 1988: 40-8.

Costa JGM, Rodrigues FFG, Sousa EO, Junior DMS, Campos AR, Coutinho HDM, De Lima SG. Composition and lavicidal activity of the essential oils of *Lantana camara* and *Lantana montevidensis. Chemistry of Natural Compounds. 2010;*46:313-315.

Cruz F, Cruz J, Lawesson JE. *Lantana camara* L., a threat to native plants and animals. Noticias de Galápagos. 1986; 43:10-1.

Dabur R, Gupta A, Mandal TK, Singh DD, Bajpai V, Gurav AM, Lavekar GS. Antimicrobial activity of some Indian medicinal plants. African Journal of Traditional, Complementary and Alternative Medicines. 2007; 4(3):313-8.

Dash GK, Suresh P, Ganapaty S. Studies on hypoglycaemic and wound healing activities of *Lantana camara* Linn. Journal of Natural Remedies. 2001; 1(2):105-10.

Day MD, Wiley CJ, Playford J, Zalucki MP. Lantana: Current management status and future prospects. *Lantana*: Current management status and future prospects. 2003.

Dubey D, Padhy RN. Antibacterial activity of *Lantana camara* L. against multidrug resistant pathogens from ICU patients of a teaching hospital. Journal of Herbal Medicine. 2013; 3(2):65-75.

Ellison CA, Evans HC. Amazon-ingly useful fungi-a biological control cornucopia? Mycologist. 1996; 10(1):11-3.

Fayaz M, Bhat MH, Fayaz M, Kumar A, Jain AK. Antifungal Activity of *Lantana camara* L. Leaf Extracts in Different Solvents against Some Pathogenic Fungal Strains. Pharmacologia, 2017; 8: 105-112.

Fichtl R, Adi A. Honeybee flora of Ethiopia. Margraf Verlag; 1994.

Florence T, Hines M, Gan D. Topical skin care formulations comprising plant extracts. *U.S. Patent* 0282194. 2012.

Forestieri AM, Monforte MT, Ragusa S, Trovato A, Iauk L. Anti-inflammatory, analgesic and antipyretic activity in rodents of plant extracts used in African medicine. Phytotherapy research. 1996; 10(2):100-6.

Francis J, Miles H, Nguyen C, Schweitzer B. Antithrombin agent derived from *Lantana camara*. *WO Patent* 98/17298. 1998.

Ganjewala D, Sam S, Khan KH. Biochemical compositions and antibacterial activities of *Lantana camara* plants with yellow, lavender, red and white flowers. EurAsian Journal of BioSciences. 2009; 3(10):69-77.

Ghisalberti EL. *Lantana camara* L. (Verbenaceae). Fitoterapia. 2000; 71(5):467-86.

Gidwani BK, Bhargava S, Rao SP, Majoomdar A, Pawar DP, Alaspure RN. Analgesic, anti-inflammatory and antihemorrhoidal activity of aqueous extract of *Lantana camara* Linn. Research Journal of Pharmacy and Technology. 2009; 2(2):378-81.

Gomes de Melo J, de Sousa Araújo TA, Thijan Nobre de Almeida e Castro V, Lyra de Vasconcelos Cabral D, Do Desterro Rodrigues M, Carneiro do Nascimento S, Cavalcanti de Amorim EL, De Albuquerque UP. Antiproliferative activity, antioxidant capacity and tannin content in plants of semi-arid northeastern Brazil. Molecules. 2010; 15(12):8534-42.

Gujral SS, Vasudevan P. *Lantana camara* L., a problem weed. Journal of Scientific & Industrial Research. 1983; 42(5):281-6.

Gundamaraju R, Sheeba DS, Ramesh C. Evaluation of anti-arthritic effects of *Lantana camara* var Linn. using acute model on albino rats. International Journal of Advanced Pharmaceutical Sciences. 2012; 3(5):272-7.

Howard RA. A check list of cultivar names used in the genus Lantana. Arnoldia. 1969; 29:73-109.

Howes FN. Fence and barrier plants in warm climates. Kew Bulletin. 1946; 1(2):51-87.

Imran Kazmi, Muhammad Afzal, Firoz Anwar. Extraction and isolation of novel cardioprotective glucoside from the leaves of *Lantana camara* Linn. *IN Patent* 273/DEL/2013. 2014.

Jean Bangou M, Kiendrebeogo M, Compaoré M, Coulibaly AY. Enzyme inhibition effect and polyphenols content of medicinal plant extracts from Burkina Faso. Journal of Biological Sciences. 2011; 11(1):31-8.

Kalita S, Kumar G, Karthik L, Rao KV. A Review on Medicinal Properties of *Lantana camara* Linn. Research Journal of Pharmacy and Technology. 2012; 5(6):711.

Kazmi I, Rahman M, Afzal M, Gupta G, Saleem S, Afzal O, Shaharyar MA, Nautiyal U, Ahmed S, Anwar F. Anti-diabetic potential of ursolic acid stearoyl glucoside: A new triterpenic gycosidic ester from *Lantana camara*. Fitoterapia. 2012; 83(1):142-6.

Kirtikar KR, Basu BD. Indian medicinal plants. Indian Medicinal Plants. 1918.

Lakshman SH, Kar N, Maurya V, Viswanatha GL. Analgesic and anti-inflammatory activity of topical preparation of *Lantan camara* leaves. Pharmacol Online 2008; 2008: 90-96.

Lal L. Studies on natural repellents against potato tuber moth (*Phthorimaea operculella* Zeller) in country stores. Potato Research. 1987; 30(2):329-34.

Mabberley DJ. The plant-book: A portable dictionary of the vascular plants. Cambridge University press; 1997 Jun 19.

Mahato SB, Sahu NP, Roy SK, Sharma OP. Potential antitumor agents from *Lantana camara*: Structures of flavonoid-, and phenylpropanoid glycosides. Tetrahedron. 1994; 50(31):9439-46.

Mayee R, Thosar A. Evaluation of *Lantana camara* Linn. (Verbenaceae) for antiurolithiatic and antioxidant activities in rats. International Journal of Pharmaceutical and Clinical Research. 2011; 3(1):10-4.

Medeiros LB, Rocha MD, Lima SG, Sousa Júnior GR, Citó AM, Silva DD, Lopes JA, Moura DJ, Saffi J, Mobin M, da Costa JG. Chemical constituents and evaluation of cytotoxic and antifungal activity of *Lantana camara* essential oils. Revista Brasileira de Farmacognosia. 2012; 22(6):1259-67.

Mekala S, Naresh MK, Das L, Shetty N, Amuthan A, Vulli V, Bhogireddy N. Evaluation of wound healing activity of ethanolic extract of *Lantana camara* in streptozotocin induced diabetic rats. International Journal of Pharmacy and Pharmaceutical Sciences. 2014; 6(1):631-3.

Mello FB, Jacobus D, Carvalho K, Mello JR. Effects of *Lantana camara* (Verbenaceae) on general reproductive performance and teratology in rats. Toxicon. 2005; 45(4):459-66.

Misra N, Sharma M, Raj K, Dangi A, Srivastava S, Misra-Bhattacharya S. Chemical constituents and antifilarial activity of *Lantana camara* against human lymphatic filariid Brugia malayi and rodent filariid *Acanthocheilonema viteae* maintained in rodent hosts. Parasitology Research. 2007; 100(3):439-48.

Munir AA. A taxonomic review of *Lantana camara* L. and *L. montevidensis* (Spreng.) Briq. (Verbenaceae) in Australia. Journal of the Adelaide Botanic Garden. 1996: 1: 1-27.

Munsif S, Khan MA, Ahmad MU, Zafar M, Shah GM, Shaheen NI. Leaf epidermal anatomy as an aid to the identification of genera Lantana, Verbena and Vitex of family Verbenaceae from Pakistan. Journal of Agriculture & Social Sciences. 2007; 3:43-6.

Nayak BS, Raju SS, Eversley M, Ramsubhag A. Evaluation of wound healing activity of *Lantana camara* L. – A preclinical study. Phytotherapy Research: An International Journal Devoted to Pharmacological and Toxicological Evaluation of Natural Product Derivatives. 2009; 23(2):241-5.

Nayak BS, Raju SS, Ramsubhag A. Investigation of wound healing activity of *Lantana camara* L. in Sprague dawley rats using a burn wound model. International Journal of applied Research in Natural Products. 2008; 1(1):15-9.

Naz R, Bano A. Phytochemical screening, antioxidants and antimicrobial potential of *Lantana camara* in different solvents. Asian Pacific Journal of Tropical Disease. 2013; 3(6):480-6.

Ngwewondo A, Wang M, Manfo FP, Samje M, Ganin's JN, Ndi E, Andersen RJ, Cho-Ngwa F. Filaricidal properties of *Lantana camara* and *Tamarindus indica* extracts, and Lantadene A from *L. camara* against *Onchocerca ochengi* and Loa loa. PLoS neglected tropical diseases. 2018; 12(6):e0006565.

Njoroge P, Bennun LA, Lens L. Habitat use by the globally endangered Hinde's Babbler *Turdoides hindei* and its sympatric relative, the Northern Pied Babbler *T. hypoleucus*. Bird Conservation International. 1998; 8(1):59-65.

Nour AH, Khan M, Sulaiman AZ, Batool T, NOUR AH, Khan MM, Kormin F. *In vitro* anti-acetyl cholinesterase and antioxidant activity of selected Malaysian plants. Asian Journal of Pharmaceutical and Clinical Research. 2014; 7(3):93-7.

O'Neill MJ, Lewis JA, Noble HM, Holland S, Mansat C, Farthing JE, Foster G, Noble D, Lane SJ, Sidebottom PJ, Lynn SM. Isolation of translactone-containing triterpenes with thrombin inhibitory activities from the leaves of *Lantana camara*. Journal of Natural Products. 1998; 61(11):1328-31.

Parsons WT, Parsons WT, Cuthbertson EG. Noxious weeds of Australia. CSIRO publishing; 2001.

Patil SP, Kumbhar ST. Evaluation of terpene-rich extract of *Lantana camara* L. leaves for antimicrobial activity against mycobacteria using Resazurin Microtiter Assay (REMA). Beni-Suef University Journal of Basic and Applied Sciences. 2018.

Pereira JM, Barreto RW, Ellison CA, Maffia LA. *Corynespora cassiicola* f. sp. lantanae: A potential biocontrol agent from Brazil for *Lantana camara*. Biological Control. 2003; 26(1):21-31.

Pérez Zamora CM, Torres CA, Nuñez MB. Antimicrobial activity and chemical composition of essential oils from Verbenaceae species growing in south America. Molecules. 2018; 23(3):544.

Priyanka N, Joshi PK. A review of *Lantana camara* studies in India. International Journal of Scientific and Research Publications. 2013; 3(10):1-1.

Qamar F, Begum S, Raza SM, Wahab A, Siddiqui BS. Nematicidal natural products from the aerial parts of *Lantana camara* Linn. Natural Product Research. 2005; 19(6):609-13.

Rajashekar Y, Bakthavatsalam N. A process of biofumigant from leaves of *Lantana camara* against stored grain insect pests. *IN Patent* 4227/CHE/2012. 2013.

Ram HM, Mathur G. Flower-insect interaction in pollination. Proceedings: Animal Sciences. 1984; 93(4):359-63.

Rosacia WZ, Achivar AN, Avanzado MB. Lantana and Hagonoy: Poisonous weeds prominent in rangeland and grassland areas. Research Information Series on Ecosystems. 2004; 1:16(2).

Saleh M, Kamel A, Li X, Swaray J. Antibacterial triterpenoids isolated from *Lantana camara*. Pharmaceutical Biology. 1999; 37(1):63-6.

Salinas O. Inventor; Salinas, Ofelia, assignee. Scalp and hair care product and process of preparing same. United States patent US 5,665,342. 1997.

Sam SM, Jacobs IE, Johnny II, Udosen IR, Mensah SI. *In vitro* antioxidant activity of methanolic leaf extracts of *Tridax procumebens* L., *Lantana camara* L. & *Tithonia diversifolia* (Hemsl) A. Gray. found in parts of Niger-delta, Nigeria. Global Journal of Research on Medicinal Plants and Indigenous Medicine. 2018 Mar 1;7(3):27-33.

Sanders RW. *Lantana sect. camara* (Verbenaceae) in Hispaniola: Novelties and notes. Moscosoa: Contribuciones cientificas del Jardin Botanico Nacional Dr. Rafael M. Moscoso. 1989.

Saxena M, Saxena J, Khare S. A brief review on: Therapeutical values of *Lantana camara* plant. International Journal of Pharmacy and Life Sciences. 2012; 3(3):1-9.

Scott LJ, Graham GC, Hannan Jones M, Yeates DK. DNA profiling resolves the limited importance of flower colour in defining varieties of *Lantana camara*. Electrophoresis. 1997; 18(9):1560-3.

Sen S. Pharmacognostic and anti-hyperglycemic evaluation of *Lantana camara* (L.) var. aculeate leaves in alloxan-induced hyperglycemic rats. International Journal of Research in Pharmaceutical Sciences. 2016; 1(3):247-52.

Sharma M, Sharma PD, Bansal MP, Singh J. Lantadene A-induced apoptosis in human leukemia HL-60 cells. Indian Journal of Pharmacology. 2007; 39(3):140.

Sharma OP, Makkar HP, Dawra RK, Negi SS. A review of the toxicity of *Lantana camara* (Linn) in animals. Clinical Toxicology. 1981; 18(9):1077-94.

Sharma OP, Makkar HP, Dawra RK. A review of the noxious plant *Lantana camara*. Toxicon. 1988; 26(11):975-87.

Sharma OP, Singh A, Sharma S. Levels of lantadenes, bioactive pentacyclic triterpenoids, in young and mature leaves of *Lantana camara* var. aculeata. Fitoterapia. 2000; 71(5):487-91.

Sharma P. Natural products of the Lantane plant: the present and prospects. Journal of Scientific and Industrial Research. 1989; 48(10):471-8.

Shonu J, Priyank I, Amit J, Dubey BK. Pharmacognostic and phytochemical evaluation and antipyretic activity of leaves of *Lantana camara* Linn. International Journal of Biomedical and Advance Research. 2011; 2(8):270-80.

Smith GC, Aridis J, Lees N. Radio-tracking revealed home ranges of black-breasted button-quail *Turnix melanogaster* in remnant vine scrub between hoop pine plantation and agriculture. Emu. 1998; 98(3):171-7.

Sousa EO, Colares AV, Rodrigues FFG, Campos AR, De Lima SG, Costa JGM. Effect of collection time on essential oil composition of *Lantana camara* Linn (Verbenaceae) growing in Brazil Northeastern. Records of Natural Products. 2009*;* 4:31-37.

Sousa EO, Costa JG. Genus Lantana: Chemical aspects and biological activities. Revista Brasileira de Farmacognosia. 2012; 22(5):1115-80.

Sousa EO, Rodrigues FFG, Coutinho HDM, Campos AR, De Lima SG, Costa JGM 2011. Chemical composition and aminoglycosides synergistic effect of *Lantana montevidensis* Briq. (Verbenaceae) essential oil. Rev Fitos;5:60-64.

Sousa EO, Viana AC, Rodrigues FF, Campos AR, Lima SG, Costa JG. Effect of collection time on essential oil composition of *Lantana camara* Linn (Verbenaceae) growing in Brazil Northeastern. Records of Natural Products. 2010; 4(1):31.

Sousa EO. Costa. JG M. Genus Lantana: Chemical aspects and biological activities. Brazilian Journal of Pharmacognosy. 2012; 22:1155-80.

Sreeramulu A, Arunakumari M, Reddy PL. Antifungal Activity of Wild Sage (*Lantana camara*) against *Colletotrichum falcatum. International Journal* of *Current* Microbiology and *Applied* Sciences. 2017; 6(2):1847-52.

Srivastava SK, Khan K, Khanuja SPS. A process for the isolation of oleanolic acid from the roots of *Lantana camara*. *IN Patent* 534/DEL/2003. 2009.

Stirton CH. Some thoughts on the polyploid complex *Lantana camara* L. (Verbenaceae). *In*: Proceedings of the Second National Weeds Conference of South Africa. 1977 (pp. 321-340).

Suthar S, Sharma P. Vermicomposting of toxic weed—*Lantana camara* biomass: Chemical and microbial properties changes and assessment of toxicity of end product using seeds bioassay. Ecotoxicology and Environmental Safety. 2013; 95:179-87.

Swamy MK, Arumugam G, Kaur R, Ghasemzadeh A, Yusoff MM, Sinniah UR. GC-MS based metabolite profiling, antioxidant and antimicrobial properties of different solvent extracts of Malaysian *Plectranthus amboinicus* leaves. Evidence-Based Complementary and Alternative Medicine. 2017; 2017.

Swamy MK, Sinniah UR, Akhtar MS. *In vitro* pharmacological activities and GC-MS analysis of different solvent extracts of *Lantana camara* leaves collected from tropical region of Malaysia. Evidence-Based Complementary and Alternative Medicine. 2015; 2015.

Swamy MK, Sinniah UR. Phytochemical profile and *in vitro* α-amylase inhibitory potential of different solvent extracts of *Lantana camara*. Bangladesh Journal of Pharmacology. 2015; 10(4): 962-3.

Thakur M, Mukhtar A, Thakur RK. Lantana weed (*Lantana camara* var. aculeata Linn.) and its possible management through natural insect pests in India. Indian Forester. 1992; 118(7):466-88.

Thamotharan G, Sekar G, Ganesh T, Sen S, Chakraborty R, Kumar SN. Antiulcerogenic effects of *Lantana camara* Linn. leaves On *in vivo* test models in rats. Asian Journal of Pharmaceutical and Clinical Research. 2010; 3(3):57-60.

Venkatachalam T, Kumar VK, Selvi PK, Maske AO, Anbarasan V, Kumar PS. Antidiabetic activity of *Lantana camara* Linn fruits in normal and streptozotocin-induced diabetic rats. Journal of Pharmaceutical Research. 2011; 4(5):1550-2.

Vennila V, Kayalvizhi N. *In vitro* anti arthritic activity of flowers of *Lantana camara* (l.) Against egg albumin and bovine serum albumin. World Journal of Pharmacy and Pharmaceutical Sciences. 2016; 5(5):1141-8.

Verma DK, Singh SK, Tripathi V. A rare antibacterial flavone glucoside from *Lantana camara*. Indian drugs. 1997; 34(1):32-5.

Verma RK, Verma SK. Phytochemical and termiticidal study of *Lantana camara* var. aculeata leaves. Fitoterapia. 2006; 77(6):466-8.

Virendra Kumar D, Akhilesh Chandra P, Dash AP. A new botanical formulation for mosquito control. *IN Patent* 2405/DEL/2007.2009.

Vyas N, Argal A. Antiurolithiatic activity of extract and oleanolic acid isolated from the roots of *Lantana camara* on zinc disc implantation induced urolithiasis. ISRN pharmacology. 2013; 2013.

Weiss MR. Floral color changes as cues for pollinators. *In:* VI International Symposium on Pollination 288 1990 Aug 27 (pp. 294-298).

Yadav SB, Tripathi V. A new triterpenoid from *Lantana camara*. Fitoterapia. 2003; 74(3): 320-1.

10

Medicinal Plants and Their Compounds with Anticancer Properties

BARBI GOGOI[1,2], MARINE HUSSAIN[1,2], SYEDA TABASSUM TASFIA[1], KRISHNAKHI BORAH[1], BABITA JOSHI[2] AND SIDDHARTHA PROTEEM SAIKIA[1*]

ABSTRACT

Medicinal plants have engrossed huge attention due to their diverse range of biological and therapeutic properties. Evidences have been documented from decades on the potential of medicinal plants in various traditional, complementary, and alternative systems of medicine, especially for the treatment of chronic diseases. Naturally occurring plants metabolites, such as polyphenols, brassinosteroids and taxols helps to maintain the health and vitality of individuals without any side effects. Cancer is globally considered as an invariable battle with lots of developments in its cures and preventative therapies including chemotherapy, surgery, radiotherapy and the recent use of natural products. The common cancer treatments, chemotherapy can uses various adverse side effects, strain and damage the patient's physical condition. Although, several medicines are accessible in the market to treat various types of cancers, however, no drug is found to be fully effective. Plant-derived phytochemicals have proved very efficient and safe in the treatment and management of various cancers to some extent. In fact, the medicinal plants are easily available, cheaper and possess no toxicity as compared to the chemotherapeutic drugs. Thus, the various combinations

[1] Medicinal Aromatic and Economic Plants Group, Biological Sciences & Technology Division (BSTD), CSIR-North East Institute of Science & Technology, Jorhat 785006, Assam, India.
[2] Academy of Scientific and Innovative Research (AcSIR), CSIR-North East Institute of Science and Technology, Jorhat-785006, Assam, India.
**Corresponding author:* siddhartha@neist.res.in; spsaikia@gmail.com

of active components of these plants after isolation and identification can be further assessed for their synergistic effects. The present chapter addresses the significance and innovative ways of using medicinal plants and their phytochemicals in anticancer therapy. In addition to the mechanism of action of important phytocompounds, their future prospects in the treatment of cancer and other related diseases are highlighted.

Key words: Cancer, Medicinal plants, Chemotherapeutic drugs, Taxol.

1. INTRODUCTION

Cancer is a life threatening disease, and represents as one of the major issues to the mankind. Hence, there is a requirement of an effective strategy for its antidote. It is characterized by an uncontrolled proliferation of normal cells. The genetic alterations within cells and tissues, transforms the normal cells into malignant cells. These genetic alterations include mutations in DNA repair genes, tumor suppressor genes, and genes involve in the cell growth/ metabolism. Both external factors and internal factors can cause cancer. There are several types of cancers in human beings. Among them, the lung cancer is highly reported in men followed by breast cancer in women. Various medicines are available to treat cancer, but no drug is found to be fully potent and safe. The major problem in the cancer therapy is the toxicity of the established drugs.

As plants are the repository for novel chemical compounds, it provides a promising line for research on cancer. Generally, populations that consume a high level of natural products have a reduced incidence of cancer. So, it made a necessary attempt to study on plants-based bioactive compounds and their potentials in the treatment of cancer. Moreover, many researchers have proved that the plant derived products are a revolutionizing this area as they are natural, ecofriendly, low-cost, and less harmful as compared with the conventional medicines. Carcinogenesis is a complicated phenomenon that involves many signaling pathways. Plant derived compounds are selective in their roles and act specifically only on tumor cells without the affecting normal cells. These phytocompounds are considered as important candidates for anticancer drug development due to their multiple actions on target sites due to their high chemical diversity. However, the cancer research is still in progress towards obtaining very effective candidates from these plant resources. In this chapter, effort has been made to comprehensively discuss on various plant derived bioactive compounds and their contribution in cancer therapies. Also, the mechanisms of action of major anticancer compounds are highlighted.

2. CONTRIBUTION OF MEDICINAL PLANTS TO MODERN MEDICINES

Medicinal plants have been an intrinsic part of the Indian, Chinese and Arabian primitive culture as medicine and their applicability even dates back to the times of archaic humans (Solecki, 1975). In the 18th century, the knowledge about plant derived compounds developed, but attempts to indentify the active ingredients from plants were ineffectual. In the early 19th century, the term 'pharmacognosy' was conceived by Johann Adam Schmid (1759-1809), but the first move came when it became distinct that the pharmaceutical properties of plants are due to different molecules that can be isolated and identified. Another successful creation in the medicinal plants field was the development of methods to study the pharmacological effect of natural products. The 20th century saw the combination of ethnobotanical, phytochemical and pharmacological studies, which allowed a new approach to the study plant-based derived compounds and their properties, and ultimately lead to the development of chemically defined drugs. These provides a huge structural diversity (Clardy and Walsh, 2004), and advanced techniques for isolation, structure clarification, screening and combinatorial synthesis (Ganesan, 2002; Steinbeck, 2004), have led to regeneration of plant products as a source of novel drugs and opened up new opportunity for drug development.

2.1. Economic demands for medicinal plants

Several clinical proven drugs have been successfully passed clinical trial tests, and are being used in modern medicines, while, many lead molecules derived from plant compounds are in the pipeline or under different phases of clinical trials. Thus, resources and plant compounds are becoming more popular in the process of drug discovery. Their non-toxic effects on normal cells and their cytotoxic effects on cancer cells put them in high demand. Many plant species have been explored mainly from the developing countries, where herbal therapies are executed widely, and people rely upon medicinal plants for their primary healthcare and treatments (Ochwang *et al.,* 2014). According to the estimates of the World Health Organization (WHO) in 2007, the plant-derived drugs trade was worth US$100 billion, and is expected to reach US$5 trillion by 2050. There is a large demand for medicinal plants in the developing countries, which is setting a high pressure on the plant habitats. Many medicinal plants are cultivated from wild populations for informal trade, but this type of cultivation is not modulated (Zschocke *et al.,* 2000). With a rapid population growth, deforestation and increasing urbanization the protection of medicinal plants is becoming a major threat and conservation of these plants is vital (Parveen *et al.,* 2013). When wild medicinal plants are harvested only definite parts of the plant are used in treatments. Isolating only segments of a plant may damage the plant and reduce its survival (Zschocke *et al.,* 2000). To increase the viability of medicinal plants, utilization of all segments of the plant including the stem, leaf, root and bark should be involved in the treatment. Other methods of conservation include conservation of germ plasm; cryopreservation; preserving biological sample in liquid nitrogen and tissue culture etc. These preservation techniques will permit for industrial utilization in developed countries (Parveen *et al.,* 2013). In the developed regions, such as Europe, and parts of India and China, some of the medicinal plants are being cultivated on a large scale to meet up with the ever increasing demands for plant based compounds (Zschocke *et al.,* 2000). Overall, it suggests the fact that medicinal plants are economically valued due to their therapeutical significance and thus, there is a dire need of their proper maintenance.

3. ROLE OF MEDICINAL PLANTS COMPOUNDS WITH ANTI-CANCER PROPERTIES

Since ancient decades, medicinal plants have been used in folk medicines and many plants are consumed for their health benefits. According to the WHO, some plant-based treatments are considered as the main source of medicine for various therapeutic purposes (Rao *et al.,* 2017). Secondary metabolites in plants contain three main groups; terpenoids, phenolics and diverse alkaloids (Kabera *et al.,* 2014; Delgoda and Murray, 2017). Several new cytotoxic secondary metabolites are being isolated from plants every year, and constitute a source of new opportunities to explore in order to fight against cancer. Additionally, phytochemicals can be regarded as an excellent leads for the development of anticancer drugs. The modifications of phytocompounds chemical structure can increase their anticancer properties, and improve their absorption, distribution, metabolism and excretion properties with a decreased toxicity and side effects (Guo, 2017). Some of the medicinal plants with anticancer properties and their major bioactive compounds effecting on various cancer types are mentioned in Table 1. Herein, we will list some of the important compounds of plants with their anticancer properties. A few of them are in the current clinical use, while others are in different stages of clinical trials.

3.1. Polyphenols

Polyphenols can inhibit or alter protein regulation which may contribute in the survival of cancer cells. Polyphenolic compounds like flavonoids, resveratrol, tannins, curcumin, and gallocatechins are considered as

Table 1: List of anticancer medicinal plants with their phytochemical compounds.

Plant	***Phytochemicals***	***Type of cancer***	***Reference(s)***
Peganum harmala	Harmine	Breast cancer	Ayoob *et al.* (2017)
Curcuma longa	Curcumin, ascorbic acid	Leukemia, gliobl-astoma and colon cancer	Ooko *et al.* (2017)
Allium wallichii	Steroids, terpenoids, flavonoids, reducing sugars and glycosides	Prostate cancer, breast cancer, cervical cancer	Bhandari *et al.* (2017)
Artemisia annua	Artemisinin	Liver, breast and pancreatic cancer	Efferth (2017)
Debregeasia saeneb	Tannins	Internal tumors	Tariq *et al.* (2017)
Camellia sinensis	Epicatechingallate, picatechin, epigallocatechin	Lung, bladder,skin, prostate and breast cancer	Kumari *et al.* (2017)
Paeonia suffruticosa	Polysaccharides (HBSS, CHSS, DASS, and CASS	Prostate, colon, human breast, and cervical cancer	Zhang *et al.* (2017)
Herba epimedii	Icariin, icaritin, icariside II	Prostate, lung, kidney and gastric cancer	Yong *et al.* (2017)
Crocus sativus	Crocetin	Hippocampal cell death and lung cancer	Hoshyar and Mollaei (2017)
Ziziphus jujuba	Linoleic acids, triterpenoids	Breast cancer, human Jurkat leukemia T cells	Hoshyar and Mollaei (2017)
Ocimum sanctum	Eugenol, orientin, vicenin	Breast, liver and fibrosarcoma cancer	Preethi and Padma (2016)
Ginkgo biloba	Ginkgetin, ginkgolide A & B	Hepatocarcinoma, ovary, prostate, colon and liver cancer	Xiong *et al.* (2016)
Camellia sinensis	Theabrownin	Lung cancer	Wu *et al.* (2016)
Ziziphus mauritiana	α-linolenic acid, Methyl stearate	Leukemia, human cervical and liver cancer	Beg *et al.* (2016)
Solanum nigrum	Solamargine, solasonine	Breast, liver, lung and skin cancer	Al Sinani *et al.* (2016)
Vigna unguiculata	Black-eyed-pea trypsin/ Chymotr-ypsin inhibitor	Human breast cancer	Mehdad *et al.* (2016)
Ziziphus spina-christi	Doxorubicin, spinanine A, rutnine, quercetin	Lung cancer and breast cancer	Jaradat *et al.* (2016)
Glycyrrhiza glabra	Licochalcone-A, licoagrochalcone	Prostate, breast, lung, stomach and kidney cancer	Zhang *et al.* (2016)

Table 1: *(Contd...)*

Table 1: (*Contd...*)

Plant	*Phytochemicals*	*Type of cancer*	*Reference(s)*
Elusine coracana	Ragi bifunctional inhibitor	Myeloid leukemia cell and K562 cell line	Srikanth and Chen (2016)
Psoralea corylifolia	Psoralidin	Stomach and prostate cancer	Pahari *et al.* (2016)
Xanthium strumarium	Xanthatin	Lymphocytic leukemia and liver cancer	Thangapazham *et al.* (2016)
Nigella sativa	Thymoquinone	Colon, prostate, breast and pancreas cancer	Tu *et al.* (2016)
Ocimum sanctum	Eugenol, orientin, vicenin	Breast, liver and fibrosarcoma	Preethi and Padma (2016)
Moringa oleifera	Moringa oleifera protease inhibitor (MoPI)	Abdominal cancer	Srikanth and Chen (2016)
Glycine max	Bowman-Birk inhibitors	Colorectal, prostate and colon cancer	Srikanth and Chen (2016)
Bauhinia variegata	Kaempferol glucoside	Breast, lung and liver cancer	Tu *et al.* (2016)
Withania somnifera	Withaferin A, D	Breast, cervix, prostate and colon cancer	Lee *et al.* (2016)
Psoralea corylifolia	Biochanin, corylifolia, psoralea	Lung, osteosarcoma,fibrosarcoma and liver cancer	Pahari *et al.* (2016)
Moringa oleifera	Niazinine A	Blood cancer	Srikanth and Chen (2016)
Bleekeriavitensis	Elliptinium	Myelogenous leukemia and breast cancer	Lauritano *et al.* (2016)
Combretum caffrum	Combretastatins	Colon, and leukemia and lung cancer	Lauritano *et al.* (2016)
Aegle marmelos	Lupeol	Lymphoma, melanoma, leukemia and breast cancer	Wal *et al.* (2015)
Zingiber officinale	Gingerol	Ovary, cervix, colon, liver and urinary caner	Rastogi *et al.* (2015)
Sylibum marianum	Silibinin	Lung, liver, skin, colon and prostate cancer	Tsai *et al.* (2015)
Capsicum annuum	Luteolin	Colorectal cancer	Osman *et al.* (2015)
Colchicum autumnale	Colchicine	Hodgkin's lymphoma, chronic granulocytic leukemia	Lin *et al.* (2015)

Table 1: (*Contd...*)

Table 1: *(Contd...)*

Plant	*Phytochemicals*	*Type of cancer*	*Reference(s)*
Aegle marmelos	Skimmianine	Liver cancer	Mukhija *et al.* (2015)
Boswellia serrata	Boswellic acid	Prostate cancer	Garg and Deep (2015)
Passiflora caerulea	Chrysin	Colorectal cancer	Leon *et al.* (2015)
Plumbago zeylanica	Plumbagin	Liver, fibrosarcoma, leukemia and breast cancer	Yan *et al.* (2015)
Curcuma longa	Curcumin	Colon adenocarcinoma	Vallianou *et al.* (2015)
Alstonia scholaris	Omethylmacralstonine, talcarpine, villalstonine, pleiocarpamine	Lung cancer	Singh (2015)
Podophyllum peltatum	Podophyllotoxin	Non-small cell lung carcinoma	Choi tum *et al.* (2015)
Andrographis paniculata	Andrographolide	Colon cancer	Osman *et al.* (2015)
Podophyllum hexandrum	Podophyllotoxin	Breast, ovary, lung, liver, bladder and testis cancer	Liu *et al.* (2015)
Betula utilis	Betulinic acid	Melanomas	Krol *et al.* (2015)
Panax ginseng	Panaxadiol	Human colon cancer	Wang *et al.* (2015)
Panax pseudoginseng	Panaxadiol	Human colon cancer	Wang *et al.* (2015)
Annona crassiflora	Caffeic acid, sinapic acid, rutin	Glioma, renal, ovary cancer, lymphoid melanoma	Formagio *et al.* (2015)
Capsicum annuum	Luteolin	Colorectal cancer	Osman *et al.* (2015)
Zingiber officinale	6-Shogaol, Gingerol	Ovary cancer Colon, breast and ovarian cancer	Ghasemzadeh *et al.* (2015) Rastogi *et al.* (2015)
Curcuma longa	Curcumin	Breast, lung, colon, prostate esophagus, liver and skin	Perrone *et al.* (2015)
Oldenlandia diffusa	Ursolic acid	Lungs, ovary, uterus, stomach, liver, colon, rectum and brain cancer	Wozniak *et al.* (2015)
Argemone gracilenta	Argemonine and berberine	B-cell lymphoma, leukemia	Leyva-Peralta *et al.* (2015)
Berberis vulgaris	Berberine, cannabisin	Breast, prostate and liver cancer	Pierpaoli *et al.* (2015)
Broussonetia papyrifera	2S-abyssinone verubulin	Glioblastoma and brain cancer	Pang *et al.* (2014)
Glycyrrhiza uralensis	Isoliquiritigenin	Human lung cancer	Jung *et al.* (2014)

Table 1: *(Contd...)*

Table 1: (*Contd...*)

Plant	***Phytochemicals***	***Type of cancer***	***Reference(s)***
Boerhavia diffusa	Punarnavine	Malignant melanoma cancer	Mishra *et al.* (2014)
Vitis vinifera	Procyanidins	Human colon cancer	Cheah *et al.* (2014)
Polygonum cuspidatum	Procyanidins	Colorectal, skin and liver	Ali and Braun (2014)
Morinda citrifolia	Damnacanthal	Lung cancer, sarcomas	Aziz *et al.* (2014)
Aristolochia fontanesii	Aqueous extract	Breast cancer	Benarba and Meddah (2014)
Panax ginseng	Panaxadiol,	Breast, ovary, lung, prostate and colon cancer	Du *et al.* (2013) panaxatriol
Argemone mexicana	Pancorine, argenaxine, higenamine, angoline	Gall bladder and breast cancer	Brahmachari *et al.* (2013)
Dioscorea collettii	Dioscin	Liver and human gastric cancer	Hu *et al.* (2013)
Tabernaemontana divaricata	Cononitarine B, Conophylline	Liver, lung, breast and colon cancer	Bao *et al.* (2013)
Nelumbo nucifera	Neferine	Liver cancer	Yoon *et al.* (2013)
Lavatera cashmeriana	Lavatera cashmeriana protease inhibitors (LC-pi I, II, III)	Leukemia, lung, colon cancer	Rakashanda *et al.* (2013)
Carissa spinarum	Alkaloids, saponins, tannins, flavonoids	Nasopharyngeal carcinoma	Sahreen *et al.* (2013)
Tabebuia impetiginosa	Beta-Lapachone, Lapachol Beta-lapachone	Pancreatic cancer	Umadevi *et al.* (2013)
Annona squamosa	Bullatacin	Liver cancer	Biba *et al.* (2013)
Nothapodytes foetida	Acetylcamptothecin, Camptothecin, Scopolectin	Inhibitor of DNA topoisomerase found in cancerous cells	Umadevi *et al.* (2013)
Azadirachta indica	Limonoids, Nimbolide	Breast, lung, stomach, prostate skin and colon cancer, malignant lymphoma, malignant melanoma and leukaemia	Umadevi *et al.* (2013)
Andrographis paniculata	Andrographolide	Breast, ovary, stomach, colon, prostate, and kidney cancer, nasopharynx malignant melanoma and leukaemia.	Umadevi *et al.* (2013)
Bauhinia variegata	Cyanidinglucoside, malvidin glucoside, peonidin glucoside	Cancers of breast, lung, liver, oral cavity, larynx and	Umadevi *et al.* (2013)

Table 1: (*Contd...*)

Table 1: *(Contd...)*

Plant	*Phytochemicals*	*Type of cancer*	*Reference(s)*
	and kaempferol glucoside	malignant ascites	
Bryophyllum pinnatum	Bryophyllin A	Cervical cancer	Mahata *et al.* (2012)
Catharanthus roseus	Vinblastine, vincristine	Breast, ovary, cervix, lung, rectum and testis cancer	Keglevich *et al.* (2012)
Centella asiatica	Asiatic acid	Melanoma, glioblastoma, breast	Heidari *et al.* (2012)
Viscum album	Viscumin, digallic acid	Breast, cervix, ovary, stomach, colon, kidney, lung cancer	Bhouri *et al.* (2012)
Leea indica	Gallic acid	Ehrlich ascites carcinoma	Raihan *et al.* (2012)
Liriodendron tulipifera	Costunolide, tulipinolide, liriodenine, germacranolide	KB (Oral cancer), HT29 cell line	Wang *et al.* (2012)
Cicer arietinum	Bowman-Birk-type	Breast and prostate protease cancer	Magee *et al.* (2012)
Calvatia caelata	Laccases (Enzymes)	Liver, breast cancer	Xu *et al.* (2012)
Amoora rohituka	Amooranin	Lymphocytic leukemia	Chan *et al.* (2011)
Conyza canadensis	Conyzapyranone A and B	Epidermoid carcinoma	Csupor-Loffler *et al.* (2011)
Vitex negundo	Chrysoplenetin	Human pancreatic cancer	Awale *et al.* (2011)
Tylophora indica	Tylophorine	Breast cancer	Kaur *et al.* (2011)
Croton macrobotrys	Corydine, salutaridine	Leukemia and lung cancer	Motta *et al.*,(2011)
Clausena lansium	Clausenalansamid A and B	Gastric, liver cancer	Maneerat *et al.* (2011)
Solanum lycopersicum	Lycopene	Prostate and colon cancer	Hahm *et al.* (2011)
Syzygium cumini	Kaempferol-7-Omethylether	Leukemia	Afify *et al.* (2011)
Coccinia grandis	(CG) protease inhibitors	Colon cancer	Satheesh and Murugan (2011)
Cannabis sativa	Cannabinoid	Lung, pancreas, breast, prostate and colorectal cancer	Appendino *et al.* (2011)
Sylibum marianum	Silymarin	Colorectal cancer	Colombo *et al.* (2011)
Enterolobium contortisiliquum	Enterolobium, contortisiliquum trypsin inhibitor	Gastric and breast cancer	Nakahata *et al.* (2011)
Linum usitatissimum	Cyanogenic glycosides	Breast cancer	Sakarkar and Deshmukh (2011)

Table 1: *(Contd...)*

Table 1: (*Contd...*)

Plant	*Phytochemicals*	*Type of cancer*	*Reference(s)*
Tylophora indica	Tylophorine	Breast cancer	Kaur *et al.* (2011)
Allium sativum	Allylmercaptocysteine, allicin	Lymphoma, cervix cancer	Karmakar *et al.* (2011)
Bacopa monnieri	Stigmasterol	Liver cancer	Ghosh T *et al.* (2011)
Plumbago zeylanica	Plumbagin	Blood and skin cancer	Checker *et al.* (2010)
Peristrophe bicalyculata	β-Caryophyllene, α-zingiberene	Breast cancer	Ogunwande *et al.* (2010)
Stevia rebaudiana properties	Labdanesclareol	Anti-tumorous and cytotoxic	Kaushik *et al.* (2010)
Camellia sinensis	Epigallocatechin gallate	Brain, prostate, cervical and bladder cancer	Das *et al.* (2010)
Lens culinaris	Lentil (Lens culinaris trypsin inhibitor)	Human colon cancer	Caccialupi *et al.* (2010)
Vaccinium macrocarpon	Hydroxycinnamoylursolic acid	Cervical, prostate cancer	El-Shemy *et al.* (2010)
Phaseolus vulgaris	Tepary bean protease inhibitor	Lukemia L1210 and lymphoma MBL2	Sun *et al.* (2010)
Berberis vulgaris	Berberine cancers	Breast, liver, colon	De Bono *et al.* (2010)
Phaseolus acutifolius	Tepary bean protease inhibitor	Leukemia L1210 and lymphoma MBL2	Sun *et al.* (2010)
Withania somnifera	Adriamycin and fluorouracil	Human cervical cancer cell	Yadav *et al.* (2010)
Colchicum autumnale	Colchicine	Multiple solid tumors	Atkinson *et al.* (2010)
Butea monosperma	Butrin, (7,30,40-trihydroxyflavanone 7,30-diglucoside)	Liver cancer	Choedon *et al.* (2010)
Actaea racemosa	Actein	Liver and breast cancer	Einbond *et al.* (2009)
Smilax chinensis	Tannin, saponins and flavonoid	Sarcoma-180 and	Madhuri and Pandey ascites sarcoma (2009)
Vitis vinifera	Cyanidin	Colon cancer	Lim and Park (2009)
Hibiscus mutabilis	Lectin	Liver, breast cancer	Lam and Ng (2009)
Gossypium hirsutum	Gossypol	Breast, stomach, liver, prostate and bladder cancer	Zhan *et al.* (2009)
Actaea racemosa	Actein	Liver and breast cancer	Einbond *et al.* (2009)
Pyrus malus	Quercetin, procyanidin	Colon cancer	Madhuri and Pandey (2009)

Table 1: (*Contd...*)

Table 1: (*Contd...*)

Plant	***Phytochemicals***	***Type of cancer***	***Reference(s)***
Vitex agnus-castus	Vitex or luteolin	Human uterine, ovarian, cervical and breast cancer	Imai *et al.* (2009)
Citrus limon	5-hydroxy-6,7,8,30, 40 pentamethoxy-flavone	Human colon cancer	Hirata *et al.* (2009)
Taxus wallichiana	Diterpenoid 2deace-toxytaxinine	Breast and kidney cancer	Reddy *et al.* (2009)
Asclepias curassavica	Asclepin, cardenolides	Liver cancer	Li *et al.* (2009)
Ardisia crenata	Ardisiacrispin	Liver cancer	Li M *et al.* (2008)
Sylibum marianum	Silymarin	Colorectal cancer and colon cancer	Ramasamy and Agarwal (2008)
Biophytum sensitivum	Alcoholic extract	Dalton's lymphoma ascites, Ehrlich ascites carcinoma	Guruvayoorappan and Kuttan (2007)
Matricaria chamomilla	Apigenin	Colorectal cancer	Srivastava and Gupta (2007)
Taxus brevifolia	Paclitaxel	Breast and ovarian cancer	Cragg and Newman (2005)
Catharanthus roseus	Vindesine	Leukemias, testicular, breast and lung cancer	Cragg and Newman (2005)
Betula Sp.	Betulinic acid	Human melanoma xenografts and	Cragg and Newman (2005) leukemia
Curcuma zedoaria	Curcumin	Colorectal cancer and B-16 melanoma cells	Seo *et al.* (2005)
Clematis manshrica	1,4-benzoquinone, 5-oethyl- embelin, 15carbon isoprenoid	Liver cancer and blood cancer	Zhao *et al.* (2005)
Glycine max inhibitor	Soybean trypsin	Human ovarian cancer	Suzuki *et al.* (2005)
Ipomoea batatas	Trypsin inhibitor protein	Promyelocytic leukemia cells	Suzuki *et al.* (2005)
Medicago scutellata	Medicago scutellata trypsin inhibitor	Human breast and cervical cancer	Lanza *et al.* (2004)
Pleurotus sajor caju	Ribonucleases	Leukemia and liver cancer	Ngai and Ng (2004)
Lentinus edodes	Lentinan	Sarcoma-180 in mice	Ngai and Ng (2004)
Calvatia caelata	Calcaelin	Breast and spleen cancer cells	Ng *et al.* (2003)
Schizophyllum commune		Schizophyllan cancer	Head and neck Smith *et al.* (2002)
Taxus brevifolia	Nab-paclitaxel	Ovarian and breast cancer	*Caruso et al.* (2000)

anticancer compounds (Azmi *et al.,* 2006). These polyphenolic compounds act as natural antioxidants, and when supplied through the diet can improve individual's health and reduce the risk of cancers (Apostolou *et al.,* 2013). Mechanisms of polyphenols include the initiation of apoptosis through regulating copper ions mobilization that are bound to chromatin, and inducing DNA fragmentation.

Moreover, plant polyphenols can interfere with proteins which are present in cancer cells to promote their growth. For example, curcumin treated cancer cells of various cancer types have shown the suppression of the Tumour Necrosis Factor (TNF) expression through their interaction with various stimuli (Gupta *et al.,* 2014). Some examples of polyphenols (Fig. 1) with their anticancer effect are described in details below.

3.1.1. *Resveratrol*

Resveratrol is found in mulberries, peanuts, grapes, bilberries and blueberries. Resveratrol suppresses the action of Vascular endothelial growth factor (VEGF) protein by reducing Mitogen activated protein (MAP) kinase phosphorylation, and up-regulates p53 as well as Bcl-2 associated X proteins, and down-regulates Matrix metalloproteinases (MMP)s, Nuclear factor kappa B cells (NFkB), Activator protein-1 (AP-1), B cell lymphoma 2 (Bcl-2), cyclins, cyclin dependent kinases, cytokines and cyclooxygenase (COX-2) to destroy

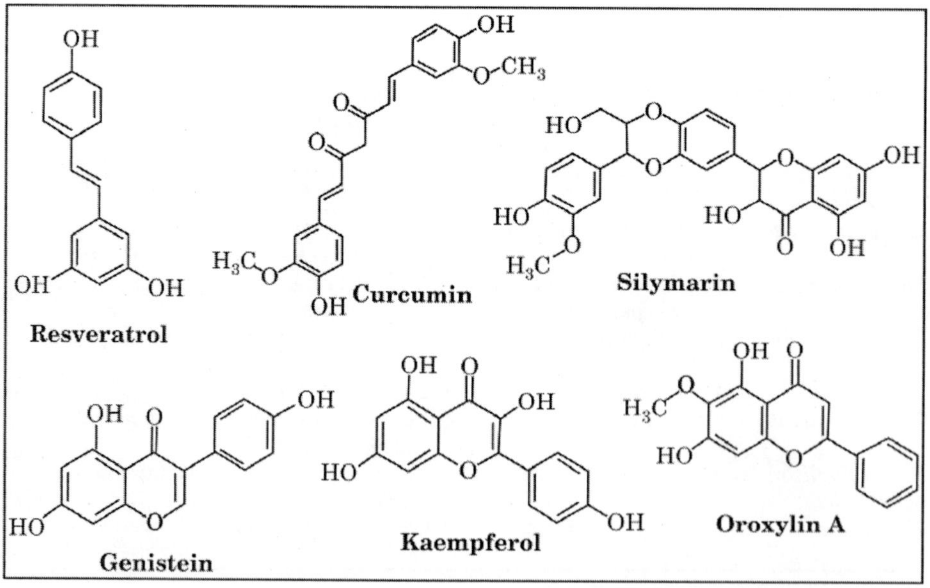

Fig. 1: *(Contd...)*

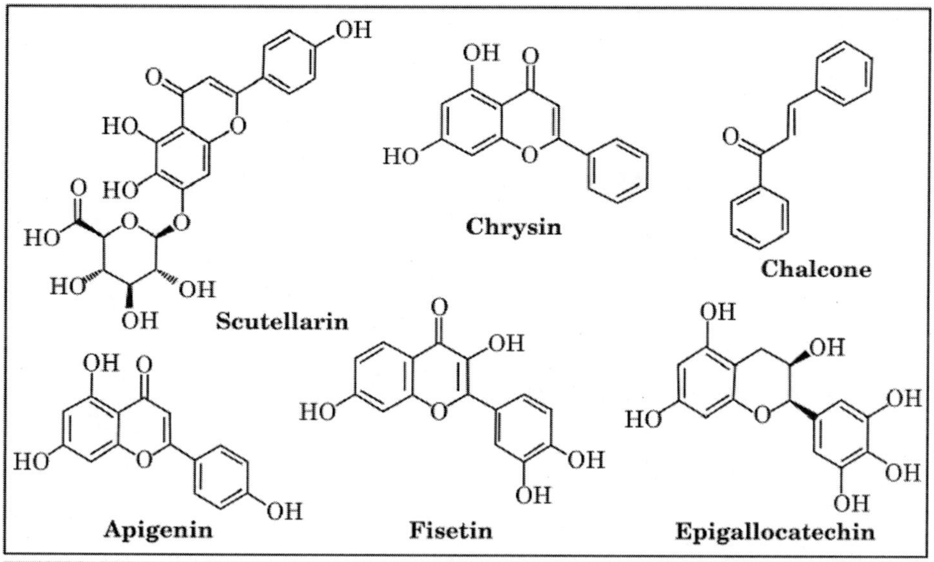
Scutellarin
Chrysin
Chalcone
Apigenin
Fisetin
Epigallocatechin

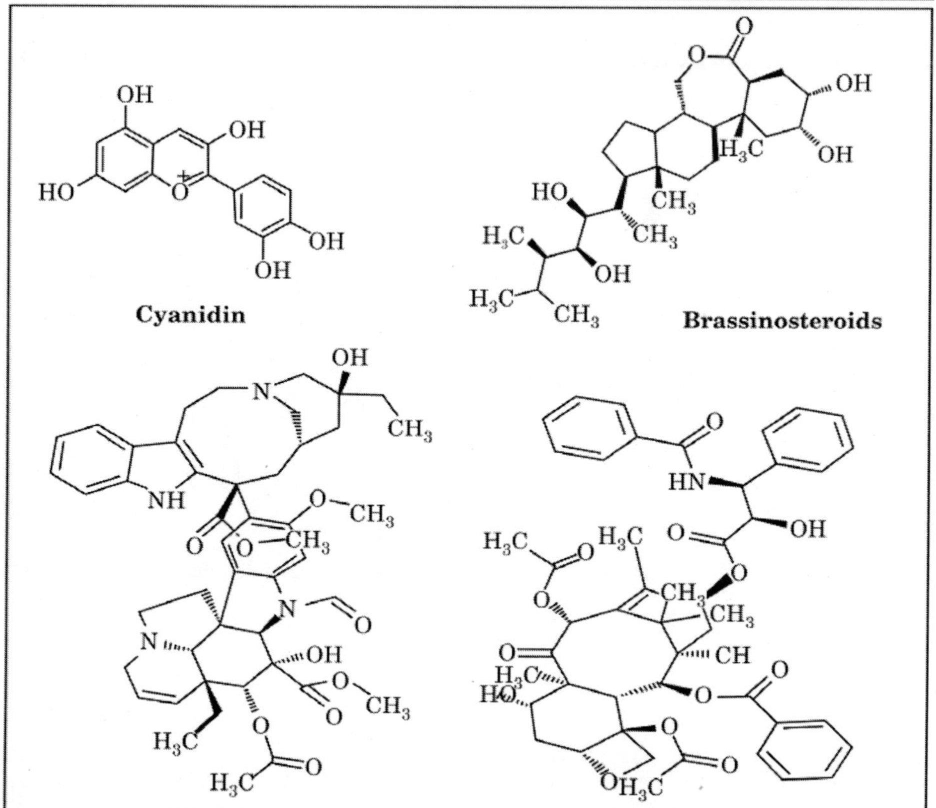
Cyanidin
Brassinosteroids
Vincristine
Paclitaxel

Fig. 1: (*Contd...*)

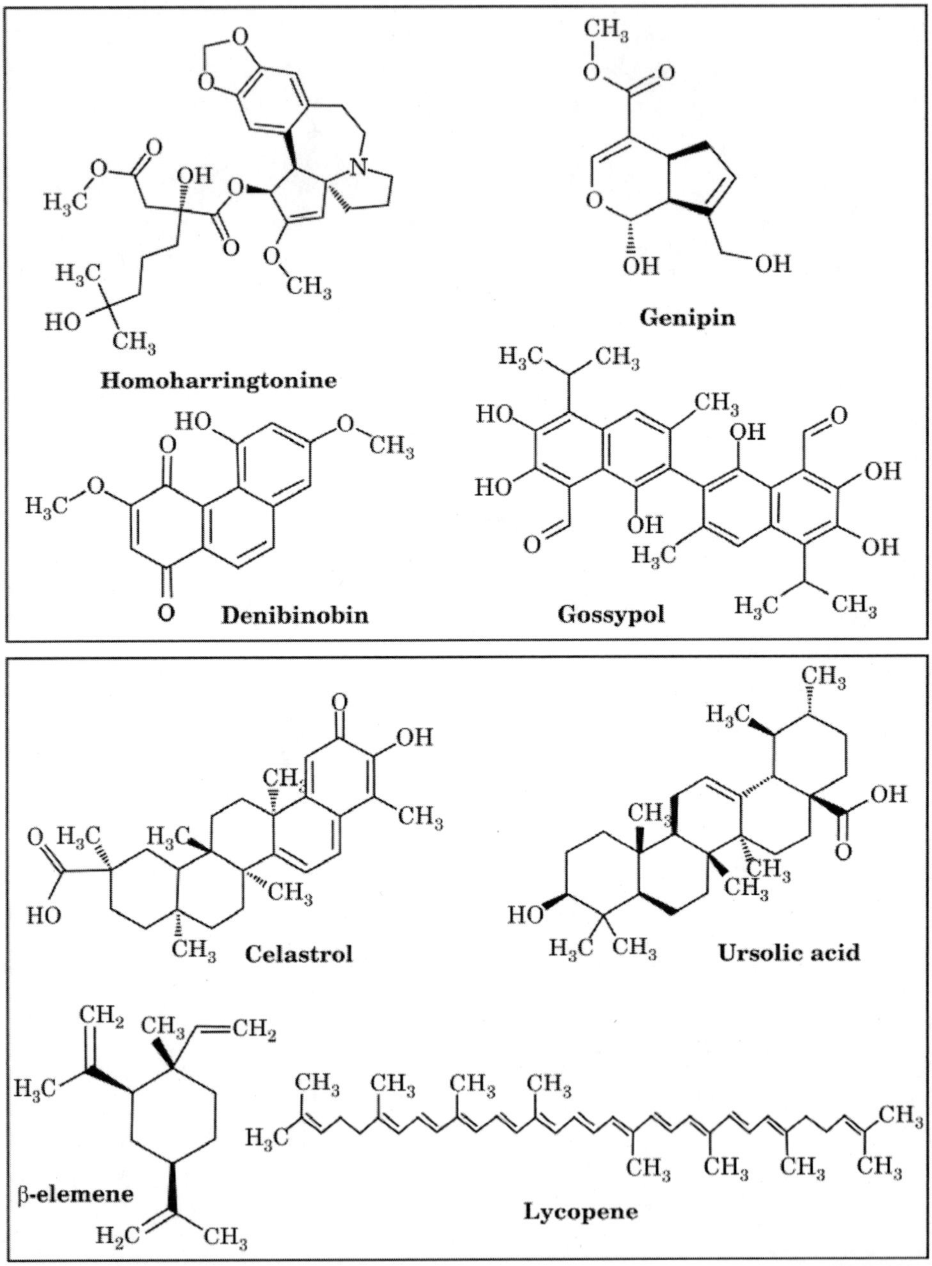

Fig. 1: *(Contd...)*

wide range of cancer types, including liver, pancreatic, breast, colorectal, lungs and prostate cancers (Patel *et al.,* 2010; Varoni *et al.,* 2016).

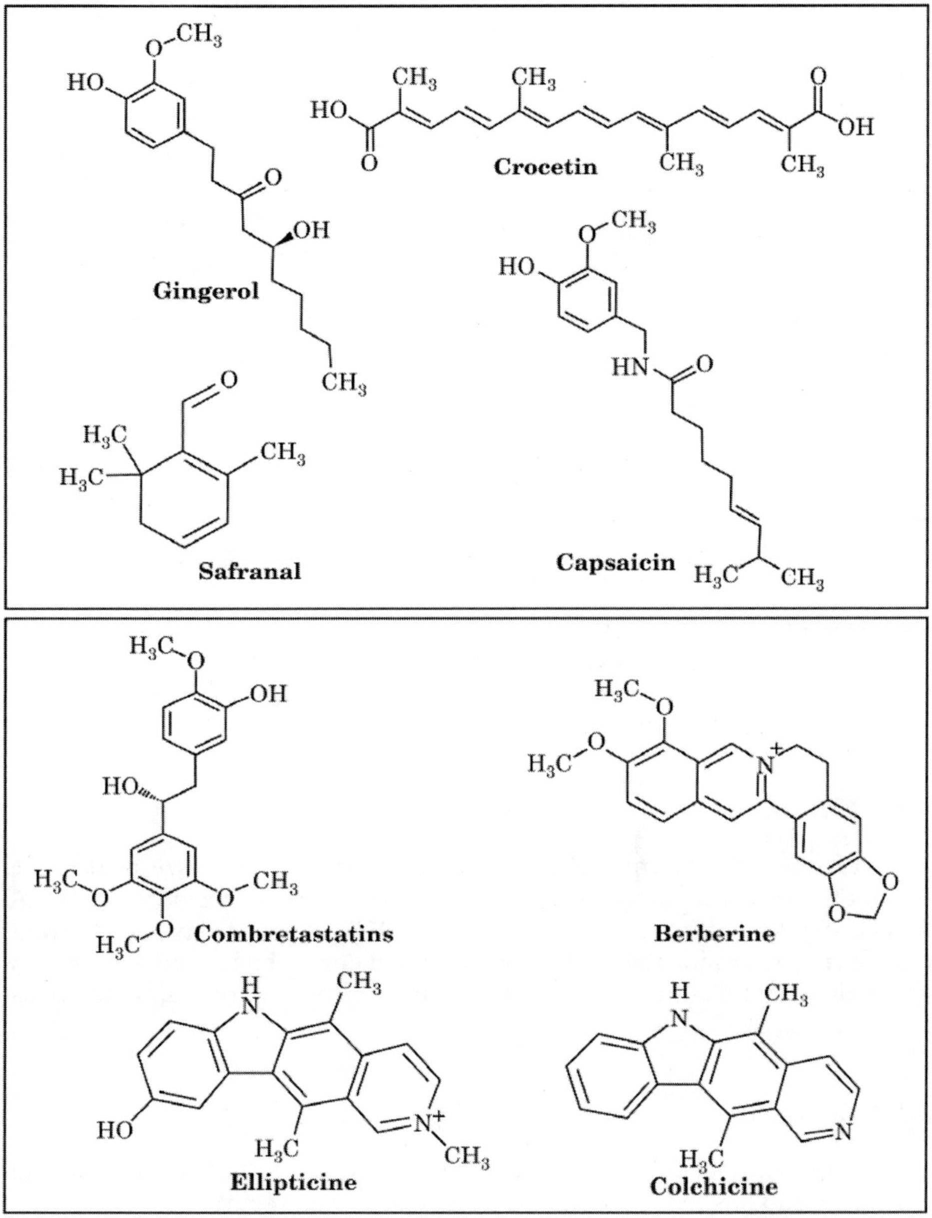

Fig. 1: *(Contd...)*

3.1.2. *Curcumin*

Curcumin is a lead compound extracted from *Curcuma longa* inhibits the growth of human glioblastoma cells, upregulates the expressions of different gene products *i.e.,* p16, p21 and p53, Bax protein, ETS oncogenic family,

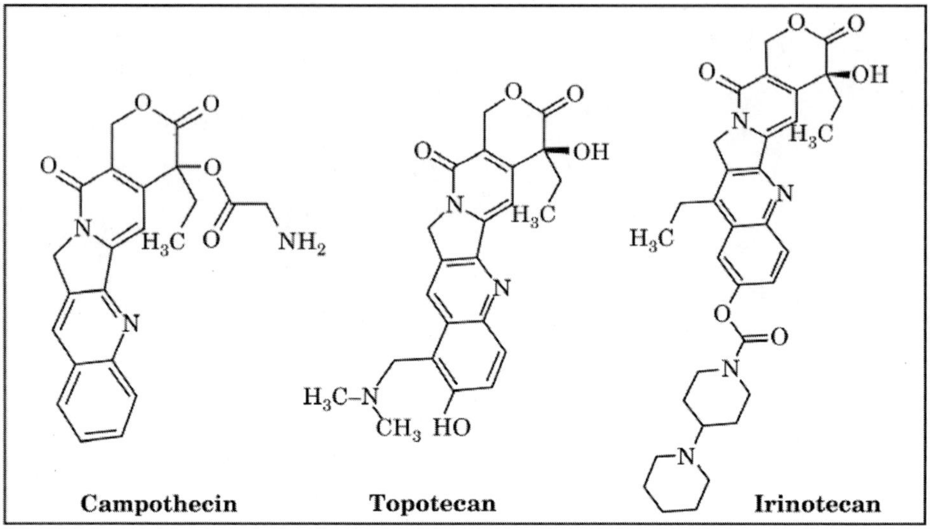

Fig. 1: Phytochemical structures of medicinal plants.

extracellular signal regulated kinase, early growth response protein, c-Jun N-terminal kinase, and caspase enzymes, and decreases the level of Bcl-2, mTOR, p65, protein kinase B, retinoblastoma protein, NF-kB, and cyclin D1 proteins (Vallianou *et al.,* 2015).

3.1.3. *Silymarin*

Silymarin is a flavolignan obtained from *Silybum marianum* contains a blend of anticancer compounds, such as silydianin, silychristin, silybin A and B, and isosilybin (A and B) (Lee *et al.,* 2016). Silymarin is used to treat colorectal cancer mutually with paclitaxel and doxorubicin, and also acts on cyclin dependent kinases (CDKs) to induce cell cycle arrest and apoptosis (Thorn *et al.,* 2011).

3.1.4. *Genistein*

Genistein is an isoflavone isolated from soybeans, lentils, beans and chickpeas and has proapoptotic function against colorectal cancer (Marin *et al.,* 2015). Genistein can also up-regulate the expression of pro-apoptotic proteins, upregulate expression of antioxidant enzymes, such as glutathione peroxidase, and inhibits NF-kb and topoisomerase II enzymes (Ganai and Farooqi, 2015).

3.1.5. *Kaempferol*

Kaempferol, an anticancer agent isolated from plants, such as propolis, black tea, grapefruit and broccoli. Kaempferol acts by activating the expression of caspase-3 enzyme, p53 gene and its products against colorectal cancer (HT-29) cells (Lee *et al.* 2014; Gutierrez-del-Rio *et al.,* 2016).

3.1.6. *Oroxylin flavone*

Oroxylin A isolated from the *Scutellariae radix* is reported to down-regulate the expression of COX-2 and iNOS genes, block IkB degradation to inhibit the activation of LPS-induced by NF-kB (Chen *et al.,* 2004). Oroxylin A together with 5-FU is also used to treat colorectal cancer. It is also reported that Oroxylin A induces carcinogenesis through an increased ROS generation and increased ROS generation (Ha *et al.,* 2012).

3.1.7. *Scutellarin glycoside*

Scutellarin is considered as a promising anticancer agent, and is commonly isolated from *Scutellaria barbata* and *Scutellaria altissima*. It exhibits the suppression of cancer cell proliferation, upregulation of caspase- 3, 9, and Bax/Bcl-2 ratio in prostate cancer (Gao *et al.,* 2017), induces apoptosis in liver carcinoma, human colorectal cancer by regulating the p53 gene product (Yang *et al.,* 2017).

3.1.8. *Chrysin*

Chrysin (5,7-dihydroxyflavone) found in propolis, honey, blue passion flower and chamomile is reported to posses antitumor effects against different cancer cell lines, such as DU145 and PC-3 with minimal side effects (Kasala *et al.,* 2015; Renuka *et al.,* 2016). This flavone also arrested cell cycle at G2/ M phase, cleaves DNA, increase ROS production and lipid peroxidation, stimulates MAPK, ERK1/2 and P38 proteins and concealed the profusion of S6, AKT, PI3K, P90RSK and P70S6K proteins in the prostate cancer cells (Ryu *et al.,* 2017).

3.1.9. *Chalcone*

Chalcone is also an anticancer flavonoid of fruits and vegetables. It is used for the treatment of colon, lung, breast, liver and prostate cancers. Its mechanisms of action is based on the activation of different caspases (caspase-8, 9, 12 enzymes), upregulation of the expression of proapoptotic proteins, and by decreasing the anti-apoptotic Bcl-2 gene expression (Das and Manna, 2016).

3.1.10. *Apigenin*

Apigenin, a flavonoid is identified in different fruits and vegetables, such as celery, chamomile and parsley. It possesses low toxicity and non-mutagenecity. It brings anticancer activity by inducing apoptosis, targeting the leptin/leptin receptor pathway, activating caspase dependent extrinsic apoptosis pathway, inhibiting signal transducer and activator of transcription 3 (STAT3) signaling pathways in lung cancer cells (Seo *et al.,* 2015; Bauer *et al.,* 2017).

3.1.11. *Fisetin*

Fisetin is found in plant species, such as strawberries, apple, grape and onion (Bhandari *et al.,* 2017). It is used to treat human lung cancer, where it acts by inhibiting PI3K/Akt signaling pathways (Khan *et al.,* 2012). Also, it is found to induce apoptosis in human renal carcinoma cells by means of p53-mediated up-regulation of DR5 (Min *et al.,* 2017; Bhandari *et al.,* 2017).

3.1.12. *Epigallocatechin gallate*

Epigallocatechin is the key polyphenolic constituent of green tea, and is has the capability to restore suppress tumor genes expression, such as retinoid X receptor alpha which inhibits breast cancer by binding to different target proteins, such as 70 kDa zeta-associated protein (Zap-70) (Morris *et al.,* 2016).

3.1.13. *Cyanidin glycosides F*

Cyanidin is isolated from fruits and vegetables like apples, grapes, plums, blackberry, raspberry, red berries, cranberry, red onion and red cabbage. It exhibits anticancer activity by inhibiting cell growth and division in colon cancer through gene expression of COX-2 and iNOS (Kim *et al.,* 2010). Cyanidin glycosides from red berries prevent the synthesis of COX-2 enzyme in colon cancer and sMMP-9 expression in bladder (Singh *et al.,* 2011).

3.2. Brassinosteroids

Brassinosteroids (BRs) are naturally occurring compounds in plants, and function as a signal hormone to regulate the growth and cell differentiation, stem and root cells elongation, plant senescence, disease resistance, stress tolerance. Also, they are known to possess anticancer activities (Bishop and Koncz, 2002). Two natural BRs, namely 28-homocastasterone and 24-epibrassinolide have been demonstrated with anticancer effects on various cancer cell lines and confirmed to be efficient even at micro molar concentrations (Malikova *et al.,* 2008; Steigerova *et al.,* 2010). BRs can induce responses essential for the growth inhibition and apoptosis by interacting with the cell cycle. It is reported to treat various cancer cell lines such as breast cancer, T-lymphoblastic leukaemia CEM, cervical carcinoma HeLa, Estrogen receptor, epidermal growth factor receptor and human EGFR-2, Estrogen receptor, etc. (Malikova *et al.,* 2008; Pledgie-Tracy *et al.,* 2007).

3.3. Vincristine

Vincristine is the first clinically approved plant-derived anticancer agents by the Food and Drug Administration (FDA) in 1963 (Newman and Gragg, 2016). It is a naturally-occurring alkaloid extracted from the leaves of *Catharanthus roseus* (L.) G. Don. It is used in the pediatric oncology as a chemotherapy agent and in adults; it is used against the acute lymphoblastic leukemia. The reports have mentioned that it can increase the survival rate of cancer patients upto 80% (Evans *et al.,* 1963). It is also used in the treatment of rhabdomyosarcoma, neuroblastoma, lymphomas and nephroblastoma (Moore and Pinkerton, 2009; Almagro *et al.,* 2015). Since the concentration of vincristine (and other vinca alkaloids) is low in nature, its extraction process is very expensive. To overcome the situation, negative-pressure cavitations extraction and genetic engineered enzyme manipulation and elicitors are studied to raise the metabolic pathways of vincristine biosynthesis in plant cells (Mu*et al.,* 2012; Tang and Pan, 2017). The most accepted mechanism of vincristine antitumor activity involves its interaction with tubulins and disrupts the assembly of the mitotic spindle, which in turn leads to the termination of actively-dividing cells (Wang *et al.,* 2016). Sphingomyelin/cholesterol liposomal vincristine, Marqibo® was approved by FDA in 2012 in order to treat adults with relapsed acute lymphoblastic leukemia (Velde *et al.,* 2017). Furthermore, other vincristine encapsulated formulations are tested in clinical studies against cancer such as small-cell lung cancer (ClinicalTrials.gov Identifier: NCT02566993), advanced cervical cancer (ClinicalTrials. gov Identifier: NCT02471027) and liver cancer (ClinicalTrials.gov Identifier: NCT00980460) (Yoshihara *et al.,* 2017).

3.4. Paclitaxel

Paclitaxel (a tricyclic diterpenoid) is extracted from the bark of *Taxus brevifolia* Nutt. (Pacific Yew) and marketed under the brand name, Taxol® since 1993. It is a complex molecule and has become one of the most active chemotherapeutic drugs in the new era of anticancer drug discovery (Weaver 2014; Bernabeu *et al.,* 2017). Its biosynthetic pathway starts with the precursor, geranylgeranyl diphosphate along with 19 steps regulated by numerous enzymes, but the process is still proclaimed to be vague (Howat *et al.,* 2014). The therapeutic efficiency of paclitaxel has achieved an immense success in the treatment of breast, ovarian and lung cancer (Bernabeu *et al.,* 2017). Additionally, it is effective on both solid and disseminated tumors. Its unique action of mechanism of antitumor activity is predicted to be by targeting the cancer phenotypes like cell proliferation and DNA repair (Weaver 2014). Two semi-synthetic derivatives, docetaxel and cabazitaxel were obtained by structural modifications of paclitaxel together with the structure activity relationship (SARs) and quantitative SAR (QSAR), and they are known to possess better efficacy with low risks (Xiao *et al.,* 2016). The development of multidrug resistance (MDR) has limited the efficacy of paclitaxel to treat many cancer diseases due to over expression of ABCB1 (P-glycoprotein) and ABCC10 (multidrug resistance protein 7) efflux transporters, the α-/β-tubulin mutations and/or alterations in the binding region (Barbuti and Chen, 2015). However, the improvement of new formulations and delivery system of drugs allowed paclitaxel to be used as safe anticancer agent and to conquer paclitaxel's multidrug resistance, its poor aqueous solubility, clinical neurotoxicity and neutropenia (Nehate *et al.,* 2014; Zong *et al.,* 2017). For example, Lipusu® marketed in China since 2006 that is used for treating ovarian, breast, gastric, and neck cancers (Bernabeu *et al.,* 2017). Abraxane®, also named as *nab*-paclitaxel was approved by FDA in 2005 and European Medicines Agency (EMA/99258/ 2015, EMEA/H/C/000778) in 2012 which improved the solubility of paclitaxel (Rivera and Cianfrocca, 2015). Cabazitaxel (Jevtana®) was approved in 2010 by FDA for the treatment of patients with hormone-refractory metastatic prostate cancer and tumors that are docetaxel- or paclitaxel-resistant. Paclitaxel has high demands in market due to its combinational applications with other anticancer drugs, such as ClinicalTrials.gov Identifier: NCT02379416, NCT00584857 and NCT01288261 (Gill *et al.,* 2016; Ricci *et al.,* 2017) and also in clinical trials for treating other diseases, such as psoriasis (Ehrlich *et al.,* 2004) and inhibition of botulinum neurotoxin (Dadgar *et al.,* 2013).

3.5. Homoharringtonine

Homoharringtonine was first isolated from bark of *Cephalotaxus harringtonii* (Knight ex J. Forbes) K. Koch and *Cephalotaxus fortunei* Hook. It is an alkaloid with a cephalotaxine nucleus named cephalotaxine 4-methyl-2(R)-hydroxy-2-(4-hydroxy-4-methylpentyl) succinate, and used in the traditional Chinese medicines to treat hematological malignancies (Lu and Wang, 2014). Homoharringtonine and other cephalotaxine derivatives can also be found in leaves, bark and seeds of other *Cephalotaxus* species (Kantarjian *et al.,* 2013). Homoharringtonine inhibits the elongation step of protein synthesis by binding to the A-site of 50 Sribosomal subunit, which blocks the access of charged tRNA (Gandhi *et al.,* 2014). Recently, other mechanisms have been found *i.e.,* it could affect signaling pathways, like activation of the TGF-β pathway through phosphorylation of smad3 (Chen *et al.,* 2017) and Jak-stat5 pathway by regulating tyrosine kinase phosphorylation (Li *et al.,* 2017). Homoharringtonine was approved by FDA in 2012, and is traded in the market as Synribo® for treating patients with chronic myeloid leukemia and till date it is the only commercial natural therapeutic agent to treat this disease.

Further, it is being diagnosed in 20 clinical trials such as patients with newly-diagnosed acute myelogenous leukemia (NCT01873495), myelodysplastic syndrome (NCT02159872), and relapsed/refractory acute myeloid leukemia carrying FLT3-ITD (NCT03170895), cytarabine and idarubicin (NCT02440568) and quizartinib (NCT03135054) (Seca and Pinto, 2018).

3.6. Isothiocyanate

Isothiocyanate is a potent phytochemical found in vegetables of Cruciferae family, such as watercress and broccoli. It is used for the treatment of diverse cancers, like colorectal cancer, cervical cancer, lung cancer, prostate cancer, and human T-Leukemia cells devoid of any toxic side effects (Luo *et al.,* 2017). Isothiocyanates can induce apoptosis and ROS-mediated mechanism, down regulate activated signaling cascades, arresting cell cycle at G2/M phase and modulate changes in epigenetic, inhibit cell proliferation, progression and invasion metastasis in both colorectal and prostate cancer (Pereira *et al.,* 2017).

3.7. Genipin

The natural phytochemical, Genipin is isolated from a *Gardenia jasminoides,* and used in breast cancer treatment (Shindo *et al.,* 2014). It function by regulating different protein and enzymes as caspase-3, Bax, Bcl-2, JNK, p38, MAPK. Additionally, Genipin exhibits an anti-proliferative activity by down-regulating Bcl-2 expression, and up-regulating Bax and caspase-3, pro-apoptotic signaling cascades, such as JNK and p38 MAPK in MDA-MB-231 breast cancer cells (Pons *et al.,* 2015).

3.8. Denbinobin

Denbinobin, a multifunctional phytochemical is found in stems of *Ephemerantha lonchophylla* and *Dendrobium moniliforme.* It exhibits various bioactive properties including anti-cancer, anti-angiogenesis and induce-apoptosis (Liu *et al.,* 2011). This compound acts by inhibiting metastasis of Src kinase activity, decreases iNOS and COX-2 activity in concentration-dependent manner by suppressing NF-kB activation in human breast cancer cells (Peiro *et al.,* 2014).

3.9. Gossypol

Gossypol is isolated from cotton seeds (*Gossypium hirsutum*) and *Thespesia populnea.* It has completed the phase II of clinical trials as a potential anti-cancer agent for the treatment of human breast and prostate cancer (Iqbal *et al.,* 2017). Gossypol is also used to suppress cell proliferation, induces autophagy and apoptosis in colorectal cancer (HT-29, HCT116 and RKO) cell lines (Lan *et al.,* 2015).

3.10. Celastrol

Celastrol is an anticancer compound, isolated from the bark of *Tripterygium wilfordii.* It inhibits heat shock proteins (Hsp90 ATPase activity) by blocking their interface with its cochaperone (Cdc37), and induces apoptosis *via* caspase-3 enzyme in ovary (OVCAR-8), lung 95-D and prostate cancer cells (Zhu *et al.,* 2010). Several studies have suggested that Celastrol can induce apoptosis and cell cycle arrest, inhibit angiogenesis and exhibit anti-invasive effect, autophagy by the activation of ROS/c-JNK signaling pathway, activate Fas/Fas ligand pathway in lung cancer, upregulate death receptors in breast and colon cancer and inhibit PI3K/Akt/mTOR pathway in triple negative breast cancer (Cascao *et al.,* 2017).

3.11. Ginsenosides

Six major ginsenosides (Rb1, Rb2, Rc, Rd, Re, and Rg1) constitute around 80% of the total ginsenosides in ginseng (*Panax ginseng*) roots. Researches on preclinical and clinical trial suggest that ginsenosides have anticancer activity for liver, breast, gastric, ovarian, melanoma and colon cancer (Chen *et al.,* 2016). Panaxadiol is an anticancer agent isolated from *P. ginseng* and *P. pseudo ginseng.* It has the potent anti-cancer activity against different cancer cell lines, which is mediated *via* modulating various signaling pathways (Gao *et al.,* 2013; Lee *et al.,* 2018).

3.12. Ursolic acid

Ursolic acid is a triterpenoid antioxidant compound, and found in herbal species, like rosemary and basil plants. Its plays a significant role in exhibiting pro-apoptotic effects on colorectal cancer (HCT116) cell line by reducing the level of pro-inflammatory NF-kB cytokine, pro-metastatic MMP-9 matrix metalloprotease and survival effectors Bcl-2 (Kim *et al.,* 2015; Mu *et al.,* 2018).

3.13. β-elemene

β-elemene, a sesquiterpene is isolated from *Curcuma wenyujin* (Liu *et al.,* 2011) has a wide range of effects against the drug-resistant tumors. β-elemene induces apoptosis and cell death, attenuate angiogenesis and upregulates the E3 ubiquitin ligases in gastric cancer of humans, and also restrain the proliferation of VEGF by down regulating expression of Akt phosphorylation and CD34, suppressing PI3K/Akt/mTOR, MAPK and pathway (Jiang *et al.,* 2016; Jiang *et al.,*2017).

3.14. Lycopene

Lycopene is a bright red pigment found in tomatoes, watermelons, red papayas and red carrots. It plays an important role in down-regulating Erk and Bcl-2 proteins by targeting PI3K/Akt pathway in pancreatic and stomach cancer (Kim *et al.,* 2015). It can also restrict the invasion, metastasis and proliferation of active NF-kB and JNK in human SW480 colorectal cancer, causing inflammation and suppression of COX-2, iNOS IL-1b, IL-6, and TNF-α (Cha *et al.,* 2017).

3.15. Gingerol

Gingerol is extracted from fresh rhizome of *Zingiber officinale* possess anticancer properties against breast, ovarian, pancreas and colon cancers. It is responsible for NF-kB nuclear translocation and IkBa phosphorylation *via* suppressing the expression of down-regulated iNOS and TNF-alpha (Oyagbemi *et al.,* 2010; Meng *et al.,* 2018).

3.16. Crocetin (Saffron)

Crocus sativus L. (Saffron) is rich with many potent anticancer compounds *viz.,* carotenoids, crocin, crocetin, and safranal (Pang *et al.,* 2014). It is traded as a promising anticancer agent against human lung, liver, skin, pancreatic, colorectal and breast cancers. It can also inhibits iNOS, COX-2 enzymes, reduced serum level IL-β, TNF-α, cyclin B, cyclin A and cdk2, regulate the expression of caspase-3, 8 and 9, upregulation of Bax/Bcl-2 ratio and down regulation of MMP-2 and MMP-9 expression (Hoshyar and Mollaei, 2017).

3.17. Capsaicin

Capsaicin, isolated from the red pepper possess anticancer, antimutagenic, antimetastatic, anti-angiogenic and chemo preventive functions against pancreatic, prostatic, liver, skin, leukemia, lung, bladder, colon, and endothelial cells (Kim and Moon, 2004; Clark and Lee, 2016). It can induce apoptosis in presence of p53 gene product and breast cancer apoptosis by stimulating ROS and Rac1 signaling pathways *via* p38 and c-Jun N-terminal protein kinase-1 proteins (Sarkar *et al.,* 2015).

3.18. Combretastatins

The combretastatins are isolated from *Combretum caffrum* (Combretaeae) and *Terminalia bellerica* fruit that prevent angiogenesis in tumor. Combretastatins and its derivatives are developed by National Cancer Institute (USA) has collaborated with botanical Research Institute of South Africa (Pretoria) as a potent anticancer agent. Combretastatins (A-4 CA4) is efficient against leukemia, lung cancer and colon cancers (Lauritano *et al.,* 2016; Kumar *et al.,* 2018).

3.19. Berberine

Berberine is found in the root and rhizome of *Tinospora cordifolia*, *Berberis vulgaris*, *Berberis aquifolium* and *Rhizoma coptidis* (Mantena *et al.,* 2006). Berberine plays a significant role in inducing cell cycle arrest and apoptosis in liver, breast and colorectal cancer, activates p21, p53, caspase-3 and caspase-9 and inhibits c-IAP1and Bcl-2 proteins (Xu and Zhang, 2013; Mao *et al.,* 2018).

3.20. Ellipticine

Ellipticine (topoisomerase II inhibitor) along with isoreserpiline are extracted from the stem, bark, leaf and root of *Bleekeria vitensis* and *Ochrosia elliptica*. This compound can interact with DNA and inhibits topoisomerase II in order to prevent proliferation (Stiborova *et al.,* 2015). Derivatives of ellipticine such as N-2-(diethylaminoethyl)–9–hydroxyellipticinium chloride, 2-N-methyl 9-hydroxyellipticine are used for the treatment of ependymoblastoma, leukemia, myeloma, melanoma, breast and colon cancer (Kizek *et al.,* 2012; Isah, 2016). It also used to inhibit p53 protein phosphorylation and CDK2 kinase in human lung and colon cancer.

3.21. Colchicine

Colchicine is a bioactive compound isolated from *Colchicum autumnale* (Colchicaceae), and used in the treatment of some diseases like crystal arthritis, cirrhosis, gout, etc. It stabilizes microtubule formation, induces apoptosis and permanently binds to tubulin (Negia *et al.,* 2015). Semi-synthetic derivatives of colchicines like colchicinamide, deacetylcolchicine, etc., are used for the treatment of breast, central nervous system, chronic granulocytic leukemia, melanoma and colorectal cancer with less toxicity (Xie and Zhou, 2017).

3.22. Camptothecin derivatives

Camptothecin, a plant derived phytochemical is isolated from *Camptotheca acuminata* (Nyssaceae). It is a clinically-active chemotherapeutic agent and possesses the potential activity of inhibiting topoisomerase I in several types of cancers (Kim *et al.,* 2015). Researches have suggested that the derivatives of Camptothecins like topotecan (hycamtin) and irinotecan are very effective and hence, are widely used to treat ovarian, lung and colorectal cancer (Rahier *et al.,* 2005; Fang *et al.,* 2018).

4. STRATEGIES FOR THE DEVELOPMENT OF ANTICANCER PHYTOCHEMICALS

The therapeutic potential of medicinal plants depends on quality and quantity of active phytochemicals present in them, but it varies with geographical location, age, plant parts or climate. Therefore, extensive researches are still on process in order to achieve more effective bioactive phytochemicals. The process of extracting phytochemicals from a mixture of compounds involves the combinatorial chemistry, isolation assays and bioassay-fractionation. Natural extracts from plants with a confirmed biological activity are fractionated using suitable matrices such as Superdex, Sephadex, Silica, etc., and various analytical techniques, such as mass spectrometry, nuclear magnetic resonance, high performance liquid chromatography, thin layer chromatography, fourier transform infra-red spectrophotometer, etc., are used for separation of bioactive compounds. Furthermore, different dyeing agents such as vanillin sulfuric acid are used in the detection of natural compounds. Subsequently, the purified phytochemicals are examined using *in-vitro* or *in-vivo* assays, and finally tested in clinical trials for the development of future effective anticancer drugs.

5. CONCLUSIONS AND FUTURE PERSPECTIVES

Since the dawn of human civilization, medicinal plants have been considered to be the best resource for curing various dreaded diseases. Cancer is one of the major problems in both developing and developed countries in the present days. Chemotherapy and radiation therapy causes various side effects; therefore there is a requirement for an alternative way to treat cancer. Plant-derived bioactive compounds have contributed greatly to the progress of oncology development and to clinical practice. The growing incidence of cancer and high cost, limitations in the conventional therapy and high toxicity of present anticancer drugs has created a challenge to the researchers to develop an alternative, eco-friendly and cost-effective strategy in a greener way. Plant-derived bioactive compound are expected to revolutionize cancer treatment in the next decade. Potential anticancer compounds should be further researched in clinical trials on different models for their effectiveness and toxicological documentation. Various plants like *Terminalia chebula, Moringa oleifera, Tinospora cordifolia Withania somnifera* (Ashwagandha), *Oroxylum indicum* etc. possess good immuno-modulatory and antioxidant properties leading to anticancer activity. However, extensive research work should be carried out on these medicinal plants and their compounds from isolation to anticancer activity evaluation, and their possible applications in curing other diseases. Further, toxicological studies and particularly, genotoxic profile studies of these phytocompounds against a wide range of cancers should be encouraged in future considering both *in-vitro* or *in-vivo* approaches. Moreover, the mechanism of the anticancer role has not yet been fully elucidated for many plants and needs better understanding to explore the molecular mechanism of plants based compounds in order to determine the potency of gene expression, and defective cancer causing proteins, and to identify the novel cancer biomarkers. Thus, by identifying all factors and pivotal genes related with cancer, a comprehensive map can be formed to in order to treat and reduce the risk of cancer in the future. Hence, from this chapter it can be concluded that natural products offer as a significant source of metabolites possessing high potential to decrease the growth of cancer, and hence, can be used as adjuvant with cancer treatments.

REFERENCES

Afify AE, Fayed SA, Shalaby EA, El-Shemy HA. *Syzygium cumini* (Pomposia) active principles exhibit potent anticancer and antioxidant activities. African Journal of Pharmacy and Pharmacology. 2011; 5(7): 948-56.

Al Sinani SS, Eltayeb EA, Coomber BL, Adham SA. Solamargine triggers cellular necrosis selectively in different types of human melanoma cancer cells through extrinsic lysosomal mitochondrial death pathway. Cancer Cell International. 2016; 16(1): 11.

Ali I, Braun DP. Resveratrol enhances mitomycin C-mediated suppression of human colorectal cancer cell proliferation by up-regulation of p21WAF1/CIP1. Anticancer Research. 2014; 34: 5439-46.

Almagro L, Fernandez-Perez F, Pedreno MA. Indole alkaloids from *Catharanthus roseus*: Amin S, Barkatullah HK. Pharmacology of *Xanthium* species. A review. The Journal of Phytopharmacology. 2016; 5: 126-127.

Apostolou A, Stagos D, Galitsiou E, Spyrou A, Haroutounian S, Portesis N, Trizoglou I, Hayes AW, Tsatsakis AM, Kouretas D. Assessment of polyphenolic content, antioxidant activity, protection against ROS-induced DNA damage and anticancer activity of *Vitis vinifera* stem extracts. Food and Chemical Toxicology. 2013; 61: 60–68.

Appendino G, Chianese G, Taglialatela-Scafati O. Cannabinoids: Occurrence and medicinal chemistry. Current Medicinal Chemistry. 2011; 18(7): 1085-99.

Atkinson JM, Falconer RA, Edwards DR, Pennington CJ, Siller CS, Shnyder SD, Bibby MC, Patterson LH, Loadman PM, Gill JH. Development of a novel tumor-targeted vascular disrupting agent activated by membrane-type matrix metalloproteinases. Cancer Research. 2010; 70(17): 6902-12.

Awale S, Linn TZ, Li F, Tezuka Y, Myint A, Tomida A, Yamori T, Esumi H, Kadota S. Identification of chrysoplenetin from *Vitex negundo* as a potential cytotoxic agent against PANC1 and a panel of 39 human cancer cell lines (JFCR 39). Phytotherapy Research. 2011; 25(12): 1770-5.

Ayoob I, Hazari YM, Lone SH, Khuroo MA, Fazili KM, Bhat KA. Phytochemical and cytotoxic evaluation of *Peganum harmala*: Structure activity relationship studies of harmine. Chemistry Select. 2017; 2(10): 2965-8.

Aziz A, Yusran M, Omar AR, Subramani T, Yeap SK, Ho WY, Ismail NH, Ahmad S, Alitheen NB. Damnacanthal is a potent inducer of apoptosis with anticancer activity by stimulating p53 and p21 genes in MCF7 breast cancer cells. Oncology Letters. 2014; 7(5): 1479-84.

Azmi AS, Bhat SH, Hanif S, Hadi SM. Plant polyphenols mobilize endogenous copper in human peripheral lymphocytes leading to oxidative DNA breakage: A putative mechanism for anticancer Properties. Federations of European Biochemical Societies Letters. 2006; 580:533–538.

Bao MF, Yan JM, Cheng GG, Li XY, Liu YP, Li Y, Cai XH, Luo XD. Cytotoxic indole alkaloids from *Tabernaemontana divaricata*. Journal of Natural Products. 2013, 76(8), 1406-12.

Barbuti AM, Chen ZS. Paclitaxel through the ages of anticancer therapy: Exploring its role in chemoresistance and radiation therapy. Cancers. 2015;7(4):2360-2371.

Bauer D, Redmon N, Mazzio E, Soliman KF. Apigenin inhibits TNFá/IL-1á-induced CCL2 release through IKBK-epsilon signaling in MDA-MB-231 human breast cancer cells. Plos One. 2017; 12(4): e0175558.

Beg MA, Teotia UV, Farooq S. *In vitro* antibacterial and anti-cancer activity of *Ziziphus*. Journal of Medicinal Plants. 2016; 4(5): 230-233.

Benarba B, Meddah B. Ethnobotanical study, antifungal activity, phytochemical screening and total phenolic content of Algerian *Aristolochia longa*. Journal of Intercultural Ethnopharmacology. 2014; 3(4): 150.

Bernabeu E, Cagel M, Lagomarsino E, Moretton M, Chiappetta DA. Paclitaxel: What has been done and the challenges remain ahead. International Journal of Pharmaceutics. 2017; 526(1-2): 474-495.

Bhandari J, Muhammad B, Thapa P, Shrestha BG. Study of phytochemical, anti-microbial, anti-oxidant, and anti-cancer properties of *Allium wallichii*. BMC Complementary and Alternative Medicine. 2017; 17(1): 102.

Bhouri W, Boubaker J, Skandrani I, Ghedira K, Ghedira LC. Investigation of the apoptotic way induced by digallic acid in human lymphoblastoid TK6 cells. Cancer Cell International. 2012; 12(1): 26.

Biba VS, Jeba MP, Remani P. Differential effects of *Annona squamosa* seed extracts: Antioxidant, antibacterial, cytotoxic and apoptotic study. International Journal of Pharma and Biosciences. 2013; 4: 899-907.

Bishop GJ, Koncz C. Brassionsteroids and Plant Steroid Hormone Signaling. The Plant Cell. 2002;14(suppl 1):S97-110.

Brahmachari G, Gorai D, Roy R. *Argemone mexicana*: Chemical and pharmacological aspects. Revista Brasileira de Farmacognosia. 2013; 23(3): 559-67.

Caccialupi P, Ceci LR, Siciliano RA, Pignone D, Clemente A, Sonnante G. Bowman-Birk inhibitors in lentil: Heterologous expression, functional characterisation and anti-proliferative properties in human colon cancer cells. Food Chemistry. 2010: 120(4): 1058-66.

Caruso M, Colombo AL, Fedeli L, Pavesi A, Quaroni S, Saracchi M, Ventrella G. Isolation of endophytic fungi and actinomycetes taxane producers. Annals of Microbiology. 2000; 50(1): 3-14.

Cascao R, Fonseca JE, Moita LF. Celastrol: A spectrum of treatment opportunities in chronic diseases. Frontiers in Medicine. 2017; 4: 69.

Cha JH, Kim WK, Ha AW, Kim MH, Chang MJ. Anti-inflammatory effect of lycopene in SW480 human colorectal cancer cells. Nutrition Research and Practice. 2017; 11(2): 90-6.

Chan LL, George S, Ahmad I, Gosangari SL, Abbasi A, Cunningham BT, Watkin KL. Cytotoxicity effects of *Amoora rohituka* and chittagonga on breast and pancreatic cancer cells. Evidence-Based Complementary and Alternative Medicine. 2011; 2011: 1-8.

Cheah KY, Howarth GS, Bindon KA, Kennedy JA, Bastian SE. Low molecular weight procyanidins from grape seeds enhance the impact of 5-Fluorouracil chemotherapy on Caco-2 human colon cancer cells. PLOS Pathogens. 2014; 9: e98921.

Checker R, Sharma D, Sandur SK, Subrahmanyam G, Krishnan S, Poduval TB, Sainis KB. Plumbagin inhibits proliferative and inflammatory responses of T cells independent of ROS generation but by modulating intracellular thiols. Journal of Cellular Biochemistry. 2010; 110(5): 1082-93.

Chen J, Mu Q, Li X, Yin X, Yu M, Jin J, Li C, Zhou Y, Zhou J, Suo S, Lu D. Homoharringtonine targets Smad3 and TGF-â pathway to inhibit the proliferation of acute myeloid leukemia cells. Oncotarget. 2017; 8(25): 40318.

Chen XJ, Zhang XJ, Shui YM, Wan JB, Gao JL. Anticancer activities of protopanaxadiol- and protopanaxatriol-type ginsenosides and their metabolites. Evidence-Based Complementary and Alternative Medicine. 2016; 2016: 1-19.

Chen YC, Yang LL, Lee TJ. Oroxylin A inhibition of lipopolysaccharide-induced iNOS and COX-2 gene expression *via* suppression of nuclear factor-êB activation. Biochemical Pharmacology. 2000; 59(11): 1445-57.

Choedon T, Shukla SK, Kumar V. Chemopreventive and anti-cancer properties of the aqueous extract of flowers of *Butea monosperma*. Journal of Ethnopharmacology. 2010; 129(2): 208-13.

Choi JY, Hong WG, Cho JH, Kim EM, Kim J, Jung CH, Hwang SG, Um HD, Park JK. Podophyllotoxin acetate triggers anticancer effects against non-small cell lung cancer cells by promoting cell death via cell cycle arrest, ER stress and autophagy. International Journal of Oncology. 2015; 47(4): 1257-65.

Clardy J, Walsh C. Lessons from natural molecules. Nature. 2004; 432: 829-837.

Clark R, Lee SH. Anticancer properties of capsaicin against human cancer. Anticancer Research. 2016; 36(3): 837-43.

Colombo V, Lupi M, Falcetta F, Forestieri D, D'Incalci M, Ubezio P. Chemotherapeutic activity of silymarin combined with doxorubicin or paclitaxel in sensitive and multidrug-resistant colon cancer cells. Cancer Chemotherapy and Pharmacology. 2011; 67(2): 369-79.

Cragg GM, Newman DJ. Plants as a source of anti-cancer agents. Journal of Ethnopharmacology. 2005; 100(1-2); 72-79.

Csupor-Loffler B, Hajdu Z, Zupko I, Molnar J, Forgo P, Vasas A, Kele Z, Hohmann J. Antiproliferative constituents of the roots of *Conyza canadensis*. Planta Medica. 2011; 77(11): 1183-1188.

Dadgar S, Ramjan Z, Floriano WB. Paclitaxel is an inhibitor and its boron dipyrromethene derivative is a fluorescent recognition agent for botulinum neurotoxin subtype A. Journal of Medicinal Chemistry. 2013; 56(7): 2791-803.

Das I, Das S, Saha T. Saffron suppresses oxidative stress in DMBA-induced skin carcinoma: A histopathological study. Acta Histochemica. 2010; 112(4): 317-327.

Das M, Manna K. Chalcone scaffold in anticancer armamentarium: A molecular insight. Journal of Toxicology. 2016; 2016: 1-14.

De Bono JS, Oudard S, Ozguroglu M, Hansen S, Machiels JP, Kocak I, Gravis G, Bodrogi I, Mackenzie MJ, Shen L, Roessner M. Prednisone plus cabazitaxel or mitoxantrone for metastatic castration-resistant prostate cancer progressing after docetaxel treatment: A randomised open-label trial. The Lancet. 2010; 376(9747): 1147-54.

Delgoda R, Murray JE. Evolutionary perspectives on the role of plant secondary metabolites. In Pharmacognosy: Fundamentals, Applications and Strategies, 1st ed.; Badal, S., Delgoda, R., (*eds.*); Academic Press: Oxoford, UK, 2017, 93–100.

Du GJ, Wang CZ, Qi LW, Zhang ZY, Calway T, He TC, Du W, Yuan CS. The synergistic apoptotic interaction of panaxadiol and epigallocatechin gallate in human colorectal cancer cells. Phytotherapy Research. 2013; 27(2): 272-7.

Efferth T. From ancient herb to versatile, modern drug: *Artemisia annua* and artemisinin for cancer therapy. In Seminars in Cancer Biology. 2017.

Ehrlich A, Booher S, Becerra Y, Borris DL, Figg WD, Turner ML, Blauvelt A. Micellar paclitaxel improves severe psoriasis in a prospective phase II pilot study. Journal of the American Academy of Dermatology. 2004; 50(4): 533-40.

Einbond LS, Soffritti M, Esposti DD, Park T, Cruz E, Su T, Wu HA, Wang X, Zhang YJ, Ham J, Goldberg IJ. Actein activates stress and statin associated responses and is bioavailable in SpragueDawley rats. Fundamental and Clinical Pharmacology. 2009; 23(3): 311-21.

El-Shemy HA, Aboul-Soud MA, Nassr-Allah AA, Aboul-Enein KM, Kabash A, Yagi A. Antitumor properties and modulation of antioxidant enzymes' activity by Aloe vera leaf active principles isolated *via* supercritical carbon dioxide extraction. Current Medicinal Chemistry. 2010; 17(2): 129-38.

Evans AE, Farber S, Brunet S, Mariano PJ. Vincristine in the treatment of acute leukemia in children. Cancer. 1963; 16(10): 1302-6.

Fang S, Hou Y, Ling L, Wang D, Ismail M, Du Y, Zhang Y, Yao C, Li X. Dimeric camptothecin derived phospholipid assembled liposomes with high drug loading for cancer therapy. Colloids and Surfaces B: Biointerfaces. 2018; 166:235-244.

Formagio AS, Vieira MC, Volobuff CR, Silva MS, Matos AI, Cardoso CA, Foglio MA, Carvalho JE. *In vitro* biological screening of the anticholinesterase and antiproliferative activities of medicinal plants belonging to Annonaceae. Brazilian Journal of Medical and Biological Research. 2015; 48(4): 308-315.

Ganai AA, Farooqi H. Bioactivity of genistein: A review of *in vitro* and *in vivo* studies. Biomedicine and Pharmacotherapy. 2015; 76: 30-38.

Gandhi V, Plunkett W, Cortes JE. Omacetaxine: A protein translation inhibitor for treatment of chronic myelogenous leukemia. Clinical Cancer Research. 2014; 20(7): 1735-40.

Ganesan A. Recent developments in combinatorial organic synthesis. Drug Discovery Today. 2002; 7: 47-55.

Gao C, Zhou Y, Jiang Z, Zhao Y, Zhang D, Cong X, Cao R, Li H, Tian W. Cytotoxic and chemosensitization effects of Scutellarin from traditional Chinese herb *Scutellaria altissima* L. in human prostate cancer cells. Oncology Reports. 2017; 38(3): 1491-9.

Gao JL, Lv GY, He BC, Zhang BQ, Zhang H, Wang N, Wang CZ, Du W, Yuan CS, He TC. Ginseng saponin metabolite 20 (S)-protopanaxadiol inhibits tumor growth by targeting multiple cancer signaling pathways. Oncology Reports. 2013; 30(1): 292-8.

Garg P, Deep A. Anti-cancer potential of boswellic acid: A mini review. Hygeia: Journal for Drugs and Medicines. 2015; 7(2): 18-27.

Ghasemzadeh A, Jaafar HZ, Rahmat A. Optimization protocol for the extraction of 6-gingerol and 6-shogaol from *Zingiber officinale var. rubrum* Theilade and improving antioxidant and anticancer activity using response surface methodology. BMC Complementary and Alternative Medicine. 2015; 15(1): 258.

Ghosh T, Maity TK, Singh J. Evaluation of antitumor activity of stigmasterol, a constituent isolated from *Bacopa monnieri* Linn aerial parts against Ehrlich Ascites Carcinoma in mice. Oriental Pharmacy and Experimental Medicine. 2011; 11(1): 41-9.

Gill KK, Kamal MM, Kaddoumi A, Nazzal S. EGFR targeted delivery of paclitaxel and parthenolide co-loaded in PEG-Phospholipid micelles enhance cytotoxicity and cellular uptake in non-small cell lung cancer cells. Journal of Drug Delivery Science and Technology. 2016; 36: 150-5.

Guo Z. The modification of natural products for medical use. Acta Pharmaceutica Sinica B. 2017 Yao H, Liu J, Xu S, Zhu Z, Xu J. The structural modification of natural products for novel drug discovery. Expert Opinion on Drug Discovery. 2017; 12(2); 121-40.

Gupta SC, Tyagi AK, Deshmukh-Taskar P, Hinojosa M, Prasad S, Aggarwal BB. Downregulation of tumor necrosis factor and other proinflammatory biomarkers by polyphenols. Archives of Biochemistry and Biophysics. 2014; 559: 91–99.

Guruvayoorappan C, Kuttan G. Immunomodulatory and antitumor activity of *Biophytum sensitivum* extract. Asian Pacific Journal of Cancer Prevention. 2007; 8(1): 27-32.

Gutierrez-del-Rio I, Villar CJ, Lombo F. Therapeutic uses of kaempferol: Anticancer and antiinflammatory activity. *In*: Biosynthesis, Food Sources and Therapeutic Uses. 2016; 71-101.

Ha J, Zhao L, Zhao Q, Yao J, Zhu BB, Lu N, Ke X, Yang HY, Li Z, You QD, Guo QL. Oroxylin A improves the sensitivity of HT-29 human colon cancer cells to 5-FU through modulation of the COX-2 signaling pathway. Biochemistry and Cell Biology. 2012; 90(4): 521-31.

Hahm ER, Moura MB, Kelley EE, Van Houten B, Shiva S, Singh SV. Withaferin A-induced apoptosis in human breast cancer cells is mediated by reactive oxygen species. Plos One. 2011; 6(8): e23354.

Heidari M, Heidari-Vala H, Sadeghi MR, Akhondi MM. The inductive effects of *Centella asiatica* on rat spermatogenic cell apoptosis *in vivo*. Journal of Natural Medicines. 2012; 66(2): 271-8.

Hirata T, Fujii M, Akita K, Yanaka N, Ogawa K, Kuroyanagi M, Hongo D. Identification and physiological evaluation of the components from Citrus fruits as potential drugs for anti-corpulence and anticancer. Bioorganic and Medicinal Chemistry. 2009; 17(1): 25-8.

Hoshyar R, Mollaei H. A comprehensive review on anticancer mechanisms of the main carotenoid of saffron, crocin. Journal of Pharmacy and Pharmacology. 2017; 1: 1-9.

Howat S, Park B, Oh IS, Jin YW, Lee EK, Loake GJ. Paclitaxel: Biosynthesis, production and future prospects. New Biotechnology. 2014; 31(3): 242-5.

Hu M, Xu L, Yin L, Qi Y, Li H, Xu Y, Han X, Peng J, Wan X. Cytotoxicity of dioscin in human gastric carcinoma cells through death receptor and mitochondrial pathways. Journal of Applied Toxicology. 2013; 33(8): 712-22.

Iqbal J, Abbasi BA, Mahmood T, Kanwal S, Ali B, Khalil AT. Plant-derived anticancer agents: A green anticancer approach. Asian Pacific Journal of Tropical Biomedicine. 2017; 7(12): 1129-1150

Isah T. Anticancer alkaloids from trees: Development into drugs. Pharmacognosy Reviews. 2016; 10(20): 90.

Jaradat NA, Al-Ramahi R, Zaid AN, Ayesh OI, Eid AM. Ethnopharmacological survey of herbal remedies used for treatment of various types of cancer and their methods of preparations in the West Bank-Palestine. BMC Complementary and Alternative Medicine. 2016; 16(1): 93.

Jiang Z, Jacob JA, Loganathachetti DS, Nainangu P, Chen B. β-Elemene: mechanistic studies on cancer cell interaction and its chemosensitization effect. Frontiers in Pharmacology. 2017; 8: 105.

Jung SK, Lee MH, Kim JE, Singh P, Lee SY, Jeong CH, Lim TG, Chen H, Chi YI, Kundu JK, Lee NH. Isoliquiritigenin induces apoptosis and inhibits xenograft tumor growth of human lung cancer cells by targeting both wild type and L858R/T790M mutant EGFR. Journal of Biological Chemistry. 2014; 289(52): 35839-48.

Kabera JN, Semana E, Mussa AR, He X. Plant secondary metabolites: Biosynthesis, classification, function and pharmacological properties. Journal of Pharmacy and Pharmacology. 2014; 2: 377–392.

Kantarjian HM, O'brien S, Cortes J. Homoharringtonine/omacetaxine mepesuccinate: The long and winding road to food and drug administration approval. Clinical Lymphoma, Myeloma and Leukemia. 2013; 13(5): 530-3.

Karmakar S, Roy Choudhury S, L Banik N, K Ray S. Molecular mechanisms of anti-cancer action of garlic compounds in neuroblastoma. Anti-Cancer Agents in Medicinal Chemistry (Formerly Current Medicinal Chemistry-Anti-Cancer Agents). 2011; 11(4): 398-407.

Kasala ER, Bodduluru LN, Madana RM, Gogoi R, Barua CC. Chemopreventive and therapeutic potential of chrysin in cancer: Mechanistic perspectives. Toxicology Letters. 2015; 233(2): 214-25.

Kaur R, Kapoor K, Kaur H. Plants as a source of anticancer agents. Journal of Natural Product and Plant Resources. 2011; 1(1): 119-24.

Kaushik R, Narayanan P, Vasudevan V, Muthukumaran G, Usha A. Nutrient composition of cultivated stevia leaves and the influence of polyphenols and plant pigments on sensory and antioxidant properties of leaf extracts. Journal of Food Science and Technology. 2010; 47(1): 27-33.

Keglevich P, Hazai L, Kalaus G, Szántay C. Modifications on the basic skeletons of vinblastine and vincristine. Molecules. 2012; 17(5): 5893-914.

Khan N, Afaq F, Khusro FH, Adhami VM, Suh Y, Mukhtar H. Dual inhibition of PI3K/AKT and mTOR signaling in human non-small cell lung cancer cells by a dietary flavonoid fisetin. International Journal of Cancer. Journal International du Cancer. 2012; 130(7): 1695.

Kim JE, Kwon JY, Seo SK, Son JE, Jung SK, Min SY, Hwang MK, Heo YS, Lee KW, Lee HJ. Cyanidin suppresses ultraviolet B-induced COX-2 expression in epidermal cells by targeting MKK4, MEK1, and Raf-1. Biochemical Pharmacology. 2010; 79(10): 1473-82.

Kim S, Moon A. Capsaicin-lnduced apoptosis of h-ras-transformed human breast epithelial cells is rac-dependent *via* ros generation. Archives of Pharmaceutical Research. 2004; 27(8): 845-9.

Kim SH, Kaplan JA, Sun Y, Shieh A, Sun HL, Croce CM, Grinstaff MW, Parquette JR. The Self-Assembly of Anticancer Camptothecin–Dipeptide Nanotubes: A Minimalistic and High Drug Loading Approach to Increased Efficacy. Chemistry-A European Journal. 2015; 21(1): 101-5.

Kizek R, Adam V, Hrabeta J, Eckschlager T, Smutny S, Burda JV, Frei E, Stiborova M. Anthracyclines and ellipticines as DNA-damaging anticancer drugs: Recent advances. Pharmacology and Therapeutics. 2012; 133(1): 26-39.

Krol SK, Kie³bus M, Rivero-Müller A, Stepulak A. Comprehensive review on betulin as a potent anticancer agent. BioMed Research International. 2015;2015: 1-11.

Kumar B, Sharma P, Gupta VP, Khullar M, Singh S, Dogra N, Kumar V. Synthesis and biological evaluation of pyrimidine bridged combretastatin derivatives as potential anticancer agents and mechanistic studies. Bioorganic Chemistry. 2018; 78: 130-40.

Kumari M, Pattnaik B, Rajan SY, Shrikant S, Surendra SU. EGCG-A Promis anti-cancer Phytochem. Annals of International Medical and Dental Research. 2017; 3(2): 8-10.

Lam SK, Ng TB. Novel galactonic acid-binding hexameric lectin from *Hibiscus mutabilis* seeds with antiproliferative and potent HIV-1 reverse transcriptase inhibitory activities. Acta Biochimica Polonica. 2009; 56(4): 649.

Lan L, Appelman C, Smith AR, Yu J, Larsen S, Marquez RT, Liu H, Wu X, Gao P, Roy A, Anbanandam A. Natural product (")gossypol inhibits colon cancer cell growth by targeting RNA binding protein Musashi 1. Molecular Oncology. 2015; 9(7): 1406-20.

Lanza A, Tava A, Catalano M, Ragona L, Singuaroli I, Della Cuna FS, Della Cuna GR. Effects of the *Medicago scutellata* trypsin inhibitor (MsTI) on cisplatin-induced cytotoxicity in human breast and cervical cancer cells. Anticancer Research. 2004; 24(1): 227-34.

Lauritano C, Andersen JH, Hansen E, Albrigtsen M, Escalera L, Esposito F, Helland K, Hanssen KO, Romano G, Ianora A. Bioactivity screening of microalgae for antioxidant, anti-inflammatory, anticancer, anti-diabetes, and antibacterial activities. Frontiers in Marine Science. 2016; 3: 68.

Lauritano H, Andersen JH, Hansen E, Albrigtsen M, Escalera L, Esposit F, Helland K, Hanssen K, Romano G, Lanora A. Bioactivity screening of microalgae for antioxidant, anti-inflammatory, anticancer, anti-diabetes, and antibacterial activities. Frontiers in Marine Science. 2016; 3: 68.

Lee HS, Cho HJ, Yu R, Lee KW, Chun HS, Park JH. Mechanisms underlying apoptosis-inducing effects of Kaempferol in HT-29 human colon cancer cells. International Journal of Molecular Sciences. 2014; 15(2): 2722-37.

Lee IC, Choi BY. Withaferin-A, a natural anticancer agent with pleitropic mechanisms of action. International Journal of Molecular Sciences. 2016; 17(3): 290.

Lee SJ, Lee JS, Lee E, Lim TG, Byun S. The ginsenoside metabolite compound K inhibits hormone-independent breast cancer through downregulation of cyclin D1. Journal of Functional Foods. 2018; 46: 159-66.

Leon IE, Cadavid-Vargas JF, Tiscornia I, Porro V, Castelli S, Katkar P, Desideri A, Bollati-Fogolin M, Etcheverry SB. Oxidovanadium (IV) complexes with chrysin and silibinin: anticancer activity and mechanisms of action in a human colon adenocarcinoma model. Journal of Biological Inorganic Chemistry. 2015; 20(7): 1175-91.

Leyva-Peralta MA, Robles-Zepeda RE, Garibay-Escobar A, Ruiz-Bustos E, Alvarez-Berber LP, Galvez-Ruiz JC. *In vitro* anti-proliferative activity of *Argemone gracilenta* and identification of some active components. BMC Complementary and Alternative Medicine. 2015; 15(1): 13.

Li JZ, Qing C, Chen CX, Hao XJ, Liu HY. Cytotoxicity of cardenolides and cardenolide glycosides from *Asclepias curassavica*. Bioorganic and Medicinal Chemistry Letters. 2009; 19(7): 1956-9.

Li M, Wei SY, Xu B, Guo W, Liu DL, Cui JR, Yao XS. Pro-apoptotic and microtubule-disassembly effects of ardisiacrispin (A+ B), triterpenoid saponins from *Ardisia crenata* on human hepatoma Bel-7402 cells. Journal of Asian Natural Products Research. 2008; 10(8): 729-36.

Lim DY, Park JH. Induction of p53 contributes to apoptosis of HCT-116 human colon cancer cells induced by the dietary compound fisetin. American Journal of Physiology-Gastrointestinal and Liver Physiology. 2009; 296(5): G1060-8.

Lim TK. Edible medicinal and non-medicinal plants. New York, NY, USA, Springer; 2012.

Lin X, Peng Z, Su C. Potential anti-cancer activities and mechanisms of costunolide and dehydrocostus lactone. International Journal of Molecular Sciences. 2015; 16(5): 10888-906.

Liu J, Zhang Y, Qu J, Xu L, Hou K, Zhang J, Qu X, Liu Y. β-Elemene-induced autophagy protects human gastric cancer cells from undergoing apoptosis. BMC Cancer. 2011; 11(1): 183.

Liu YQ, Tian J, Qian K, Zhao XB, Morris-Natschke SL, Yang L, Nan X, Tian X, Lee KH. Recent progress on C4 modified podophyllotoxin analogs as potent antitumor agents. Medicinal Research Reviews. 2015; 35(1): 1-62.

Lu S, Wang J. Homoharringtonine and omacetaxine for myeloid hematological malignancies. Journal of Hematology and Oncology. 2014; 7(1): 2.

Luo B, Wang J, Li X, Lu W, Yang J, Hu Y, Huang P, Wen S. New Mild and simple approach to isothiocyanates: A class of potent anticancer agents. Molecules. 2017; 22(6): 773.

Madhuri S, Pandey G. Some anticancer medicinal plants of foreign origin. Current Science. 2009;96(6):779-83.

Magee PJ, Owusu-Apenten R, McCann MJ, Gill CI, Rowland IR. Chickpea (*Cicer arietinum*) and other plant-derived protease inhibitor concentrates inhibit breast and prostate cancer cell proliferation *in vitro*. Nutrition and Cancer. 2012; 64(5): 741-8.

Mahata S, Maru S, Shukla S, Pandey A, Mugesh G, Das BC, Bharti AC. Anticancer property of *Bryophyllum pinnatum* (Lam.) Oken. leaf on human cervical cancer cells. BMC Complementary and Alternative Medicine. 2012; 12(1): 15.

Malikova J, Swaczynova J, Kolar Z, Strnad M. Anticancer and antiproliferative activity of natural brasinosteroids. Phtyochemistry. 2008; 69: 418–426.

Maneerat W, Tha-In S, Cheenpracha S, Prawat U, Laphookhieo S. New amides from the seeds of *Clausana lansium*. Journal of Medicinal Plants Research. 2011; 5(13): 2812-5.

Mantena SK, Sharma SD, Katiyar SK. Berberine. A natural product, induces G1-phase cell cycle arrest and caspase-3-dependent apoptosis in human prostate carcinoma cells. Molecular Cancer Therapeutics. 2006; 5: 296-308.

Mao L, Chen Q, Gong K, Xu X, Xie Y, Zhang W, Cao H, Hu T, Hong X, Zhan YY. Berberine decelerates glucose metabolism *via* suppression of mTOR-dependent HIF1α protein synthesis in colon cancer cells. Oncology Reports. 2018; 39(5): 2436-42.

Marin L, Miguelez EM, Villar CJ, Lombo F. Bioavailability of dietary polyphenols and gut microbiota metabolism: Antimicrobial properties. Biomed Research International. 2015; 2015: 1-18.

Mehdad A, Brumana G, Souza AA, Barbosa JA, Ventura MM, De Freitas S. A Bowman–Birk inhibitor induces apoptosis in human breast adenocarcinoma through mitochondrial impairment and oxidative damage following proteasome 20S inhibition. Cell Death Discovery. 2016; 2: 15067.

Meng B, Ii H, Qu W, Yuan H. Anticancer effects of gingerol in retinoblastoma cancer cells (RB355 Cell Line) are mediated *via* apoptosis induction, cell cycle arrest and upregulation of PI3K/Akt signaling pathway. Medical Science Monitor: International Medical Journal of Experimental and Clinical Research. 2018; 24: 1980-1987.

Min KJ, Nam JO, Kwon TK. Fisetin induces apoptosis through p53-mediated up-regulation of DR5 expression in human renal carcinoma caki cells. Molecules. 2017; 22(8): 1285.

Mishra S, Aeri V, Gaur PK, Jachak SM. Phytochemical, therapeutic, and ethnopharmacological overview for a traditionally important herb: *Boerhavia diffusa* Linn. Biomed Research International. 2014; 2014: 1-14.

Moore A, Pinkerton R. Vincristine: Can its therapeutic index be enhanced?. Pediatric Blood and Cancer. 2009; 53(7): 1180-7.

Morris J, Moseley VR, Cabang AB, Coleman K, Wei W, Garrett-Mayer E, Wargovich MJ. Reduction in promotor methylation utilizing EGCG (epigallocatechin-3-gallate) restores RXRα expression in human colon cancer cells. Oncotarget. 2016; 7(23): 35313.

Motta LB, Furlan CM, Santos DY, Salatino ML, Duarte-Almeida JM, Negri G, Carvalho JE, Ruiz AL, Cordeiro I, Salatino A. Constituents and antiproliferative activity of extracts from leaves of *Croton macrobothrys*. Revista Brasileira de Farmacognosia. 2011; 21(6): 972-7.

Mu D, Zhou G, Li J, Su B, Guo H. Ursolic acid activates the apoptosis of prostate cancer *via* ROCK/PTEN mediated mitochondrial translocation of cofilin-1. Oncology Letters. 2018; 15(3): 3202–3206.

Mu F, Yang L, Wang W, Luo M, Fu Y, Guo X, Zu Y. Negative-pressure cavitation extraction of four main vinca alkaloids from *Catharanthus roseus* leaves. Molecules 2012; 17: 8742–8752.

Mukhija M, Singh MP, Dhar KL, Kalia AN. Cytotoxic and antioxidant activity of *Zanthoxylum alatum* stem bark and its flavonoid constituents. Journal of Pharmacognosy and Phytochemistry. 2015; 4(4): 86.

Nakahata AM, Mayer B, Ries C, de Paula CA, Karow M, Neth P, Sampaio MU, Jochum M, Oliva ML. The effects of a plant proteinase inhibitor from *Enterolobium contortisiliquum* on human tumor cell lines. Biological Chemistry. 2011; 392(4): 327-36.

Nehate C, Jain S, Saneja A, Khare V, Alam N, Dhar Dubey R, N Gupta P. Paclitaxel formulations: Challenges and novel delivery options. Current Drug Delivery. 2014; 11(6): 666-86.

Newman DJ, Cragg GM. Natural products as sources of new drugs from 1981 to 2014. Journal of Natural Products. 2016; 79(3): 629-61.

Ng TB, Lam YW, Wang H. Calcaelin, a new protein with translation-inhibiting, antiproliferative and antimitogenic activities from the mosaic puffball mushroom *Calvatia caelata*. Planta Medica. 2003; 69(03): 212-7.

Ngai PH, Ng TB. A ribonuclease with antimicrobial, antimitogenic and antiproliferative activities from the edible mushroom *Pleurotus sajor-caju*. Peptides. 2004; 25(1): 11-7.

Ochwang'i DO, Kimwele CN, Oduma JA, Gathumbi PK, Mbaria JM, Kiama SG. Medicinal plants used in treatment and management of cancer in Kakamega County, Kenya. Journal of Ethnopharmacology. 2014; 151(3): 1040-55.

Ogunwande IA, Walker TM, Bansal A, Setzer WN, Essien EE. Essential oil constituents and biological activities of *Peristrophe bicalyculata* and *Borreria verticillata*. Natural Product Communications. 2010; 5(11): 1815-8.

Ooko E, Kadioglu O, Greten HJ, Efferth T. Pharmacogenomic characterization and isobologram analysis of the combination of ascorbic acid and curcumin-two main metabolites of *Curcuma longa*-in cancer cells. Frontiers in Pharmacology. 2017; 8:38.

Osman NH, Said UZ, El-Waseef AM, Ahmed ES. Luteolin supplementation adjacent to aspirin treatment reduced dimethylhydrazine-induced experimental colon carcinogenesis in rats. Tumor Biology. 2015; 36(2): 1179-90.

Oyagbemi AA, Saba AB, Azeez OI. Capsaicin: A novel chemopreventive molecule and its underlying molecular mechanisms of action. Indian Journal of Cancer. 2010; 47(1): 53.

Pahari P, Saikia UP, Das TP, Damodaran C, Rohr J. Synthesis of Psoralidin derivatives and their anticancer activity: First synthesis of Lespeflorin I1. Tetrahedron. 2016; 72(23): 3324-34.

Pang SQ, Wang GQ, Lin JS, Diao Y, Xu RA. Cytotoxic activity of the alkaloids from *Broussonetia papyrifera* fruits. Pharmaceutical Biology. 2014; 52(10): 1315-9.

Parveen S, Jan U, Kamili A. Importance of Himalayan medicinal plants and their conservation strategies. Australian Journal of Herbal Medicine. 2013; 25(2): 63.

Patel KR, Brown VA, Jones DJ, Britton RG, Hemingway D, Miller AS, West KP, Booth TD, Perloff M, Crowell JA, Brenner DE. Clinical pharmacology of resveratrol and its metabolites in colorectal cancer patients. Cancer Research. 2010; 70(19): 7392-9.

Peiro G, Ortiz-Martinez F, Gallardo A, Perez-Balaguer A, Sanchez-Paya J, Ponce JJ, Tibau A, Lopez-Vilaro L, Escuin D, Adrover E, Barnadas A. Src, a potential target for overcoming trastuzumab resistance in HER2-positive breast carcinoma. British Journal of Cancer. 2014; 111(4): 689.

Pereira LP, Silva P, Duarte M, Rodrigues L, Duarte CM, Albuquerque C, Serra AT. Targeting colorectal cancer proliferation, stemness and metastatic potential using brassicaceae extracts enriched in isothiocyanates: A 3D cell model-based study. Nutrients. 2017; 9(4): 368.

Perrone D, Ardito F, Giannatempo G, Dioguardi M, Troiano G, Lo Russo L, De Lillo A, Laino L, Lo Muzio L. Biological and therapeutic activities, and anticancer properties of curcumin. Experimental and Therapeutic Medicine. 2015; 10(5): 1615-23.

Pierpaoli E, Damiani E, Orlando F, Lucarini G, Bartozzi B, Lombardi P, Salvatore C, Geroni C, Donati A, Provinciali M. Antiangiogenic and antitumor activities of berberine derivative NAX014 compound in a transgenic murine model of HER2/neu-positive mammary carcinoma. Carcinogenesis. 2015; 36(10): 1169-79.

Pledgie-Tracy A, Sobolewski MD, Davidson NE. Sulforaphane induces cell type-specific apoptosis in human breast cancer cell lines. Molecular Cancer Therapeutics. 2007; 6(3): 1013–1021.

Pons DG, Nadal-Serrano M, Torrens-Mas M, Valle A, Oliver J, Roca P. UCP2 inhibition sensitizes breast cancer cells to therapeutic agents by increasing oxidative stress. Free Radical Biology and Medicine. 2015; 86: 67-77.

Preethi R, Padma PR. Biosynthesis and bioactivity of silver nanobioconjugates from grape (*Vitis vinifera*) seeds and its active component resveratrol. International Journal of Pharmaceutical Sciences and Research. 2016; 7(10): 4253.

Rahier NJ, Thomas CJ, Hecht SM. Camptothecin and its analogs. In: Cragg GM, Kingston DGI, New DG, editors. Anticancer agents from natural products. Taylor and Francis Group, CRC Press, Boca Raton FL. 2005, 22.

Raihan M, Tareq SM, Brishti A, Alam M, Haque A, Ali M. Evaluation of Antitumor Activity of *Leea indica* (Burm. f.) Merr. extract against Ehrlich Ascites Carcinoma (EAC) Bearing Mice. American Journal of Biomedical Sciences. 2012; 4(2): 143-152.

Rao BR, Singh K, Sastry KP, Singh CP, Kothari SK, Rajput DK, Bhattacharya AK. Cultivation technology for economicaly important medicinal plants. Advances in Medicinal Plants, Universities Press India Pvt Ltd, Hyderabad. 2007, 112-122.

Rakashanda S, Mubashir S, Qurishi Y, Hamid A, Masood A, Amin S. Trypsin inhibitors from *Lavatera cashmeriana* Camb. seeds: Isolation, characterization and *in-vitro* cytoxicity activity. International Journal of Pharmaceutical Science Invention. 2013; 2(5): 55-65.

Ramasamy K, Agarwal R. Multitargeted therapy of cancer by silymarin. Cancer Letters. 2008; 269(2): 352-62.

Rastogi N, Duggal S, Singh SK, Porwal K, Srivastava VK, Maurya R, Bhatt ML, Mishra DP. Proteasome inhibition mediates p53 reactivation and anti-cancer activity of 6-gingerol in cervical cancer cells. Oncotarget. 2015; 6(41): 43310-25.

Reddy KP, Bid HK, Nayak VL, Chaudhary P, Chaturvedi JP, Arya KR, Konwar R, Narender T. *In vitro* and *in vivo* anticancer activity of 2-deacetoxytaxinine J and synthesis of novel taxoids and their *in vitro* anticancer activity. European Journal of Medicinal Chemistry. 2009; 44(10): 3947-53.

Renuka M, Vijayakumar N, Ramakrishnan A. Chrysin, a flavonoid attenuates histological changes of hyperammonemic rats: A dose dependent study. Biomedicine and Pharmacotherapy. 2016; 82: 345-54.

Ricci F, Guffanti F, Damia G, Broggini M. Combination of paclitaxel, bevacizumab and MEK162 in second line treatment in platinum-relapsing patient derived ovarian cancer xenografts. Molecular Cancer. 2017; 16(1): 97.

Rivera E, Cianfrocca M. Overview of neuropathy associated with taxanes for the treatment of metastatic breast cancer. Cancer chemotherapy and pharmacology. 2015; 75(4): 659-70. Vrignaud P, Semiond D, Benning V, Beys E, Bouchard H, Gupta S. Preclinical profile of cabazitaxel. Drug Design, Development and Therapy. 2014; 8: 1851.

Ryu S, Lim W, Bazer FW, Song G. Chrysin induces death of prostate cancer cells by inducing ROS and ER stress. Journal of Cellular Physiology. 2017; 232(12): 3786-97.

Sahreen S, Khan MR, Khan RA, Shah NA. Estimation of flavoniods, antimicrobial, antitumor and anticancer activity of *Carissa opaca* fruits. BMC Complementary and Alternative Medicine. 2013; 13(1): 372.

Sakarkar DM, Deshmukh VN. Ethnopharmacological review of traditional medicinal plants for anticancer activity. International Journal of PharmTech Research. 2011; 3(1): 298-308.

Sarkar A, Bhattacharjee S, Mandal DP. Induction of apoptosis by eugenol and capsaicin in human gastric cancer AGS cells: Elucidating the role of p53. Asian Pacific Journal of Cancer Prevention. 2015; 16(16): 6753-9.

Satheesh LS, Murugan K. Antimicrobial activity of protease inhibitor from leaves of *Coccinia grandis* (L.) Voigt. Indian Journal of Experimental Biology. 2011; 49: 366-74.

Seca AM, Pinto DC. Plant Secondary Metabolites as Anticancer Agents: Successes in Clinical Trials and Therapeutic Application. International Journal of Molecular Sciences. 2018; 19(1): 263.

Seo HS, Jo JK, Ku JM, Choi HS, Choi YK, Woo JK, Kang SY, min Lee K, Nam KW, Park N, Jang BH. Induction of caspase-dependent extrinsic apoptosis by apigenin through inhibition of signal transducer and activator of transcription 3 (STAT3) signalling in HER2-overexpressing BT-474 breast cancer cells. Bioscience Reports. 2015; 35(6): e00276.

Seo WG, Hwang JC, Kang SK, Jin UH, Suh SJ, Moon SK, Kim CH. Suppressive effect of *Zedoariae rhizoma* on pulmonary metastasis of B16 melanoma cells. Journal of Ethnopharmacology. 2005; 101(1-3): 249-57.

Shindo S, Hosokawa Y, Hosokawa I, Ozaki K, Matsuo T. Genipin inhibits MMP-1 and MMP-3 release from TNF-α-stimulated human periodontal ligament cells. Biochimie. 2014; 107: 391-5.

Singh BN, Shankar S, Srivastava RK. Green tea catechin, epigallocatechin-3-gallate (EGCG): mechanisms, perspectives and clinical applications. Biochemical Pharmacology. 2011; 82(12): 1807-21.

Smith J, Rowan N, Sullivan R. Medicinal mushrooms: Their therapeutic properties and current medical usage with special emphasis on cancer treatments. London: Cancer Research UK; 2002.

Solecki RS. Shanidor IV. A Neanderthal flower buriel in northern Iraq. Science. 1975; 190: 880-881.

Srikanth S, Chen Z. Plant protease inhibitors in therapeutics-focus on cancer therapy. Frontiers in Pharmacology. 2016; 7: 470.

Srivastava JK, Gupta S. Antiproliferative and apoptotic effects of chamomile extract in various human cancer cells. Journal of Agricultural and Food Chemistry. 2007; 55(23): 9470-8.

Steigerova J, Oklest'kova J, Levkova L, Kolar Z, Strnad M. Brassinosteroids cause cell cycle arrest and apoptosis of human breast cancer cells. Chemico-Biological Interactions. 2010; 188: 487–496.

Steinbeck C. Recent developments in automated structure elucidation of natural products. Natural Product Reports. 2004; 21: 512-518.

Stiborova M, Cerna V, Moserova M, Mrizova I, Arlt VM, Frei E, Saez GT. The anticancer drug ellipticine activated with cytochrome P450 mediates DNA damage determining its pharmacological efficiencies: Studies with rats, hepatic cytochrome P450 reductase null (HRN™) mice and pure enzymes. International Journal of Molecular Sciences. 2015; 16: 284-306.

Sun J, Wang H, Ng TB. Trypsin isoinhibitors with antiproliferative activity toward leukemia cells from *Phaseolus vulgaris* cv "White Cloud Bean". BioMed Research International. 2010; 2010: 1-8.

Suzuki K, Yano T, Sadzuka Y, Sugiyama T, Seki T, Asano R. Restoration of connexin 43 by Bowman-Birk protease inhibitor in M5076 bearing mice. Oncology Reports. 2005; 13(6): 1247-50.

Tang K, Pan Q. Strategies for enhancing alkaloids yield in *Catharanthus roseus via* metabolic engineering approaches. *In*: *Catharanthus Roseus*: Current Research and Future Prospects; Naeem M, Aftab T, Khan M, (*eds.*), Springer International Publishing: Basel, Switzerland, 2017, 1–16.

Tariq A, Sadia S, Pan K, Ullah I, Mussarat S, Sun F, Abiodun OO, Batbaatar A, Li Z, Song D, Xiong Q. A systematic review on ethnomedicines of anticancer plants. Phytotherapy Research. 2017;31(2):202-264.

Thangapazham RL, Sharad S, Maheshwari RK. Phytochemicals in wound healing. Advances in Wound Care. 2016; 5(5): 230-41.

Thorn CF, Oshiro C, Marsh S, Hernandez-Boussard T, McLeod H, Klein TE, Altman RB. Doxorubicin pathways: Pharmacodynamics and adverse effects. Pharmacogenetics and Genomics. 2011; 21(7): 440.

Tsai CC, Chuang TW, Chen LJ, Niu HS, Chung KM, Cheng JT, Lin KC. Increase in apoptosis by combination of metformin with silibinin in human colorectal cancer cells. World Journal of Gastroenterology. 2015; 21(14): 4169.

Tu LY, Pi J, Jin H, Cai JY, Deng SP. Synthesis, characterization and anticancer activity of kaempferol-zinc (II) complex. Bioorganic and Medicinal Chemistry Letters. 2016; 26(11): 2730-4.

Umadevi M, Kumar KS, Bhowmik D, Duraivel S. Traditionally used anticancer herbs in India. Journal of Medicinal Plants Studies. 2013; 1(3): 56-74.

Vallianou NG, Evangelopoulos A, Schizas N, Kazazis C. Potential anticancer properties and mechanisms of action of curcumin. Anticancer Research. 2015; 35: 645-51.

van de Velde ME, Kaspers GL, Abbink FC, Wilhelm AJ, Ket JC, van den Berg MH. Vincristine-induced peripheral neuropathy in children with cancer: A systematic review. Critical Reviews in Oncology/Hematology. 2017; 114: 114-30.

Varoni EM, Lo Faro AF, Sharifi-Rad J, Iriti M. Anticancer molecular mechanisms of resveratrol. Frontiers in Nutrition. 2016; 3: 8.

Wal A, Srivastava RS, Wal P, Rai A, Sharma S. Lupeol as a magic drug. Pharmaceutical and Biological Evaluations. 2015;2: 142-51.

Wang CZ, Zhang Z, Wan JY, Zhang CF, Anderson S, He X, Yu C, He TC, Qi LW, Yuan CS. Protopanaxadiol, an active ginseng metabolite, significantly enhances the effects of fluorouracil on colon cancer. Nutrients. 2015; 7(2): 799-814.

Wang L, Xu GF, Liu XX, Chang AX, Xu ML, Ghimeray AK, Piao JP, Cho D. *In vitro* antioxidant properties and induced G2/M arrest in HT-29 cells of dichloromethane fraction from *Liriodendron tulipifera*. Journal of Medicinal Plants Research. 2012; 6(3): 424-32.

Wang X, Song Y, Su Y, Tian Q, Li B, Quan J, Deng Y. Are PEGylated liposomes better than conventional liposomes? A special case for vincristine. Drug Delivery, 2016; 23: 1092–1100.

Weaver BA. How Taxol/paclitaxel kills cancer cells. Molecular Biology of the Cell. 2014; 25(18): 2677-81.

Wozniak L, Skapska S, Marszalek K. Ursolic acid-a pentacyclic triterpenoid with a wide spectrum of pharmacological activities. Molecules 2015; 20: 20614-41.

Wu F, Zhou L, Jin W, Yang W, Wang Y, Yan B, Du W, Zhang Q, Zhang L, Guo Y, Zhang J. Anti-proliferative and apoptosis-inducing effect of theabrownin against non-small cell lung adenocarcinoma A549 cells. Frontiers in Pharmacology. 2016; 7: 465.

Xiao Z, Morris-Natschke SL, Lee KH. Strategies for the optimization of natural leads to anticancer drugs or drug candidates. Medicinal Research Reviews. 2016; 36(1): 32-91.

Xie S, Zhou J. Harnessing plant biodiversity for the discovery of novel anticancer drugs targeting microtubules. Frontiers in Plant Science. 2017; 8: 720.

Xiong M, Wang L, Yu HL, Han H, Mao D, Chen J, Zeng Y, He N, Liu ZG, Wang ZY, Xu SJ. Ginkgetin exerts growth inhibitory and apoptotic effects on osteosarcoma cells through inhibition of STAT3 and activation of caspase-3/9. Oncology Reports. 2016; 35(2): 1034-40.

Xu H, Zhang S. Scutellarin induced apoptosis in HepG2 hepatocellular carcinoma cells *via* a STAT3 pathway. Phytotherapy Research. 2013; 27(10): 1524-8.

Xu LN, Lu BN, Hu MM, Xu YW, Han X, Qi Y, Peng JY. Mechanisms involved in the cytotoxic effects of berberine on human colon cancer HCT-8 cells. Biocell 2012; 36: 113-20.

Yadav B, Bajaj A, Saxena M, Saxena AK. *In vitro* anticancer activity of the root, stem and leaves of *Withania somnifera* against various human cancer cell lines. Indian Journal of Pharmaceutical Sciences. 2010; 72(5): 659.

Yan CH, Li F, Ma YC. Plumbagin shows anticancer activity in human osteosarcoma (MG-63) cells *via* the inhibition of S-Phase checkpoints and down-regulation of c-myc. International Journal of Clinical and Experimental Medicine. 2015; 8(8): 14432.

Yang N, Zhao Y, Wang Z, Liu Y, Zhang Y. Scutellarin suppresses growth and causes apoptosis of human colorectal cancer cells by regulating the p53 pathway. Molecular Medicine Reports. 2017; 15(2): 929-35.

Yong YL, Tan LT, Ming LC, Chan KG, Lee LH, Goh BH, Khan TM. The effectiveness and safety of topical capsaicin in postherpetic neuralgia: A systematic review and meta-analysis. Frontiers in Pharmacology. 2017; 7: 538.

Yoon JS, Kim HM, Yadunandam AK, Kim NH, Jung HA, Choi JS, Kim CY, Kim GD. Neferine isolated from *Nelumbo nucifera* enhances anti-cancer activities in Hep3B cells: Molecular mechanisms of cell cycle arrest, ER stress induced apoptosis and anti-angiogenic response. Phytomedicine. 2013; 20(11): 1013-22.

Yoshihara H, Yoshimoto Y, Hosoya Y, Hasegawa D, Kawano T, Sakoda A, Okita H, Manabe A. Infantile fibrosarcoma treated with postoperative vincristine and dactinomycin. Pediatrics International. 2017; 59(3): 371-4.

Zhang LQ, Lv RW, Qu XD, Chen XJ, Lu HS, Wang Y. Aloesin. Aloesin suppresses cell growth and metastasis in ovarian cancer SKOV3 cells through the inhibition of the MAPK signaling pathway. Analytical Cellular Pathology. 2017; 2017: 1-6.

Zhang YY, Huang CT, Liu SM, Wang B, Guo J, Bai JQ, Fan XJ, Jia YS. Licochalcone A exerts antitumor activity in bladder cancer cell lines and mice models. Tropical Journal of Pharmaceutical Research. 2016; 15(6): 1151-7.

Zhao Y, Wang CM, Wang BG, Zhang CX. Study on the anticancer activities of the Clematis manshrica saponins *in vivo*. Zhongguo Zhong yao za zhi = Zhongguo zhongyao zazhi = China Journal of Chinese Materia Medica. 2005; 30(18): 1452-3.

Zhu H, Ding WJ, Wu R, Weng QJ, Lou JS, Jin RJ, Lu W, Yang B, He QJ. Synergistic anti-cancer activity by the combination of TRAIL/APO-2L and celastrol. Cancer Investigation. 2010; 28(1): 23-32.

Zong Y, Wu J, Shen K. Nanoparticle albumin-bound paclitaxel as neoadjuvant chemotherapy of breast cancer: A systematic review and meta-analysis. Oncotarget. 2017; 8(10): 17360.

Zschocke S, Rabe T, Taylor JL, Jäger AK, Van Staden J. Plant part substitution – a way to conserve endangered medicinal plants?. Journal of Ethnopharmacology. 2000; 71(1-2): 281-92.

11

Appraisal of Medicinal Plants for Anticancer Properties

SHALINI MANI[1]*, GEETA SWARGIARY[1] AND SAHIL SRIVASTAV[1]

ABSTRACT

Cancer is a disease, which severely effects the human population throughout the world. To cure this disease there are different synthetic anti-cancerous drugs but they are known to target these rapidly dividing cells without the adequate discrimination between normal and cancerous cells, and hence also damage the normal tissues. Thus, there is a real need for new efficient anti-cancer drugs with reduced side effects. Some medicinal plants are known for their usage in effective anticancer remedies and have been used since ages. It is mainly because, the plant produces naturally occurring secondary metabolites, and many of these metabolites are studied and proven for their medicinal significance, including cancer. Some common anti-cancerous medicinal plants are also investigated for their anti-cancerous properties as well mechanism of action of their metabolites. Thus, the use of phytochemicals seems to be very promising and their uses are escalating rapidly. The appropriate scientific study to extract these bioactive chemicals, detailed assessment for their role in anticancer treatment and clinical studies might be the appealing issue of upcoming cancer research. This chapter summarizes all the important steps and methods to validate any herbs for their potential anticancerous properties. It is explained with the help of all the approaches, which has been adopted till date for the validation of various common anticancerous herbs. This chapter may provide an overview of the comprehensive approach for studying a potential anticancerous herb. This

[1] Department of Biotechnology, Jaypee Institute of Information Technology, Noida, UP, India

**Corresponding author:* shalini.mani@jiit.ac.in

summary of the approaches may help the basic researchers in designing new technologies for the development of staple drugs for cancer treatment.

Key words: Cancer, Anti-cancerous plants, Treatment, Apoptosis, Medicine.

1. INTRODUCTION

Amongst the world's leading deathly diseases, cancer holds its second position across the globe. The characteristic feature of cancer is defined by the abnormal cells that grows uncontrollably, followed by massive invasion of other parts of the body and destruction of the entire cell community. Amidst the world's most life threatening diseases, 1 in 6 deaths is due to cancer. Also, World Health Organisation (WHO) estimated that 8.8 million people died of cancer in 2015 (WHO 2015). According to the survey, the cancer prevalence has reached to its peak in the past few decades (WHO 2015). Different sources and surveys have reported that there are 100 types of cancer governing the world population. These commonly includes the cancer of lung, stomach, liver, pancreatic, oral, colon, prostate, cervical, brain, breast, ovary and so on. The WHO statistics data for 2012 have reported that lung cancer has the highest prevalence rate in men, followed by prostate, colorectum, stomach and liver cancer. In women, the prevalence of breast cancer is very high, and then further followed by colorectum, lungs, cervical and stomach cancer. Overall, the mortality rate of lung cancer is 19.4%, which is the highest among all the types of cancers (Ferlay *et al.*, 2012).

Despite of several researches and efforts, the complete cure for cancer remains unresolved. This could be probably due to the complex nature of cancer, where the abnormal cells grow uncontrollably, and are regulated by multiple mechanisms that directly or indirectly triggers the cancer pathway. There are vivid number of treatment options like surgery, chemotherapy, radiotherapy, immunotherapy and chemically derived drugs, but these treatments carry their own side effects. The most common side effects are vomiting, nausea, weakness, fatigue and diarrhoea. For example, Tamoxifen, a synthetic drug prescribed for breast cancer had exhibited the side effects such as mood changes, fatigue and joint pain. Chemotherapy has also the potential to elevate certain cardiotoxic effects thereby increasing the chance and risk of cardiovascular diseases (Partridge *et al.*, 2001; Lorusso *et al.*, 2017). Overall, these side effects can put forth the patients to diversified stress and pain that could further harm their health conditions. Hence it necessitates to design alternative therapies that could preferably improvise the current cancer therapeutics.

2. ALTERNATIVE THERAPY FOR CANCER: HERBAL MEDICINE

While talking about the alternative treatments and therapies against cancer, the herbal medicines always remains a preference. The outcome of various studies conducted in the last few decades has widely emphasized on the plant-derived drugs from the ethno-medicinal herbs, and are being studied as an alternative therapy for cancer treatments. These herbs are natural, and can be delivered orally as part of patient's dietary intake as well. Therefore, the ethno-medicinal herbs becomes an eminent source for the naturally derived drugs as a tool for fighting against cancer. It is also noticed that Asian countries and Greece are highly rich in plethora of ethno-medicinal herbs (Manju *et al.,* 2012). Till date, more than 2439 anticancer herbs and their 3575 anticancer constituents have been studied for their anticancerous property and found to exhibit their cytotoxic nature by different cellular pathways (Cancer HSP, 2018; http://lsp.nwu.edu.cn/CancerHSP.php). Some of the common anticancerous herbs are turmeric, green tea, garlic, ashwagandha, Indian mulberry, mint, aloe vera, Asian pigeonwings, night-flowering jasmine, arjuna, madagascar periwinkle, basil, grape seed, clove, asiatic pennywort, thumbai etc. Different *in-vitro* and *in-vivo* studies stands as an evidence of confirmation for these herbs that exhibited their potential anticancerous property. For example, the anticancerous property of asiatic pennywort was studied in the following cell lines of breast cancer MCF-7MDA MB-, B6 F10, and *in-vivo* studies in the xenograft model of mouse lung cancer; thumbai (*Leucas aspera*) in HeLa cell line, madagascar periwinkle in MCF and He La cell lines *(Rai et al.,* 2014; Ruskin and Aruna, 2014; Mohan *et al.*, 2017; Wu *et al.*, 2017). Certain herbs are also studied at the patient level, which includes turmeric in *colorectal*, pancreatic, prostate, lung and breast cancer; garlic in stomach, gastric, colorectal, esophageal and prostate cancer; green tea in hormone refractory prostate cancer; and ashwagandha in breast cancer patients (Choan *et al.,* 2005; Gupta *et al.,* 2013; Biswal *et al.,* 2013; Nicastro *et al.,* 2015*)*. There are several other herbs that has been used in the ancient times for the ailment of different kinds of diseases. Those herbs have shown their significant potentials in the history, but as the time evolved, the current generation has lost its touch with most of these precious treasure of this earth. Past few decades have been a renaissance for those herbs, where the researches have started to explore the ethno-medicinal herbs for their anticancerous properties. Yet, many of them are still remaining unexplored. Table 1 highlights few important anticancerous herbs which have been reported for their potential anticancerous property and their active compounds along with their mechanism of action.

Table 1: A list of some commonly known anticancerous herbs and their mechanism of action.

Plant used	*Parts*	*Bioactive compounds*	*Mode of action*	*Cancer type*	*References*
Curcuma longa (Turmeric)	Rhizome	Curcumin (diferuloylmethane);Demethoxycurcumin; Bisdemethoxycurcumin; Turmerone; Zingiberene; Cineole; D-phellandrene; D-sabinene; Borneol	Increase expression of growth suppressor factors (such as p57 Kip2, TP53, and Rb); Reduce the proliferation *via* pathways such as NFκB, AP1, PI3K, TGF beta, JAK-STAT, MAPK, and Wnt-Betacatenin; Anti-angiogenesis; Elevate apoptosis (BAX, BIM, PUMA, BCL2, and BCL-XL)	Colon; Breast; Lungs; Prostate; Pancreatic; Stomach; Cervical; Uterine; Ovarian; Pulmonary; Gastric; Bladder; Bone; Oral and Oesophageal cancer	Vallianou *et al.* (2015); Allegra *et al.* (2017); Imran *et al.* (2017)
Aloe barbadensis (*Aloe vera*)	Leaves and gel	Aloin; Barbalion; Anthranol; Cinnamic acid; Aloetic acid; Emodin;Chrysophanic acid; Resistanol	Modulate lipid peroxidation; Increase antioxidant defence system inhibits angiogenesis of the tumor and inhibit the tumouric growth by blocking the transducer of signal and also stop the transcription 3 activation activator.	Liver, Glioma, Breast, Lung, Colorectal and Skin Cancer	Shalabi *et al.* (2015); Radha and Laxmipriya (2015)
Allium sativum (Garlic)	Bulb	Allicin; Alliin, Diallyl disulphide; Diallyl trisulfide, Allyl methyl Allyl methyl trisulfide; Allyl methane sulfonate; S- allyl cysteine; disulphide; Diallyl tetra-	Inhibit the proliferation of cancerous cells by inhibiting the expression of cyclin E; Attenuate formation of peroxide and DNA strand; ROS inhibition; Cell cycle arrest	Liver; Gastric and Colorectal cancers.	Raghu *et al.* (2012)

Table 1: (*Contd...*)

Table 1: (*Contd...*)

Plant used	***Parts***	***Bioactive compounds***	***Mode of action***	***Cancer type***	***References***
		sulfide; Allyl methyl tetrasulfide	at the G0/G1 phases;Induction of apoptosis by increased expression of Fas,Capase-3 , Bax and reduced Bcl-2 expression.		
Camellia sinensis (Green tea)	Leaves	Epigallocatechin- 3-gallate (EGCG), Catechins, Flavan-3-ol	Induction of apoptotic markers like p53 and poly- ADP- ribose polymerase cleavage; Reduced expression of beta catenin bio- markers, COX-2 and Cyclin D1; Cancer cell growth arrest	Colon; Colorectal; Prostate; Skin; Cervical; Bladder; Oral; Liver; Lung and Breast	Ullah *et al.* (2016)
Withania somnifera (Ashwagandha)	Roots and leaves	Withaferin –A; Withanolide D; Withanamides; Steroidal saponins; Withanolides; Withano sides; Withanoolide glycosides; Lignanamides; Glycowithanolides; Withanone	Reduced expression of MMP-3 and MMP-9 in cancer cells that leads to antimetastatic activity; cell growth arrest at G1 phase, tumor suppressor protein (pRB) activation; Decreased expression of nuclear factor -kappaB; Suppress the intercellular TNF; potentiate apoptotic signalling, p53- dependent apoptosis	Colon; Lung Breast; Skin; Pancreatic; Blood; Fibrosarcoma; Prostate; Cervical and cancer Neurroblasoma	Oza *et al.* (2010); Munagala *et al.* (2011); Wadhwa *et al.* (2013); Palliyaguru *et al.* (2016); Joshi *et al.* (2016)
Zingiber officinale (Ginger)	Leaf and rhizome	Quercetin; Rutin; Epicatechin; Catechin; Kaempferol; Naringenin; Salicylic acid;	Induction of apoptosis by increased expression of ATF3; cancer cell growth arrest, down-regul-	Colorectal; Ovarian; Breast; Liver; Cervical; Leukemia; Pancreatic; Colon; Gastric	Habib *et al.* (2008); Park *et al.* (2014); Akimoto *et al.* (2015)

Table 1: (*Contd...*)

Table 1: (*Contd...*)

Plant used	*Parts*	*Bioactive compounds*	*Mode of action*	*Cancer type*	*References*
		Cinnamic acid; Gingerol; Parasol and Shogaol	ation of the gene products regulated by NF-κB involved in proliferation of the cell and angiogenesis ROS mediated cell death	and Lung cancer	
Centella asiatica (Gotu-Kola)	Leaves and whole plant	Asiatic acid; Asiaticoside; Madecassoside; Quercetin; Quercitrin; Kaempferol; Apigenin; Luteolin; Naringin; Betulic acid; Chlorogenic acid; Ascorbic acid; α -Pinene and β -Pinene	Immunosuppressi-ve activity; Antioxidative activity; Inhibit proliferation of the cancer cell and induce apoptosis.	Breast; Glioblastma and Lung,	Babu *et al.* (1995); Yoshida *et al.* (2005)
Terminalia arjuna (Arjun)	Bark and leaves	Alkaloids; Tannins; Steroids; Flavonoids; Arjunine, Punicalin; Arjunetin; Lactone; Arjunolic acid and	Enhance lipid peroxidation; Increase superoxide radical levels; reduce enzyme activity; Quenching free radicals induced by the N- nitroso diethylamine; Ascorbic acid Cell growth inhibition;Apoptosis induction through effecting growth regulators;DNA damage and Expression of apoptotic proteins.	Liver; Colon and Breast cancer	Kandil and Nassar(1998); Sivalokanathan *et al.* (2006); Ahmad *et al.* (2014); Singh *et al.* (2017)
Citrus imon (Lemon)	Peel	Tang3eretin; Nobiletin; 5-demethyl-tangeretin;	Cell cycle arrest at G2/M phase by upregulation of tumor suppr-	Liver; Cervical; Breast; Colon; Lung; Skin and	Wang *et al.* (2014); Rawson *et al.* (2014)

Table 1: (*Contd...*)

Table 1: (*Contd...*)

Plant used	***Parts***	***Bioactive compounds***	***Mode of action***	***Cancer type***	***References***
		Hesperetin; Naringin; Sinensetin; Naringenin; Hesperidin; Neohesperidin; Narirutin; Eriocitrin; Didymin and Rutin	essor gene (p53) and downregulation of cdc2 & Cyclin B1; Induction of caspase -3 activation; apoptosis due to increased expressions of p53 and PPARγ and NF -κB activation supressed; Inhibition of angiogenesis by inducing cell cycle arrest	Prostate	
Mentha spicata (Mint)	Leaves	Rosmarinic acid; Rutin; Epicatechin; Luteolin and Catechin	Anti angiogenic activity; inhibition of cancer cell growth by loss of transmembrane mitochondrial potential; Modulatory actions on lipid peroxidation and anti oxidant enzymes	Breast; Leukemia; Ovarian; Cervical and Lung	Hajighasemi *et al.* (2011); Brahmi *et al.* (2017)
Morinda citrifolia (Indian mulberry)	Fruits and roots	Polysaccharide; Acubin; Damnacanthal; Asperulosidetetraacetate; Asperulosidic acid; Morindine; Morinda diol; Morindone; Morindanidrine; Narcissoside; Oleic acid; Butanoic acid	Apoptosis induction *via* mitochondrial pathway; Increased ROS production; Overexpressed p53 and caspase-3 proteins and down regulate Bcl-2,	Breast; Liver; Lung; Colorectal and Cervical	Brown (2012); Saminathan *et al.* (2013); Srinivasahan and Durairaj (2015)
Calotropis gigantea (Madar)	Root bark, roots and leaves	Cardenolides; Phytoterols; Desmosterols; Naphthalene; Terpene derivatives; Glycosides;	Chemopreventive activity; Inhibition of transcription factor NF-κB; Intracellular DNA fragmen-	Liver; Cervical and Breast cancer	Sureshkumar *et al.* (2012)

Table 1: (*Contd...*)

Table 1: (*Contd...*)

Plant used	*Parts*	*Bioactive compounds*	*Mode of action*	*Cancer type*	*References*
		Pregnanes; Saponins; Triterpenoids; Steroids and Phenylpropanoids	tation;		
Laurus nobilis (Bay leaf)	Leaves	Costunolide; α-Terpineol; Dehydrocostuslactone; α-Terpinolene; α-Pinene; Sabinene; 1,8 Cineole; p-Cymene	Cancer cell cycle arrest by regulation of cell cycle-associated regulatory factors;Generation of ROS; DNA damage; Activation of p53; Reversal of multidrug resistance; Inhibition of angiogenesis; Inhibition of metastasis and invasion	Liver, Leukemia, Breast, Ovarian; Prostatic and Bladder cancer	Saab *et al.* (2012); Lin *et al.* (2015)
Murraya koenigii (Curry leaf)	Leaves	Rutin; Quercetin; Catechin; Epicatechin; Naringin; Myricetin; Gallic acid; Ferulic acid; Vanillic acid	Activation of caspase 3 and 8; upregulation of p53 and cell proliferation repressor proteins (p27 and p2); Inhibition of 26S proteasome complex; Apoptosis induction by DNA fragmentation	Leukemia; Breast, Colorectal; Liver and Blood cancer	Ghasemzadeh *et al.* (2014); Patterson and Verghese (2015)
Cuminum cyminum (Cumin)	Seeds	Limonene; Cuminaldehyde; Cymene; Terpenoids; α- and β-pinene; 1, 8-cineole; o-and p -cymene; α- and γ-terpinene; Safranal and Linalool	Chemopreventive and anti carcinogenic activity; Modulate lipid peroxidation; metabolize antioxidant enzymes	Liver; Prostate; Colon; Ovarian; Lung; Stomach and Cervical	Prakash and Gupta (2014); Singh *et al.* (2017)
Tinospora cordifolia	Stem and	Berberine; tinosporin; Diterp-	DNA damage; Increase in the	Colon; Skin; Lung;	Saha and Ghosh (2012);

Table 1: (*Contd...*)

Table 1: (*Contd...*)

Plant used	*Parts*	*Bioactive compounds*	*Mode of action*	*Cancer type*	*References*
(Giloy)	leaves	enoid lactones, Glycosides, Sesquiterpenoid, Aliphatic compounds, Phenolics, Polysaccharides; Tinosporide, Tinosporaside, Cordifolide, Cordifol, Heptacosanol, Clerodane fura noditerpene, Diterpenoidfuranol actonetinosporidine, Columbin and β-sitosterol	expression of Bax (proapoptotic gene) and decrease in expression of Bcl-2 (anti-apoptotic gene); Antiangiogenic activity; Lipid peroxidation	Lymphoma; Breast; Prostate; Oral; Cervical and Brain	Mishra and Kaur (2013)
Moringa oleifera (Drumstick)	Leaves; bark and seeds	Isopropyl isothiocyanate; D-allose; Cetene;Eugenol, dibutyl phthalate, 2-chloropropionic acid; 5-eicosene; 1-butanamine, 1-dodecene, 2-decenal, 3-tetradecene, 2-tetradecene, 1-octadecene, hexadecanoic acid, 10-octadecenoic acid, and Heptadecanoic Acid	Induction of apoptosis; Interfere with the signal transduction cascade and inhibit the cancer cell proliferation; Cell cycle arrest at G2/M phase	Liver; Breast; Colorectal; Lung; Ovarian and Prostate cancer	Al-Asmari *et al.* (2015); Jung *et al* (2015); Zayas-Viera (2016)
Jatropha curcas (Jatropha)	Root; leaves and latex	Gallic acid; Pyrogallol; Rutin; Myricetin; Daidzein; Apigenin; Glycosides; Vitexin; Isovitexin; Stigmasterol; β-sitosterol;	Antimetastatic activity; Induction of apoptosis through overexpression of PKCδ; PKC, serine protease and caspase-3/CPP32 activation	Breast; Liver; Cervical; Skin; Leukemia; Bladder; Prostate and Gastric cancer	Oskoueian *et al.* (2011); Oskoueian *et al.* (2011)

Table 1: (*Contd...*)

Table 1: (*Contd...*)

Plant used	*Parts*	*Bioactive compounds*	*Mode of action*	*Cancer type*	*References*
		Ellagic acid; Quercetin; Coumaric acid; Benzoic acid and Salicylic acid.			
Andrographis paniculata (Green chiretta)	Leaves	Andrographolide	Cell cycle arrest and apoptosis of the cancer cell at G1 phase; Induce p27 expression that mainly inhibits CDK; Inhibit protein synthesis by DNA damage; Activation of p53 tumour suppresser gene, caspase 8, pro-apoptotic Bcl-2 family protein	Laryngeal; Breast; Skin; Colorectal and Colon cancer	Rajagopal *et al.* (2003); Ahmad *et al.* (2014)
Catharanthus roseus (Madagascar periwinkle)	Roots; stem; leaves; flowers and whole plant	Catharicine; Calmodulin; Vindioline; Quercetin; Carosidine; Vincaline; Vinpocetine; Virosine; Vinosidine; Zeatin; Vinorelbine; Vinflunine; Vinaspine; Indole-3-acetic acid; Malvidine; Serpentine	Inhibit resistance to multi-drug response;Cancer cell proliferation arrest through binding to tubulin; Slow down the transition from metaphase to anaphase that results in blockage of cancer cells in mitosis and hence apoptosis is induced.	Breast; Leukemia Neuroblastoma; Ovary; Lung; Bladder and Colon cancer	Arora *et al.* (2010); Sain and Sharma (2013)
Azadirachta indica (Neem)	Leaves	Nimbolide; Limonoids; Azadirachtin; Nimbin; Nimbinin; Nimbidinin and Nimbidic acid	tumour invasion inhibition; Angiogenesis inhibition; Prevent procarcinogen activation and oxidative DNA damage; inhibit	Breast; Leukemia and Prostate cancer	Mahapatra *et al.* (2011); Arumugam *et al.* (2014); Alzohairy (2016)

Table 1: (*Contd...*)

Table 1: (*Contd...*)

Plant used	***Parts***	***Bioactive compounds***	***Mode of action***	***Cancer type***	***References***
			angiogenesis induced by VEGF; upregulate antioxidants and the enzymes that detoxify carcinogens; upregulate p53 and Bax (proapoptotic proteins);		
Phyllanthus emblica (Indian gooseberry)	Fruits	Ellagic acid; Corilagin; Gallic acid; Quercetin; Pyrogallol; Chebulagic acid	Inhibit PI3K and proliferation of the cancer cell; Cell death *via* induction of autophagy; Inhibition of transcription factor NF-kappaB; Increase ROS; Downregulate the expression of AP-1 Protein Components	Colon; Prostate; Lung; Gastric; Cervical; Leukemia; Ovarian; Breast and Liver cancer	Mahata *et al.* (2013); Zhao *et al.* (2015)
Ocimum sanctum (Basil)	Roots; seeds and leaves	Eugenol;Eugenic acid; Ursolic acid; Carvacrol; Linalool; Limatrol; Caryophyllene; Estragol; Rosmarinic acid; Propanoic acid; Apigenin; Isothymusin; Isothymonin	Reduce cell proliferation; Increased intracellular ROS; mitochondrial membrane potential alteration and apoptosis; inhibition of metabolic activation of the carcinogen;	Colon; Lung; Neuroblastoma and Oral cancer	Pattanayak *et al.* (2010); Shivpuje *et al.*(2015); Sridevi *et al.* (2016)
Plumbago zeylanica (Chitraka)	Roots; seeds and leaves	Plumbagin; Elliptinone, Zeylanone, Sistostero; Suberosin; Seselin; Psoralen; 3-Chloroplumbagin; Saponaretin; Xanthyletin	Inhibit cancer cell growth; Modulate lipid peroxidation; Cell cycle arrest at G2/M phase	Colon; Breast; Leukemia; Lung Prostate,	Ganesan and Gani (2013); Jain *et al.* (2014)

Table 1: (*Contd...*)

Table 1: (*Contd...*)

Plant used	*Parts*	*Bioactive compounds*	*Mode of action*	*Cancer type*	*References*
Solanum nigrum (Black nightshade)	Leaves	Solamargine; Solasonine; Solanin; Quercetin	Apoptosis induction; Activation of caspase-3 and ROS production results in cell cycle arrest at G2/M phase; Mitochondria mediated apoptosis	Breast; Melanoma; Endometrial; Cervical and Colorectal cancer	Chavan *et al.* (2013); Lai *et al.* (2016)
Clitoria ternatea L. (Blue-bellvine)	Roots; flowers; seeds and leaves	4-bromoquinuclidine;Pentanal;Acetic acid; Mome inositol; cyclohexen; hirsutene; 1-methyl4-(1-methylethylideme); cyano	Decreased lipid peroxidation; Increased malonndialdehyde level; Increased antioxidant activity	Lymphatic cancer;Lung, Breast; Liver; Prostate; Cervical and Ovarian	Jacob and Latha (2012); Neda *et al.* (2013)
Wedelia chinensis (Creeping-oxeyes)	Whole plant	Apigenin; Wedelolactone; Indole-3-carboxyaldehyde; Luteolin	Activation of tumour suppressor p53; Induction of cell cycle arrest at G1 phase; Induce apoptosis; suppression of NF-κB activation pathway	Prostate Cancer	Lin *et al.*(2007)
Nyctanthes arbor-tristis (Night Jasmine) Ascorbic acid; Crocetin;	Flowers; leaves and fruits	Nicotiflorin; Quercetin; Anthocyanin; Apigenin; Tan-nic acid; proliferation Loganin; Diterpene-Nyctanthin;	Antioxidant and antiproliferative activity; Inhibition of the cancer cell	Colorectal; Breast; Leukemia; Retinoblastoma	Kumari *et al.* (2012); Khanapur *et al.* (2014); Gulshan *et al.* (2015)
		Nyctanthine; Nyctanthoside	Induction of apoptosis *via*		
Rubia cordifolia (Indian madder)	Roots	Rubidianin; Rubiadin; Rosemary acids; Purpurin; Alizarin and	caspase 3 activation	Histolytic lymphoma; Leukemia and Cervical cancer	Patel *et al.* (2010); Tiwari *et al.* (2012)

Table 1: (*Contd...*)

Table 1: (*Contd...*)

Plant used	*Parts*	*Bioactive compounds*	*Mode of action*	*Cancer type*	*References*
		Xanthopurpurin			
Cannabis sativa (Cannabis)	Leaves	Cannabinoids; Cannabidiol; Δ9-tetrahydrocanna binol; Cannabi chromene and Cannabigerol	Inhibition of angiogenesis and metastasis reduction; Cell growth inhibition; Apoptosis induction; AKT inhibition and cell cycle arrest promoted; Activation of the CDK inhibitory proteins p21 and p27;	Glioma; Pancreatic; Melanoma; Lung; Hepatic, Leukemia; Skin, Breast; Neuroblastoma and Prostate cancer	Guzman (2003); Velasco *et al.* (2016)

3. STUDY OF SOME COMMON ANTI-CANCEROUS PLANTS AND THEIR PHYTOCOMPOUNDS

Scientific literatures are enriched with a plethora of information about the study and uses of some common anti-cancerous herbs. Most of these herbs are known to possess their unique phytocompounds that are responsible for their anti-cancerous nature. Many of these anti-cancerous herbs exhibit their medicinal potentials against different types of cancer by triggering the specific pathways that play a crucial role in the cell death. Some important anti-cancerous herbs and their compounds are mentioned below.

3.1. *Curcuma longa*

Curcumin is a natural pigment that is extracted from turmeric or *Curcuma longa*. Curcumin is a one of the major bioactive compound of turmeric, which is extensively studied to have different pharmacological activities like anti-bacterial, anti-oxidant and anti-cancerous properties (Reddy and Lokesh, 1992). Curcumin is extracted from the rhizomes of turmeric. Generally, alcohols are preferred for extraction of Curcumin. The different organic solvents used for the extraction are acetone, ethanol, methanol and isopropanol at 60°C for extraction time of 1hr. After the organic solvent extraction, it was seen that the weight of Curcumin extracted with ethanol was the highest as compared to that extracted in other solvents like acetone, methanol and isopropanol (Kwon and Chung, 2015). The extraction temperature was maintained by using a water bath, and mixed every 20 minutes using a vortex mixer. After vortexing the supernatant was recovered by filtering it through Whatman's filter paper, and then ethanol was completely removed by the evaporation. Then, the extract collected was subjected to High Performance Liquid Chromatography (HPLC) analysis for the quantitative determination.

Various studies suggest the role of Curcumin as an effective chemopreventive agent in the treatment of different types of cancer. Curcumin is used in the treatment of different cell lines of prostate adenocarcinoma. Curcumin induces apoptosis in metastatic prostate cancer cell line (LNCaP), human prostate cancer cell line (PC-3) and another human prostate cancer cell line (DU145) and triggered formation of vacuoles in cytoplasm of metastatic prostate cancer cell line PC-3M (Lee *et al.,* 2015). It was also reported from the above study that Curcumin treatments increased the expression of endoplasmic reticulum markers *i.e.,* CHOP and Bip/GRP78, and an autophagic marker, LC3-II. Another study investigated the effect of Curcumin on human liver cancer cell line, HepG2. On exposure of HepG2 cell lines with Curcumin, it was seen that Curcumin induced damages to both nuclear DNA as well as mitochondrial DNA, but the extent of damage was more severe in mitochondrial DNA. The reason behind this was the imbalance in the potential across the mitochondrial membrane which led to increase in the cytosolic concentration of Cytochrome C and triggered intrinsic mitochondrial dependent pathway in cancer cells (Cao *et al.,* 2007). It has been reported that Curcumin is responsible for decreasing the level of expression of p53 gene and Estrogen receptor in case of Estrogen positive breast cancer (Hallman *et al.,* 2017).

3.2. *Vitis vinifera*

Resveratrol is a polyphenol, which is naturally occurring in the skin of grapes (*Vitis vinifera*), blueberries, raspberries and mulberries. It is produced by the plants in response to injury such as exudation of cell sap due to mechanical injury like cut in leaves or stems or in response to attack by pathogenic organisms like bacteria and fungi. Currently, studies suggest that resveratrol can be used for the treatment of cancer, cardiovascular diseases, neurological disorders and diabetes (Berman *et al.,* 2017). Resveratrol is very commonly found in the skin of grapes and berries. This phenolic compound is extracted from the skin of grapes by the accelerated solvent extraction using ethanol. Both dry and wet grape pomace may be subjected to the extraction procedure, and in a study, it was observed that the yield of resveratrol was two times higher with wet pomace as compared to dry grape pomace. The yield of resveratrol obtained was about 70%. Also, it was seen that the dry pomace extract containing resveratrol showed a better radical scavenging activity in cancer cells than wet pomace (Rajha *et al.,* 2014). The temperature (70°C) of extraction should be maintained, because a very high temperature results in the formation of toxic by-products like furanic compounds (furfural, hydroxymethylfurfural) due to the degradation of natural sugars present in fruits. HPLC is usually performed to analyse the phenolic content yield of resveratrol, but before this the grape pomace has to be subjected to the purification step by passing through 0.2 µm syringe filter (Rajha *et al.,* 2014).

Resveratrol is reported to be as an effective chemopreventive agent against different types of cancer in humans. This phytocompound exerts its chemopreventive activity by targeting mitochondria and triggering apoptosis. The action of resveratrol was studied on two different bladder carcinoma cell lines, BTT739 and T24 (Lin *et al.,* 2012). According to them, resveratrol treatment significantly reduced cell viability through induced apoptosis, and the pattern was observed to be both time as well as dose dependent. Also, the markers of intrinsic mitochondrial dependent pathway of apoptosis were recognised by release of Cytochrome C and activities of caspase 3 and 9. It has been also reported that Resveratrol is responsible for inhibiting growth of Estrogen receptor positive breast cancer cells by up regulating the expression of HER-2 gene and by decreasing the expression of Estrogen receptor (Andreani *et al.,* 2017).

3.3. *Zingiber officinale*

Gingerol is an active component derived from fresh ginger (*Zingiber officinale*). Gingerol is normally extracted as a pungent yellow oil, but can also be converted into crystalline solid under low melting temperature. Gingerol has been reported to exhibit anti-oxidant, analgesic, anti-pyretic, anti-inflammatory and anti-tumorigenic activities (Shukla and Singh, 2007; Oyagbemi *et al.,* 2010). Gingerol has also been known to show anti-inflammatory response by decreasing the level of expression of inducible nitric oxide synthase and TNF-α (Lee *et al.,* 2014).

For the extraction of Gingerol, the ginger was sliced into small pieces, and they were dried using hot air, and converted into powder form using a high speed grinder. The dried powder was then sieved and fractionated, subjected to supercritical fluid extraction to obtain a molecular distillation residue. High-speed counter-current chromatography (HSCCC) technique was used for the extraction and purification of 6-gingerol from molecular distillation residue by using bi-phase solvent system composed of n-hexane-ethyl-acetate-methanol and water. Once the target compound was isolated, its analysis was carried out by HPLC analysis (Gan *et al.,* 2016).

Gingerol possess superior and potent anti-carcinogenic property. It has been used in treatment of various types of cancers like hepatoma, breast cancer, grade four brain tumours or glioblastoma. In human hepatoma G2 cell line, 6-gingerol has been shown to induce apoptosis through Lysosomal-Mitochondrial Axis (Yang *et al.,* 2012). In this study, it was observed that the release of lysosomal enzyme, Cathepsins D worked along with the effector caspases to carry out the release of mitochondrial Cytochrome C. Hence, cell death occurred due to mitochondria based intrinsic apoptotic pathway. Another study shows that Gingerol acts as a sensitizing agent, and it induces TNF-alpha-related-apoptosis-inducing-ligand (TRAIL)-mediated apoptosis of glioblastoma cells, which were resistant to apoptosis by TRAIL signalling. Likewise, in a wide range of tumour cell types the cellular apoptosis is mediated by Tumour Necrosis Factor (TNF)-related apoptosis- inducing ligand (TRAIL) (Lee *et al.,* 2014). In case of TRAIL-resistant glioblastoma, the mechanism behind TRAIL-mediated apoptosis is that the TRAIL binds to the death receptor (DR (4/5)), and on binding to the receptor, it induces receptor trimerization, which causes the recruitment of a downstream signalling molecules, such as Fas-associated proteins with the inner cytosolic death domain (FADD) of the receptor and this eventually leads to activation of caspase cascade (caspases 8, 9, 10 and 3) to transmit signals further into the nucleus of tumour cells. The sensitizing effects of Gingerol on death receptor were studied on the following glioblastoma cell lines U87, U343, and T98G. It has been reported that [10]-Gingerol is responsible for inhibiting the growth of triple negative breast cancer and prevents metastasis to other organs like lung, bone and brain by significantly increasing the level of expression of caspase 3 (Martin *et al.,* 2017).

3.4. *Crocus sativus*

Saffron is used as a popular spice all over the world for its colouring and flavouring properties. Saffron is obtained from the dried stigmas of *Crocus sativus* flowers. Saffron consists of a number of carotenoid derivatives, which have been reported to have nutraceutical properties and of medicinal importance. The main bioactive compounds that are extracted from saffron are crocins, picrocrocins and safranals. The bioactive component, which is a matter of interest in this chapter is crocins, because it possess a number of nutraceutical properties like antioxidant (Chen *et al.,* 2008), neuroprotective (Ochiai *et al.,* 2004), anti-depressive (Wang *et al.,* 2010), anti-tumour and anti-carcinogenic (Abdullaev and Espinosa-Aguirre, 2004).

In order to meet the increasing market demand of plant derived bioactive components having nutraceutical properties, it is important to employ techniques which can help in efficient downstream processing and scalability of such bioactive metabolites. The optimal yield of crocins extracted from dried saffron stigma was obtained by solid-liquid extraction using mixtures of ethanol: water and methanol: water. The crocin extracted was recovered from *Crocus sativus* in ethanol-potassium phosphate aqueous two-phase system (Montalvo-Hernández *et al.,* 2012). Analysis of crocinis done by HPLC with Diode-Array Detection (HPLC-DAD).

The anti-cancerous effect and mechanism of action of crocin obtained from saffron was studied on human breast cancer cell line (MCF-7). Through immunoblot studies it was revealed that there was time dependent decline in the expression of anti-apoptotic markers like bcl-2 and an increase in the expression of pre-apoptotic markers like Bax in crocin treated MCF-7 cell line. Crocin treatment showed an enhanced effect on DNA damage in a dose and time dependent manner (Bakshi *et al.,* 2016).

3.5. *Cnidium monnieri*

Osthol is a chemically derived compound from coumarin. Coumarin is a natural organic substance found in a variety of plants like *Cnidium monnieri, Leptadenia reticulata*. This compound has been shown to suppress the tumour movements and tissue invasion in many ways in different types of cancers like prostate cancer, breast cancer and glioblastoma. Osthol is known to show diverse biological properties like anti-tumour, anti-inflammatory and neuroprotective (Chao *et al.,* 2010). Osthol, a coumarin derivative is extracted from the fruits and leaves of *Cnidium monnieri* and *Leptadenia reticulata* respectively. The fruits are dried and converted into a fine powder form using a motor grinder and is stored at room temperature. About 95% ethanol is used as the extraction solvent in the process. Osthol was extracted and quantified by using accelerated solvent extraction and HPLC coupled with photodiode array, electrospray ionisation ion trap tandem mass spectrometry and time of flight mass spectrometry (Gao *et al.,* 2013).

Osthol is known to prevent angiogenesis in cancer cases by sequestering the binding of ligand to vascular endothelial growth factor (VEGF) receptor present on cancer cells. VEGF-A is a most critical angiogenic regulator and acts as a specific mediator of angiogenesis in many types of cancer. Osthol, when binds to VEGF receptor leads to inactivation of different signalling pathways in cancer like Akt signalling pathway, ERK pathway and a number of Focal Adhesion Kinases. Finally, the lack of angiogenesis makes cancer cells deprived of nutrients and oxygen due to very limited blood supply and leads to apoptosis (Yang *et al.,* 2013). Another study shows that Osthol prevents epithelial-to-mesenchymal transition (EMT) in case of GBM8401 cells, thereby preventing the glioma cells to infiltrate other healthy brain cells. EMT plays an important role in progression of cancer since it leads to metastasis and this morphological change in cancer cells is induced by a number of growth factors like IGF-1 (Kahlert *et al.,* 2012). In IGF-1 induced GBM8401 cells, epithelial markers were down regulated and the mesenchymal markers were up regulated thereby leading to EMT. However, when such cells were treated with Osthol there was a reversal in morphological effect where epithelial markers were now up regulated and mesenchymal were down regulated. Real time PCR studies demonstrated that Osthol is capable of preventing growth and proliferation of GBM8401 cells by inhibiting IGF-1 induced EMT by blocking the PI3 kinase pathway (Lin *et al.*, 2014). Osthol is known for its role in treatment of Esophageal squamous cell carcinoma (ESCC). Osthol inhibits ESCC cell proliferation in time and dose dependent manner. Application of Osthol also leads to cell cycle arrest in G2/M phase and apoptosis of ESCC (Zhu *et al.*, 2018).

4. CELLULAR AND MOLECULAR MARKERS TO STUDY APOPTOSIS IN CANCER CELLS

As mentioned earlier, different anti-cancerous herbs constitute various kinds of phytocompounds, and mostly these compounds are the secondary metabolites of those plants. Depending upon their chemical nature, they may be predominantly soluble in different solvents, such as methanol, ethanol or water. Thus, to check, if any herbs is having a potential anti-cancerous property, it is fundamental to initially prepare the extract of different plant parts using different solvents, and subsequently these extracts will be checked for their cytotoxicity. Different steps that are followed to study the cellular and molecular markers of the cancer cells in response to their treatment with different extracts are illustrated in Fig. 1.

4.1. To study changes in cell membrane integrity in cancer cells undergoing apoptosis

Cancer cells, when treated with cytotoxic drugs undergo programed cell death or apoptosis. Early apoptosis initiates with changes in cell shape, size and finally leading to the fragmentation and abrupt decrease in the amount of DNA content in drug treated cancer cells. The apoptotic cells lose their membrane integrity, and there will be membrane blabbing, irregular shape of membrane, and shrinkage in cell size. Such changes occur in the cell membrane due to translocation of phosphatidylserine residues present on the inner layer of cell membrane to the outer cell surface. To study the morphological changes in such cancer cells, Annexin V/ FITC kit can be used, where Annexin V is used as a stain, which has high binding affinity towards the exposed phosphatidylserine residue present on the outer surface of drug treated cancer cells. Upon binding with Annexin V, apoptosis can be studied in a time dependent manner using a flow cytometer (Zhang *et al.*, 2017). Morphological changes in cancer cells undergoing apoptosis can also be studied by Acridine Orange (AO) and Propidium Iodine (PI) double staining method. Acridine Orange (AO) is an intercalating dye which can enter the cell membrane of both living and dead cells and on entering inside the cells

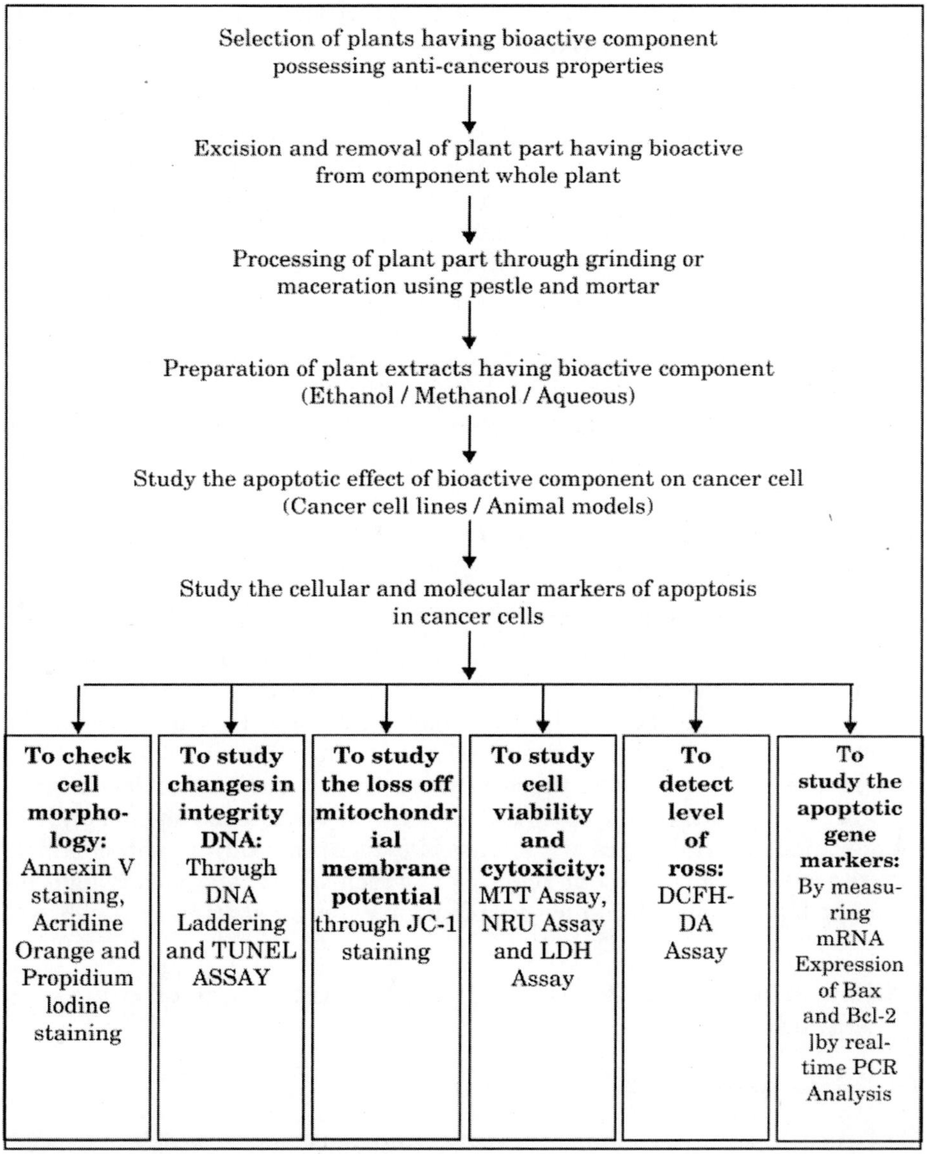

Fig. 1: Schematic diagram showing the systematic work plan to assess the anti-cancerous nature of a selected medicinal plant.

dye binds to the DNA. When observed under a microscope the nucleus of the cell upon binding with the dye gives green fluorescence. The second dye Propidium Iodine (PI) can only enter dead cells having poor or complete loss of membrane integrity; this dye will stain all dead nucleated cells to generate red fluorescence (Fani *et al.,* 2016).

4.2. To study changes in DNA structure in cancer cells undergoing apoptosis

Cancer cells, when undergo apoptosis there is excessive fragmentation and condensation of DNA finally leading to DNA laddering. This occurs due to increased production of Reactive Oxygen Species (ROS) in which there is a degradation of DNA in a ladder like pattern. Such DNA fragments can be visualized by staining with Ethidium Bromide on the Agarose Gel after electrophoretic process. It is seen that instead of getting intact DNA bands of definite length, we get a DNA ladder of multiple overlapping DNA bands of varying length (Arora and Tandon, 2015). Likewise, TUNEL (Terminal deoxynucleotidyl transferase dUTP nick end labelling) Assay is carried out to study DNA fragmentation by tagging the 3' hydroxyl end of double stranded broken DNA fragments generated during apoptosis (Arora and Tandon, 2015).

4.3. To study loss of mitochondrial membrane potential in cancer cells undergoing apoptosis

JC-1 (5,5',6,6'- tetrachloro 1,1',3,3'- tetramethyl benzimidazolyl carbocyanine iodide) dye is used to determine the change in mitochondrial membrane potential. The monomeric form of this dye has emission maxima at a wavelength of 529 nm. At higher concentrations, this dye forms red fluorescent J- aggregates with emission maxima at a wavelength of 590 nm. In the case of cancer, there is more hyperpolarized mitochondrial membrane potential (Forrest, 2015). Due to an altered mitochondrial membrane potential, there is a release of cytochrome C from mitochondria into the cytosol, this cytosolic release of Cytochrome C acts as a trigger for caspases 9 and 3, which induce apoptosis in cancer cells (Liu *et al.,* 2018).

4.4. To study cell viability and cytotoxic effect of drugs on cancer cells

4.4.1. *MTT assay*

MTT Assay is a mitochondrial based cytotoxicity assay, which is used to measure the cell viability or cell death due to the effect of chemotherapy drugs on cancer cells. This assay is based on reduction of 3-[4, 5-dimethylthiazole-2-yl] - 2, 5- diphenyltetrazolium bromide (MTT) dye to purple coloured insoluble product called MTT- formazon. This dye is reduced in the presence of mitochondrial succinate dehydrogenase enzyme. The MTT dye is reduced or taken up by only living cells, dead cells do not take MTT dye due lack of cellular metabolism, no presence of succinate dehydrogenase. Absorbance of formazon crystals in solution is measured at a wavelength of 570 nm using a spectrophotometer (Patravale *et al.,* 2012).

4.4.2. *NRU assay*

Neutral Red Uptake (NRU) is a lysosome based cytotoxicity assay, which is used to measure cell viability or cytotoxic effect of drugs on cancer cells. Neutral Red is a weak cationic dye, which penetrates the lysosomal membrane through non-ionic passive diffusion mechanism and accumulates inside the lysosome of viable cells by hydrophobic interaction with the phosphate group of lysosomal matrix (Repetto *et al.,* 2008). The dead cells fail to take up NRU dye because dead cells are not able to maintain a pH gradient inside the lysosome matrix which is essential for retaining the dye. Once the cells take up the dye, dye is then recovered from viable cells using an acidic ethanol solution, the absorbance of solubilized dye is measured using a spectrophotometer.

4.4.3. *LDH cytotoxicity assay*

Lactate Dehydrogenase (LDH) is an enzyme which is naturally present in all living cells. Whenever there is damage or loss of integrity of the cell membrane due to effect of chemotherapeutic drugs, this enzyme is released into the surrounding tissue. Therefore, in cells growing in cell culture media, detecting the levels of Lactate Dehydrogenase can conclude on the cell injury or damage, hence LDH level acts as a cell death marker.

The relative amount of viable and non-viable cells present within the cell culture medium can be identified and quantitated by measuring the level of enzyme LDH using either a colorimetric or fluorometric LDH cytotoxicity assay. Both these colorimetric and fluorometric assay are carried out for detection of cell toxicity, studying cell death, viability or proliferation and is suitable for high throughput screening. LDH Assay acts as an alternative to 51Cr release cytotoxicity essay due to its simplicity, reliability and accuracy (Fani *et al.,* 2016).

4.5. Detection of level of ROS Production in cancer cells undergoing apoptosis

Reactive Oxygen Species (ROS) are produced in all living cells as a result of cell signalling and homeostasis. ROS are produced and abolished in biological system on a regular basis due to different metabolic activities. An abnormal increase is seen in production of ROS due to mitochondrial membrane damage, apoptosis and cell death. The intracellular levels of ROS can be measured and detected using 2',7' dichlorofluorescein diacetate (DCFH-DA)

(Salcher *et al.*, 2014). This particular dye acts as a probe which is trapped within the cells and is easily oxidized to fluorescent dichlorofluorescein (DCF). This DCFH-DA assay is used to measure the ability of cytotoxic drugs to prevent formation of DCF in most of the types of cancer cells. DCFH-DA assay is done to measure and quantify the levels of intracellular hydrogen peroxide as well as oxidative stress in cells.

4.6. Detection of gene and protein expression of apoptotic markers

In cancer cells it is generally seen there is expression of Bcl 2 family of proteins. Some of the proteins are pro-apoptotic in nature like Bax and some of them are anti-apoptotic like Bcl-2. It is seen that when cancer cells are treated with chemotherapeutic drugs which exert their cytotoxic effect on cells, the expression of pro-apoptotic and anti-apoptotic markers is altered. It is the balance or ratio between the expressions of these two markers decides the fate of cancer cells, whether they would live and proliferate or would undergo apoptosis or programmed cellular death. In drug treated cancer cells the anti-apoptotic markers are supposed to be down regulated whereas pre-apoptotic marker expression is up regulated. The mRNA expression of Bax and Bcl-2 can be measured in drug treated cancer cells by real-time PCR analysis (Singh *et al.*, 2015). The advantages of going for real-time PCR over conventional PCR technique is that we can find the exact copy number of gene expressing our protein of interest in real time through calculating threshold cycle number known as C_T value.

5. CONCLUSIONS AND FUTURE DIRECTION

In conclusion, a large number of plants hold tremendous potential to cure the different lethal conditions including cancer. However it is equally important to adopt a correct approach to investigate their anti-cancerous properties and further elucidate their mechanism of action. Different plants carry the anti-cancerous compound of different chemical nature hence it is recommended to be very careful while selective extraction of these compounds for their further study/uses. Extract preparation should be followed for the confirmation of their anti-cancerous properties using various molecular biology/biochemical approaches. After confirmation of the anti-cancerous nature of the extract, the specific compound responsible for anti-proliferative activities must be identified. Future holds tremendous scope to study and investigate more number of anti-cancerous herbs and their mechanism of action. It will be great if the synthetic drugs can be replaced or get co-administered along with these natural compounds to reduce the side effects caused during the cancer therapy.

REFERENCES

Abdullaev FI, Espinosa-Aguirre JJ. Biomedical properties of saffron and its potential use in cancer therapy and chemoprevention trials. Cancer Detection and Prevention. 2004; 28(6): 426-32.

Ahmad MS, Ahmad S, Arshad M, Afzal M. *Andrographis paniculata* Miracle Herbs for cancer treatment: *In vivo* and *in vitro* studies against Aflatoxin B1 Toxicity. Egyptian Journal of Medical Human Genetics. 2014; 15(2): 163-71.

Ahmad MS, Ahmad S, Gautam B, Arshad M, Afzal M. *Terminalia arjuna*, a herbal remedy against environmental carcinogenicity: An *in vitro* and *in vivo* study. Egyptian Journal of Medical Human Genetics. 2014; 15(1): 61-7.

Akimoto M, Iizuka M, Kanematsu R, Yoshida M, Takenaga K. Anticancer effect of ginger extract against pancreatic cancer cells mainly through reactive oxygen species-mediated autotic cell death. PloS One. 2015; 10(5).

Al-Asmari AK, Albalawi SM, Athar MT, Khan AQ, Al-Shahrani H, Islam M. *Moringa oleifera* as an anti-cancer agent against breast and colorectal cancer cell lines. PloS One. 2015; 10(8): e0135814.

Allegra A, Innao V, Russo S, Gerace D, Alonci A, Musolino C. Anticancer activity of curcumin and its analogues: Preclinical and clinical studies. Cancer Investigation. 2017; 35(1): 1-22.

Alzohairy MA. Therapeutics role of *Azadirachta indica* (Neem) and their active constituents in diseases prevention and treatment. Evidence-Based complementary and alternative medicine. 2016; 2016: 1-11.

Andreani C, Bartolacci C, Wijnant K, Crinelli R, Bianchi M, Magnani M, Hysi A, Iezzi M, Amici A, Marchini C. Resveratrol fuels HER2 and ERα-positive breast cancer behaving as proteasome inhibitor. Aging. 2017; 9(2): 508.

Arora RA, Malhotra PO, Mathur AK, Mathur AR, Govil CM, Ahuja PS. Anticancer alkaloids of *Catharanthus roseus*: Transition from traditional to modern medicine. Herbal Medicine: A Cancer Chemopreventive and Therapeutic Perspective. Jaypee Brothers Medical Publishers Pvt. Ltd, New Delhi, India. 2010, pp. 292-310.

Arora S, Tandon S. DNA fragmentation and cell cycle arrest: A hallmark of apoptosis induced by *Ruta graveolens* in human colon cancer cells. Homeopathy. 2015; 104(1): 36-47.

Arumugam A, Agullo P, Boopalan T, Nandy S, Lopez R, Gutierrez C, Narayan M, Rajkumar L. Neem leaf extract inhibits mammary carcinogenesis by altering cell proliferation, apoptosis, and angiogenesis. Cancer Biology and Therapy. 2014; 15(1): 26-34.

Babu TD, Kuttan G, Padikkala J. Cytotoxic and anti-tumour properties of certain taxa of Umbelliferae with special reference to *Centella asiatica* (L.) Urban. Journal of Ethnopharmacology. 1995; 48(1): 53-7.

Bakshi HA, Hakkim FL, Sam S. Molecular mechanism of crocin induced caspase mediated MCF-7 cell death: *In vivo* toxicity profiling and *ex vivo* macrophage activation. Asian Pacific Journal of Cancer Prevention. 2016; 17: 1499-506.

Berman AY, Motechin RA, Wiesenfeld MY, Holz MK. The therapeutic potential of resveratrol: A review of clinical trials. NPJ Precision Oncology. 2017; 1(1): 35.

Biswal BM, Sulaiman SA, Ismail HC, Zakaria H, Musa KI. Effect of *Withania somnifera* (Ashwagandha) on the development of chemotherapy-induced fatigue and quality of life in breast cancer patients. Integrative Cancer Therapies. 2013; 12(4): 312-22.

Brahmi F, Hadj-Ahmed S, Zarrouk A, Bezine M, Nury T, Madani K, Chibane M, Vejux A, Andreoletti P, Boulekbache-Makhlouf L, Lizard G. Evidence of biological activity of *Mentha species* extracts on apoptotic and autophagic targets on murine RAW264. 7 and human U937 monocytic cells. Pharmaceutical Biology. 2017; 55(1): 286-93.

Brown AC. Anticancer activity of *Morinda citrifolia* (Noni) fruit: A review. Phytotherapy Research. 2012; 26(10): 1427-40.

Cancer HSP: Anticancer Herbs database of Systems Pharmacology, Retrieved on 30 May 2018; http://lsp.nwu.edu.cn/CancerHSP.php

Cao J, Liu Y, Jia L, Zhou HM, Kong Y, Yang G, Jiang LP, Li QJ, Zhong LF. Curcumin induces apoptosis through mitochondrial hyperpolarization and mtDNA damage in human hepatoma G2 cells. Free Radical Biology and Medicine. 2007; 43(6): 968-75.

Chao J, Lu TC, Liao JW, Huang TH, Lee MS, Cheng HY, Ho LK, Kuo CL, Peng WH. Analgesic and anti-inflammatory activities of ethanol root extract of *Mahonia oiwakensis* in mice. Journal of Ethnopharmacology. 2009; 125(2): 297-303.

Chavan SS, Damale MG, Shamkuwar PB, Pawar DP. Traditional medicinal plants for anticancer activity. International Journal of Current Pharmaceutical Research. 2013; 5(4): 50-4.

Chen Y, Zhang H, Tian X, Zhao C, Cai L, Liu Y, Jia L, Yin HX, Chen C. Antioxidant potential of crocins and ethanol extracts of *Gardenia jasminoides* ELLIS and *Crocus sativus* L.: A relationship investigation between antioxidant activity and crocin contents. Food Chemistry. 2008; 109(3): 484-92.

Choan E, Segal R, Jonker D, Malone S, Reaume N, Eapen L, Gallant V. A prospective clinical trial of green tea for hormone refractory prostate cancer: An evaluation of the complementary/alternative therapy approach. Urologic Oncology. 2005; 23(2): 108-113.

Fani S, Kamalidehghan B, Lo KM, Nigjeh SE, Keong YS, Dehghan F, Soori R, Abdulla MA, Chow KM, Ali HM, Hajiaghaalipour F. Anticancer activity of a monobenzyltin complex C1 against MDA-MB-231 cells through induction of Apoptosis and inhibition of breast cancer stem cells. Scientific Reports. 2016; 6: 389-92.

Ferlay J, Soerjomataram I, Dikshit R, Eser S, Mathers C, Rebelo M, Parkin DM, Forman D, Bray F. Cancer incidence and mortality worldwide: Sources, methods and major patterns in GLOBOCAN 2012. International Journal of Cancer. 2015; 136(5): E359-86.

Forrest MD. Why cancer cells have a more hyperpolarised mitochondrial membrane potential and emergent prospects for therapy. bioRxiv. 2015; 1: 1-42. doi: https://doi.org/10.1101/025197

Gan Z, Liang Z, Chen X, Wen X, Wang Y, Li M, Ni Y. Separation and preparation of 6-gingerol from molecular distillation residue of Yunnan ginger rhizomes by high-speed counter-current chromatography and the antioxidant activity of ginger oils *in vitro*. Journal of Chromatography B. 2016; 1011: 99-107.

Ganesan K, Gani SB. Ethnomedical and pharmacological potentials of *Plumbago zeylanica* L – A review. American Journal of Phytomedicine and Clinical Therapy. 2013; 1: 313-7.

Gao F, Hu Y, Ye X, Li J, Chen Z, Fan G. Optimal extraction and fingerprint analysis of *Cnidii fructus* by accelerated solvent extraction and high performance liquid chromatographic analysis with photodiode array and mass spectrometry detections. Food Chemistry. 2013; 141(3): 1962-71.

Ghasemzadeh A, Jaafar HZ, Rahmat A, Devarajan T. Evaluation of bioactive compounds, pharmaceutical quality, and anticancer activity of curry leaf (*Murraya koenigii L.*). Evidence-based Complementary and Alternative Medicine. 2014; 2014: 1-8.

Gulshan B, Suri KA, Parul G. A comprehensive review on *Nyctanthes arbor-tristis*. International Journal of Drug Delivery and Research. 2015; 7(1): 183-93.

Gupta SC, Patchva S, Aggarwal BB. Therapeutic roles of curcumin: Lessons learned from clinical trials. The AAPS journal. 2013; 15(1): 195-218.

Guzman M. Cannabinoids: Potential anticancer agents. Nature Reviews Cancer. 2003; 3(10): 745.

Habib SH, Makpol S, Hamid NA, Das S, Ngah WZ, Yusof YA. Ginger extract (*Zingiber officinale*) has anti-cancer and anti-inflammatory effects on ethionine-induced hepatoma rats. Clinics. 2008; 63(6): 807-13.

Hajighasemi F, Hashemi V, Khoshzaban F. Cytotoxic effect of *Mentha spicata* aqueous extract on cancerous cell lines *in vitro*. Journal of Medicinal Plants Research. 2011; 5(20): 5142-7.

Hallman K, Aleck K, Dwyer B, Lloyd V, Quigley M, Sitto N, Siebert AE, Dinda S. The effects of turmeric (curcumin) on tumor suppressor protein (p53) and estrogen receptor (ERα) in breast cancer cells. Breast Cancer: Targets and Therapy. 2017; 9: 153.

Imran M, Ullah A, Saeed F, Nadeem M, Arshad MU, Suleria HA. Cucurmin, anticancer, & antitumor perspectives: A comprehensive review. Critical Reviews in Food Science and Nutrition. 2017; 1: 1-23.

Jacob L, Latha MS. Anticancer activity of *Clitoria ternatea* Linn. Against dalton's lymphoma. International Journal of Pharmacognosy and Phytochemical Research. 2012; 4(4): 207-12.

Jain P, Sharma HP, Basri F, Baraik B, Kumari S, Pathak C. Pharmacological Profiles of Ethno-Medicinal Plant: *Plumbago zeylanica L.* - A Review. International Journal of Pharmaceutical Science Review and Research. 2014; 24: 157-63.

Joshi K, Tavhare S, Panara K, Kumar P, Karra N. Studies of Ashwagandha *Withania somnifera* Dunal. International Journal of Pharmaceutical and Biological Archive. 2016; 7(1): 1-11.

Jung IL, Lee JH, Kang SC. A potential oral anticancer drug candidate, *Moringa oleifera* leaf extract, induces the apoptosis of human hepatocellular carcinoma cells. Oncology Letters. 2015; 10(3): 1597-604.

Kahlert UD, Maciaczyk D, Doostkam S, Orr BA, Simons B, Bogiel T, Reithmeier T, Prinz M, Schubert J, Niedermann G, Brabletz T. Activation of canonical WNT/α-catenin signalling enhances *in vitro* motility of glioblastoma cells by activation of ZEB1 and other activators of epithelial-to-mesenchymal transition. Cancer Letters. 2012; 325(1): 42-53.

Kandil FE, Nassar MI. A tannin anti-cancer promotor from *Terminalia arjuna*. Phytochemistry. 1998; 47(8): 1567-8.

Khanapur M, Avadhanula RK, Setty OH. *In vitro* antioxidant, antiproliferative, and phytochemical study in different extracts of *Nyctanthes arbor-tristis* flowers. BioMed research international. 2014; 2014: 1-10.

Kumari TS, Madhuri TS, Charya MS, Rao KS. Antioxidant and anticancer activities of *Nyctanthes arbor-tristis*. International Journal of Pharmacy and Pharmaceutical Sciences. 2012; 4(4): 452-4.

Kwon HL, Chung MS. Pilot-scale subcritical solvent extraction of curcuminoids from *Curcuma longa* L. Food Chemistry. 2015; 185: 58-64

Lai YJ, Tai CJ, Wang CW, Choong CY, Lee BH, Shi YC, Tai CJ. Anti-cancer activity of *Solanum nigrum* (AESN) through suppression of mitochondrial function and epithelial-mesenchymal transition (EMT) in breast cancer cells. Molecules. 2016; 21(5): 553.

Lee DH, Kim DW, Jung CH, Lee YJ, Park D. Gingerol sensitizes TRAIL-induced apoptotic cell death of glioblastoma cells. Toxicology and Applied Pharmacology. 2014; 279(3): 253-65.

Lee WJ, Chien MH, Chow JM, Chang JL, Wen YC, Lin YW, Cheng CW, Lai GM, Hsiao M, Lee LM. Nonautophagic cytoplasmic vacuolation death induction in human PC-3M prostate cancer by curcumin through reactive oxygen species-mediated endoplasmic reticulum stress. Scientific Reports. 2015; 5: 104-20.

Lin FM, Chen LR, Lin EH, Ke FC, Chen HY, Tsai MJ, Hsiao PW. Compounds from *Wedelia chinensis* synergistically suppress androgen activity and growth in prostate cancer cells. Carcinogenesis. 2007; 28(12): 2521-9.

Lin X, Peng Z, Su C. Potential anti-cancer activities and mechanisms of costunolide and dehydrocostus lactone. International Journal of Molecular Sciences. 2015; 16(5): 10888-906.

Lin X, Wu G, Huo WQ, Zhang Y, Jin FS. Resveratrol induces apoptosis associated with mitochondrial dysfunction in bladder carcinoma cells. International Journal of Urology. 2012; 19(8): 757-64.

Lin YC, Lin JC, Hung CM, Chen Y, Liu LC, Chang TC, Kao JY, Ho CT, Way TD. Osthole inhibits insulin-like growth factor-1-induced epithelial to mesenchymal transition *via* the inhibition of PI3K/Akt signaling pathway in human brain cancer cells. Journal of Agricultural and Food Chemistry. 2014; 62(22): 5061-71.

Liu D, Perfettini JL, Brenner C. Mitochondrial Regulation of Cell Death. *In*: Mitochondrial Biology and Experimental Therapeutics. 2018, Springer, Cham. pp. 75-90.

Lorusso D, Bria E, Costantini A, Di Maio M, Rosti G, Mancuso A. Patients' perception of chemotherapy side effects: Expectations, doctor–patient communication and impact on quality of life–An Italian survey. European Journal of Cancer Care. 2017; 26(2): e12618.

Mahapatra S, Karnes RJ, Holmes MW, Young CY, Cheville JC, Kohli M, Klee EW, Tindall DJ, Donkena KV. Novel molecular targets of *Azadirachta indica* associated with inhibition of tumor growth in prostate cancer. The AAPS journal. 2011; 13(3): 365-77.

Mahata S, Pandey A, Shukla S, Tyagi A, Husain SA, Das BC, Bharti AC. Anticancer activity of *Phyllanthus emblica* Linn. (Indian gooseberry): Inhibition of transcription factor AP-1 and HPV gene expression in cervical cancer cells. Nutrition and Cancer. 2013; 65(sup1): 88-97.

Manju K, Jat RK, Anju G. A review on medicinal plants used as a source of anticancer agents. International Journal of Drug Research and Technology. 2012; 2(2): 177-183.

Martin AC, Fuzer AM, Becceneri AB, da Silva JA, Tomasin R, Denoyer D, Kim SH, McIntyre KA, Pearson HB, Yeo B, Nagpal A. [10]-gingerol induces apoptosis and inhibits metastatic dissemination of triple negative breast cancer *in vivo*. Oncotarget. 2017; 8(42): 72260.

Mishra R, Kaur G. Aqueous ethanolic extract of *Tinospora cordifolia* as a potential candidate for differentiation based therapy of glioblastomas. PLoS One. 2013; 8(10): e78764.

Mohan A, Nair SV, Lakshmanan VK. *Leucas aspera* nanomedicine shows superior toxicity and cell migration retarded in prostate cancer cells. Applied Biochemistry and Biotechnology. 2017; 181(4): 1388-400.

Montalvo-Hernández B, Rito-Palomares M, Benavides J. Recovery of crocins from saffron stigmas (*Crocus sativus*) in aqueous two-phase systems. Journal of Chromatography A. 2012; 1236: 7-15.

Munagala R, Kausar H, Munjal C, Gupta RC. Withaferin A induces p53-dependent apoptosis by repression of HPV oncogenes and upregulation of tumor suppressor proteins in human cervical cancer cells. Carcinogenesis. 2011; 32(11): 1697-705.

Neda GD, Rabeta MS, Ong MT. Chemical composition and anti-proliferative properties of flowers of *Clitoria Ternatea*. International Food Research Journal. 2013; 20(3): 1229-34.

Nicastro HL, Ross SA, Milner JA. Garlic and onions: Their cancer prevention properties. Cancer Prevention Research. 2015; 8(3): 181-9.

Ochiai T, Ohno S, Soeda S, Tanaka H, Shoyama Y, Shimeno H. Crocin prevents the death of rat pheochromocytoma (PC-12) cells by its antioxidant effects stronger than those of α-tocopherol. Neuroscience Letters. 2004; 362(1): 61-4.

Oskoueian E, Abdullah N, Ahmad S, Saad WZ, Omar AR, Ho YW. Bioactive compounds and biological activities of *Jatropha curcas L.* kernel meal extract. International Journal of Molecular Sciences. 2011; 12(9): 5955-70.

Oskoueian E, Abdullah N, Saad WZ, Omar AR, Ahmad S, Kuan WB, Zolkifli NA, Hendra R, Ho YW. Antioxidant, anti-inflammatory and anticancer activities of methanolic extracts from *Jatropha curcas Linn.* Journal of Medicinal Plants Research. 2011; 5(1): 49-57.

Oyagbemi AA, Saba AB, Azeez OI. Molecular targets of [6]-gingerol: Its potential roles in cancer chemoprevention. Biofactors. 2010; 36(3): 169-78.

Oza VP, Parmar PP, Kumar S, Subramanian RB. Anticancer properties of highly purified L-asparaginase from *Withania somnifera L.* against acute lymphoblastic leukemia. Applied Biochemistry and Biotechnology. 2010; 160(6): 1833-40.

Palliyaguru DL, Singh SV, Kensler TW. *Withania somnifera:* From prevention to treatment of cancer. Molecular Nutrition and Food Research. 2016; 60(6): 1342-53.

Park GH, Park JH, Song HM, Eo HJ, Kim MK, Lee JW, Lee MH, Cho KH, Lee JR, Cho HJ, Jeong JB. Anti-cancer activity of Ginger *(Zingiber officinale)* leaf through the expression of activating transcription factor 3 in human colorectal cancer cells. BMC Complementary and Alternative Medicine. 2014; 14(1): 408.

Partridge AH, Burstein HJ, Winer EP. Side effects of chemotherapy and combined chemohormonal therapy in women with early-stage breast cancer. JNCI Monographs. 2001; 30: 135-42.

Patel PR, Raval BP, Karanth HA, Patel VR. Potent antitumor activity of *Rubia cordifolia.* International Journal of Phytomedicine. 2010; 2(1): 44-6.

Patravale V, Dandekar P, Ratnesh J. 4–Nanotoxicology: Evaluating toxicity potential of drug-nanoparticles. Nanoparticulate Drug Delivery Perspectives on the Transition from Laboratory to Market. 2012

Pattanayak P, Behera P, Das D, Panda SK. *Ocimum sanctum* Linn. A reservoir plant for therapeutic applications: An overview. Pharmacognosy Reviews. 2010; 4(7): 95.

Patterson J, Verghese M. Anticancer and Toxic Effects of Curry Leaf *(Murraya koenigii)* Extracts. Journal of Pharmacology and Toxicology. 2015; 10(2): 49-59.

Prakash E, Gupta DK. Cytotoxic activity of ethanolic extract of *Cuminum cyminum* Linn against seven human cancer cell line. Universal Journal of Agricultural Research. 2014; 2(1): 27-30.

Radha MH, Laxmipriya NP. Evaluation of biological properties and clinical effectiveness of *Aloe vera*: A systematic review. Journal of Traditional and Complementary Medicine. 2015; 5(1): 21-6.

Raghu R, Lu KH, Sheen LY. Recent research progress on garlic as a potential anticarcinogenic agent against major digestive cancers. Journal of Traditional and Complementary Medicine. 2012; 2(3): 192-201.

Rai N, Agrawal RC, Khan A. *Centella asiatica* extract exhibit anticancer activity against different types of tumours. International Journal of Pure and Applied Bioscience. 2014; 2: 122-7.

Rajagopal S, Kumar RA, Deevi DS, Satyanarayana C, Rajagopalan R. Andrographolide, a potential cancer therapeutic agent isolated from *Andrographis paniculata*. Journal of Experimental therapeutics and Oncology. 2003; 3(3): 147-58.

Rajha HN, Ziegler W, Louka N, Hobaika Z, Vorobiev E, Boechzelt HG, Maroun RG. Effect of the drying process on the intensification of phenolic compounds recovery from grape pomace using accelerated solvent extraction. International Journal of Molecular Sciences. 2014; 15(10): 18640-58.

Rawson NE, Ho CT, Li S. Efficacious anti-cancer property of flavonoids from citrus peels. Food Science and Human Wellness. 2014; 3(3-4): 104-9.

Reddy AC, Lokesh BR. Studies on spice principles as antioxidants in the inhibition of lipid peroxidation of rat liver microsomes. Molecular and Cellular Biochemistry. 1992; 111(1-2): 117-24.

Repetto G, Del Peso A, Zurita JL. Neutral red uptake assay for the estimation of cell viability/cytotoxicity. Nature Protocols. 2008; 3(7): 1125

Ruskin S, Aruna SR. *In vitro* and *in vivo* antitumor activity of *Catharanthus roseus*. International Research Journal of Pharmaceutical and Applied Sciences. 2014; 4: 1-4.

Saab AM, Tundis R, Loizzo MR, Lampronti I, Borgatti M, Gambari R, Menichini F, Esseily F, Menichini F. Antioxidant and antiproliferative activity of *Laurus nobilis* L. (Lauraceae) leaves and seeds essential oils against K562 human chronic myelogenous leukaemia cells. Natural Product Research. 2012; 26(18): 1741-5.

Saha S, Ghosh S. *Tinospora cordifolia:* One plant, many roles. Ancient Science of Life. 2012; 31(4): 151.

Sain M, Sharma V. *Catharanthus roseus* (An anti-cancerous drug yielding plant). A Review of Potential Therapeutic Properties. Internatonal Journal of Pure and Applied Biosciences. 2013; 1(6): 139-42.

Salcher S, Hagenbuchner J, Geiger K, Seiter MA, Rainer J, Kofler R, Hermann M, Kiechl-Kohlendorfer U, Ausserlechner MJ, Obexer P. C10ORF10/DEPP, a transcriptional target of FOXO3, regulates ROS-sensitivity in human neuroblastoma. Molecular Cancer. 2014; 13(1): 224.

Saminathan M, Rai RB, Dhama K, Tiwari R, Chakraborty S, Amarpal, Ranganath GJ, Kannan K. Systematic review on anticancer potential and other health beneficial pharmacological activities of novel medicinal plant *Morinda citrifolia* (Noni). International Journal of Pharmacology. 2013; 9(8): 462-92.

Shalabi M, Khilo K, Zakaria MM, Elsebaei MG, Abdo W, Awadin W. Anticancer activity of *Aloe vera* and *Calligonum comosum* extracts separetely on hepatocellular carcinoma cells. Asian Pacific Journal of Tropical Biomedicine. 2015; 5(5): 375-81.

Shukla Y, Singh M. Cancer preventive properties of ginger: A brief review. Food and Chemical Toxicology. 2007; 45(5): 683-90

Shivpuje P, Ammanangi R, Bhat K, Katti S. Effect of *Ocimum sanctum* on Oral Cancer Cell Line: An *in vitro* Study. The Journal of Contemporary Dental Practice. 2015; 16(9): 709-14.

Singh L, Pushker N, Saini N, Sen S, Sharma A, Bakhshi S, Chawla B, Kashyap S. Expression of pro apoptotic Bax and anti apoptotic Bcl 2 proteins in human retinoblastoma. Clinical and Experimental Ophthalmology. 2015; 43(3): 259-67.

Singh RP, Gangadharappa HV, Mruthunjaya K. *Cuminum cyminum* – A popular spice: An updated review. Pharmacognosy Journal. 2017; 9(3): 292-301.

Singh S, Verma SK, Kumar S. Analysis of anti-cancer potential of *Terminalia arjuna*. International Journal of Advanced Scientific Research and Management. 2017; 2(11): 82-88.

Sivalokanathan S, Ilayaraja M, Balasubramanian MP. Antioxidant activity of *Terminalia arjuna* bark extract on N-nitrosodiethylamine induced hepatocellular carcinoma in rats. Molecular and Cellular Biochemistry. 2006; 281(1-2): 87.

Sridevi M, John B, Yamini K. Anticancer effect of *Ocimum-sanctum* ethanolic extract in non-small cell lung carcinoma cell line. International Journal of Pharmacy and Pharmaceutical Sciences. 2016; 8(4): 242-6.

Srinivasahan V, Durairaj B. *In vitro* cytotoxic and apoptotic activity of polysaccharide rich *Morinda citrifolia* fruit on MCF-7 cells. Asian Journal of Pharmaceutical and Clinical Research. 2015; 8(2): 190-193.

Sureshkumar P, Senthilraja P, Kalavathy S. *In-Silico* Docking Analysis of *Calotropis gigantea* (L.) R. Br Derived Compound against Anti-Cervical Cancer Activity. World Research Journal of Computer-Aided Drug Design. 2012;1 (1): 9-12.

Tiwari S, Upadhyaya R, Shroti R, Upadhyaya ST. *Rubia cordifolia* root extract induces apoptosis in cancer cell line. Science Secure Journal of Biotechnology. 2012; 1: 39-42.

Ullah N, Ahmad M, Aslam H, Tahir MA, Aftab M, Bibi N, Ahmad S. Green tea phytocompounds as anticancer: A review. Asian Pacific Journal of Tropical Disease. 2016; 6(4): 330-6.

Vallianou NG, Evangelopoulos A, Schizas N, Kazazis C. Potential anticancer properties and mechanisms of action of curcumin. Anticancer Research. 2015; 35(2): 645-51.

Velasco G, Sánchez C, Guzmán M. Anticancer mechanisms of cannabinoids. Current Oncology. 2016; 23(Suppl 2): S23.

Wadhwa R, Singh R, Gao R, Shah N, Widodo N, Nakamoto T, Ishida Y, Terao K, Kaul SC. Water extract of Ashwagandha leaves has anticancer activity: Identification of an active component and its mechanism of action. PLoS One. 2013; 8(10): e77189.

Wang L, Wang J, Fang L, Zheng Z, Zhi D, Wang S, Li S, Ho CT, Zhao H. Anticancer activities of citrus peel polymethoxyflavones related to angiogenesis and others. BioMed Research International. 2014; 2014: 1-10.

Wang Y, Han T, Zhu Y, Zheng CJ, Ming QL, Rahman K, Qin LP. Antidepressant properties of bioactive fractions from the extract of *Crocus sativus* L. Journal of Natural Medicines. 2010; 64(1): 24.

Wu T, Geng J, Guo W, Gao J, Zhu X. Asiatic acid inhibits lung cancer cell growth *in vitro* and *in vivo* by destroying mitochondria. Acta Pharmaceutica Sinica B. 2017; 7(1): 65-72.

Yang G, Wang S, Zhong L, Dong X, Zhang W, Jiang L, Geng C, Sun X, Liu X, Chen M, Ma Y. 6 Gingerol Induces Apoptosis through Lysosomal Mitochondrial Axis in Human Hepatoma G2 Cells. Phytotherapy Research. 2012; 26(11): 1667-73.

Yang HY, Hsu YF, Chiu PT, Ho SJ, Wang CH, Chi CC, Huang YH, Lee CF, Li YS, Ou G, Hsu MJ. Anti-cancer activity of an osthole derivative, NBM-T-BMX-OS01: Targeting vascular endothelial growth factor receptor signaling and angiogenesis. PloS One. 2013; 8(11): e81592.

Yoshida M, Fuchigami M, Nagao T, Okabe H, Matsunaga K, Takata J, Karube Y, Tsuchihashi R, Kinjo J, Mihashi K, Fujioka T. Antiproliferative constituents from Umbelliferae plants VII. Active triterpenes and rosmarinic acid from *Centella asiatica.* Biological and Pharmaceutical Bulletin. 2005; 28(1): 173-5.

Zayas-Viera MD. Anticancer Effect of *Moringa oleifera* Leaf Extract in Human Cancer Cell Lines. Journal of Health Disparities Research and Practice. 2016; 9(5): 102.

Zhang X, Huo L, Jin H, Han Y, Wang J, Zhang Y, Lai X, Le Z, Zhang J, Hua Z. Anti-cancer activity of Annexin V in murine melanoma model by suppressing tumor angiogenesis. Oncotarget. 2017; 8(26): 42602.

Zhao T, Sun Q, Marques M, Witcher M. Anticancer properties of *Phyllanthus emblica* (Indian gooseberry). Oxidative Medicine and Cellular Longevity. 2015; 2015: 1-7.

Zhu X, Li Z, Li T, Long F, Lv Y, Liu L, Liu X, Zhan Q. Osthol inhibits the PI3K/AKT signalling pathway *via* activation of PTEN and induces cell cycle arrest and apoptosis in esophageal squamous cell carcinoma. Biomedicine and Pharmacotherapy. 2018; 102: 502-9.

12

Chemistry, Bioactivities and Biotechnological Production of Rosmarinic Acid

HARI GAJULA, VADLAPUDI KUMAR[1]*, POORNIMA D VIJENDRA[1], RAJASHEKAR JARUBANDI[1], TORANKUMAR SANNABOMMAJI[1] AND GIRIDHARA BASAPPA[1]

ABSTRACT

Polyphenols are plant secondary metabolites that greatly benefit human health. There are many unique polyphenols present in plants, and are collectively known as phytochemicals. Among them, rosmarinic acid is one of the polyphenols found in a variety of plants. Rosmarinic acid is a dimer of caffeic acid and 3,4–dihydroxyphenyllactic acid, that are joined together by an ester linkage and is known as a phenylpropanoid. It occurs very commonly in many plant species belonging to the families of Lamiaceae and Boraginaceae, especially in the subfamily Nepetoideae. Apart from these, it has also identified in some ferns and hornwort species. The enzymes involved in the synthesis of rosmarinic acid have been well characterized at the biochemical level, and its synthesis starts with the aromatic amino acids, phenylalanine and tyrosine, however biologically, it is formed from the 4-coumaroyl-4-hydroxyphenyllactate. It is one of the highly valued natural compounds with many bioactivities including anti-inflammatory, antibacterial, antiviral and antioxidant properties. Due to low production in the parent plants, there have been some plant cell culture techniques optimized to enhance its production. In this chapter, the structure, sources, biosynthesis and rosmarinic acid production through biotechnological approaches are discussed in detail. Also, the chapter highlights on its various biological activities.

[1] Department of Biochemistry, Davangere University, Shivagangothri, Davangere-577002 Karnataka, India
Corresponding author: veeke2012@gmail.com

Key words: Rosmarinic acid, Polyphenol, Caffeic acid, Biological activities.

1. INTRODUCTION

Plants synthesize a wide variety of compounds in response to defense activities, and are called as secondary metabolites possess medicinal activities. From many decades, mankind is mainly dependent on several types of natural drugs to cure various diseases. Since last two decades, almost 71% of new drugs used in the current market are directly or indirectly derived from natural products (Newman and Cragg, 2012). Thus, plant derived natural products have been greatly contributing in the development of modern medicines.

Rosmarinic acid is one of the natural phenolic compounds produced by a variety of plants. It exhibits wide ranging biological activities and helps to improve human health. Rosmarinic acid is widely distributed in Lamiaceae family of medicinal plants (Petersen, 2013), for example *Melissa officinalis, Rosmarinus officinalis* L., *Mentha* spp., previously, many authors have explained the occurrence, structure and importance of rosmarinic acid for its significant biological activities (Petersen *et al.,* 2003). However, the production of rosmarinic acid in these plants is observed to be very low, and the chemical synthesis of this compound is time consuming and expensive. To overcome from its supply crises, many scientists have adopted various protocols for the enhancement of rosmarinic acid in plant cell tissue cultures (Khojasteh *et al.*, 2014). These approaches offer a controlled production system, which ensures the continuous production and stable supply of rosmarinic acid without any alternation in the quality and yield. Because of its wide range of biological properties, it is highly valued in the pharmaceutical industries towards human care and health.

The objectives of the present chapter is to describe the chemical structure, biosynthesis, and biological activities of rosmarinic acid. Also, possible biotechnological approaches to over produce rosmarinic acid in plant cell tissue cultures and its extraction and isolation from these cultures are discussed in detail.

2. SOURCES OF ROSMARINIC ACID

Rosmarinic acid is found most notably in many plant species that belong to the families of Lamiaceae and Boraginaceae, especially in the subfamily, Nepetoideae. Apart from these, it has also identified in some ferns (Hausler *et al.*, 1992) and hornwort species (Takeda *et al.,* 1990). Some of the important plants that are rich in rosmarinic acid are *Salvia officinalis* L.,

Thymus vulgaris L., *Rosmarinus officinalis,* from which, for the first time, rosmarinic acid was isolated (Scarpati and Oriente, 1958). Later, it was found to occur in other medicinal plants, such as *Ocimum basilicum* L., *Salvia miltiorrhiza*, *Origanum majorana*, *Mentha arvensis* L., *Melissa officinalis*, and *Perilla frutescens*.

3. STRUCTURE OF ROSMARINIC ACID

Structure of rosmarinic acid is illustrated in Fig. 1, which is a dimer of caffeic acid and 3,4-dihydroxyphenyllactic acid. Interestingly, rosmarinic acid is synthesized from phenyl alanine and tyrosine. Phenyl alanine contributes the caffeic acid, while tyrosine contributes to the 3,4-dihydroxyphenyllactic acid. These two acids, together form a polyphenol, called rosmarinic acid. In 1970, Ellis and Towers experimentally proved the involvement of these two aromatic amino acids in rosmarinic acid biosynthesis using radiolabelled amino acids in mentha plants.

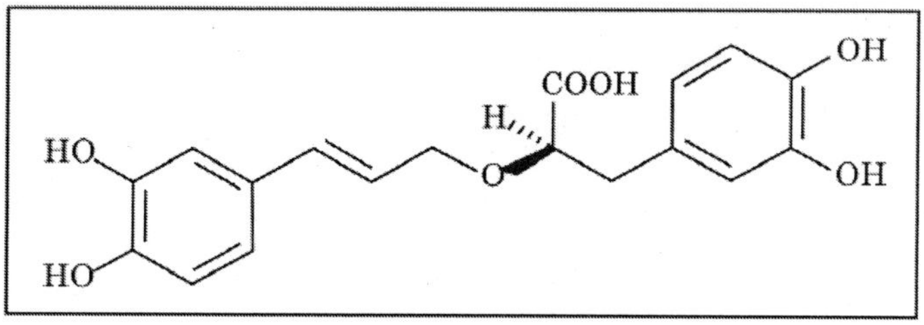

Fig. 1: Structure of rosmarinic acid.

4. ROSMARINIC ACID BIOSYNTHESIS

Phenylalanine and tyrosine are the end products of the Shikimate pathway. From phenylalanine and tyrosine, rosmarinic acid biosynthesis proceeds *via* a series of side-chain modifications and ring modifications to yield rosmarinic acid. The complete biosynthetic pathway of rosmarinic acid is illustrated in Fig. 2.

4.1. Synthesis of rosmarinic acid through phenylalanine derived pathway

4.1.1. *Deamination of L-phenylalanine to trans-cinnamic acid*

Phenylalanine ammonia lyase (PAL: EC Number: 4.3.1.24) catalyzes the deamination of L-phenylalanine to *trans*-cinammic acid and ammonia, which is the first enzyme to be involved in the phenylpropanoid pathway.

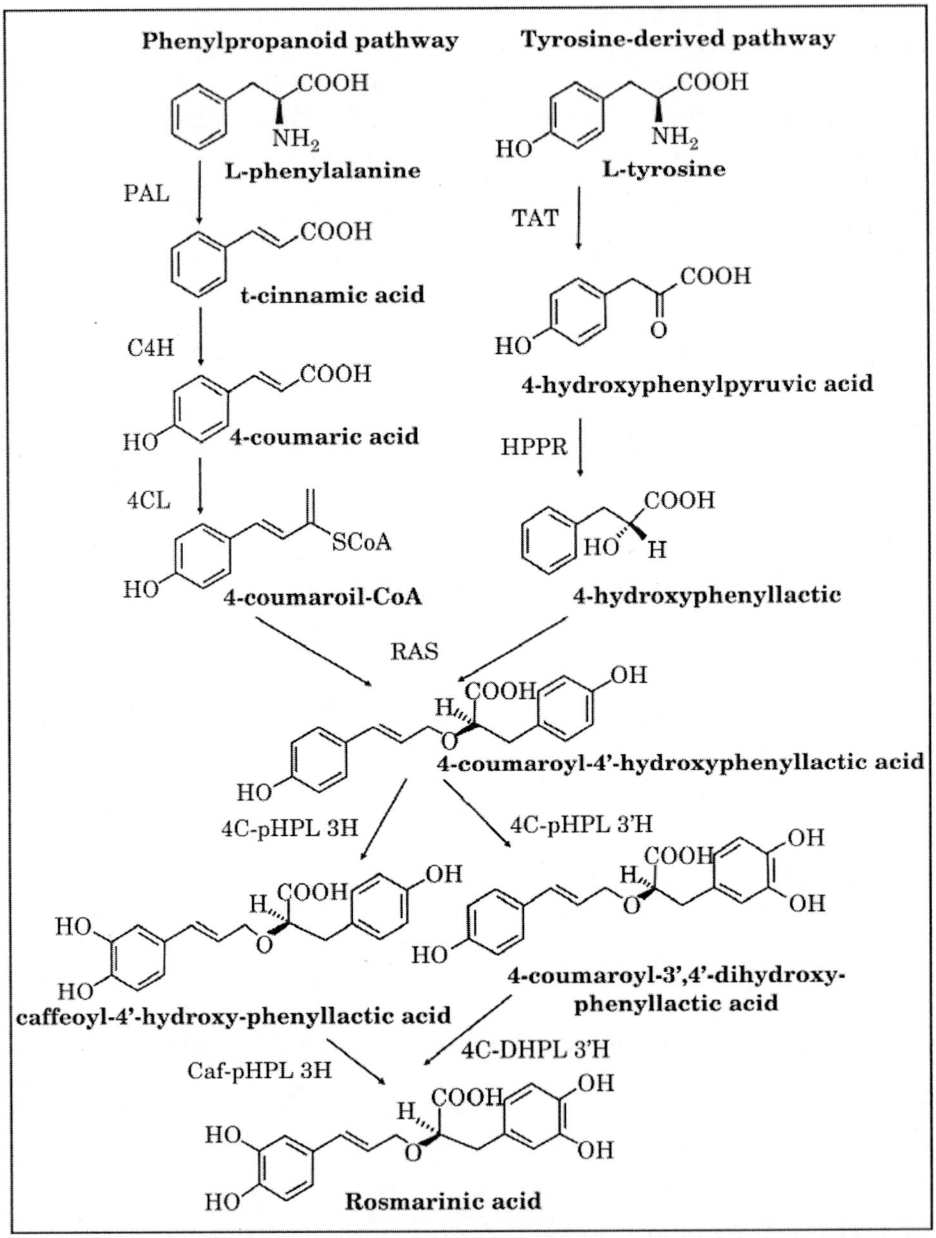

Fig. 2: Rosmarinic acid biosynthesis pathway-PAL: phenylalanine ammonia lyase, C4H:cinammic acid 4-hydroxylase, 4 CL: 4-coumaric acid CoA ligase, TAT: tyrosine aminotransferase, HPPR: hydroxyphenylpyruvate reductase, RAS: rosmarinic acid synthase, 4C-pHPL-3/3'-H: 4-coumaroyl-4'-hydroxyphenyllactate 3/3' hydroxylase(s), Caf-pHPL 3'H caffeoyl-4'-hydroxyphenyllactate 3'-hydroxylase,4C-DHPL 3H: 4-coumaroyl-3',4'-dihydoxyphenyllactate 3-hydroxylase

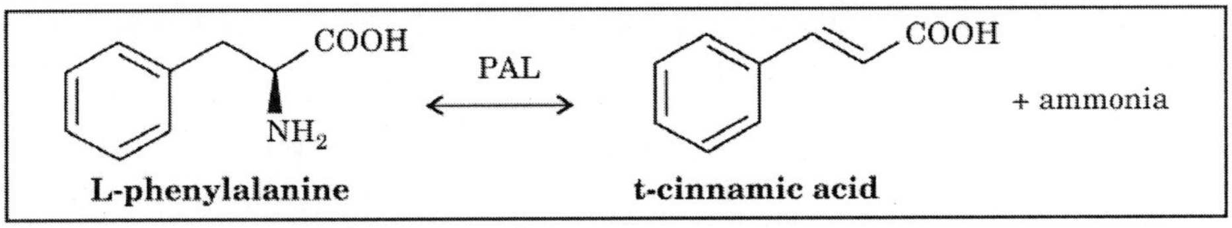

4.1.2. *Hydroxylation of trans-cinnamic acid to 4-coumaric acid*

This reaction is mediated by the cinnamic acid 4-hydroxylase (EC Number:1.14.13.11) which is a cytochrome p-450 dependent enzyme, which introduces the para-hydroxyl group into the aromatic ring of *trans*-cinnamic acid to yield the 4-coumaric acid (also known as p-coumarate) to mediate this, cinnamic acid 4-hydroxylase (C4H) depends on the NADPH and molecular oxygen.

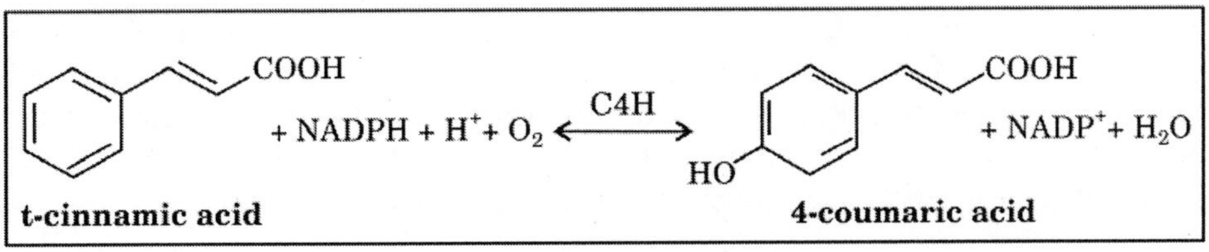

4.1.3. *4-coumaric acid to 4-coumaroyl-CoA*

For the synthesis of cinnamic acid esters, an activated cinnamic acid is essential, and this is mediated by the enzyme, 4-coumaric acid CoA ligase (4 CL) (EC Number: 6.2.1.12) with coenzyme A in an ATP dependent reaction that forms the CoA thioester, 4-coumaroyl CoA.

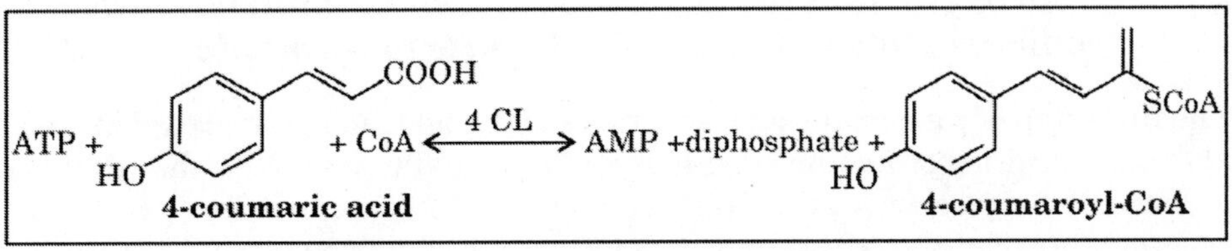

4.2. Synthesis of rosmarinic acid through tyrosine derived pathway

4.2.1. *Transamination of L-tyrosine to 4-hydroxyphenylpyruvic acid*

Transamination of L-tyrosine to 4-hydroxyphenylpyruvic acid and glutamate will be catalyzed by the enzyme tyrosine aminotransferase (TAT) (*EC Number: 2.6.1.5)*

4.2.2. *Reduction of 4-hyroxyphenylpyruvic acid to 4-hydroxyphenyl lactate*

Later, the NADPH-dependent hydroxyphenylpyruvate reductase (HPPR) reduces the 4-hydroxyphenylpyruvic acid to form 4-hydroxyphenyl lactate

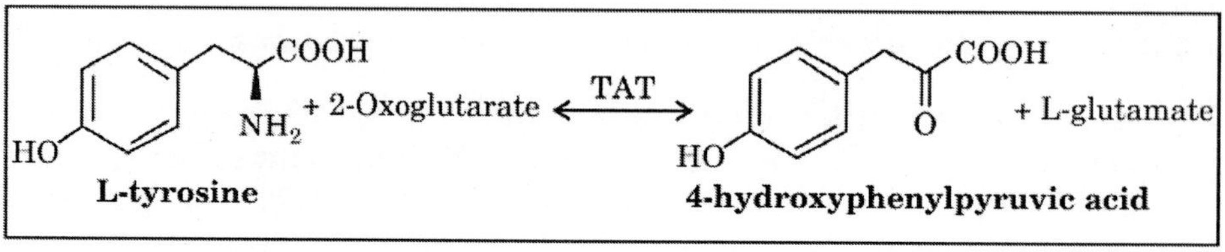

4.2.3. *Ester formation between 4-Hydroxyphenyl lactate and 4-Coumaryol CoA (rosmarinic acid synthase: ester formation)*

4-hydroxyphenyl lactate and 4-coumaryol CoA are the two precursors that are synthesized from L-phenyl alanine and L-tyrosine, that are combined together by an ester linkage and form the 4-coumaryl-4'-hydroxyphenyllactic acid with the help of enzyme rosmarinic acid synthase (RAS) (EC Number: 2.3.1.140).

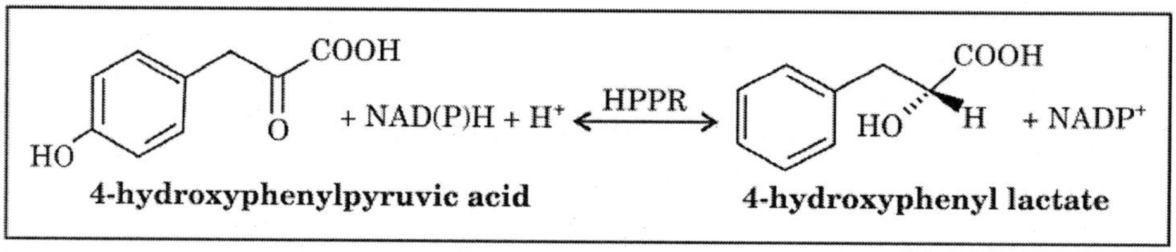

4.2.4. *Hydroxylations at 3 and 3' of the aromatic rings (4-coumaroyl-4'-hydroxyphenyllactate to rosmarinic acid)*

The final step of rosmarinic acid synthesis is the addition of hydroxyl groups at 3 and 3' position of 4-coumaroyl-4'-hydroxyphenyllactate. With the addition of these hydroxyl groups, the final product rosmarinic acid is formed. These reactions are catalyzed by hydroxycinnamoyl-4'hydroxyphenyllactate 3'-hydroxylase (4C-pHPL-3'-H) (EC Number: 1.14.13) it catalyzes both the

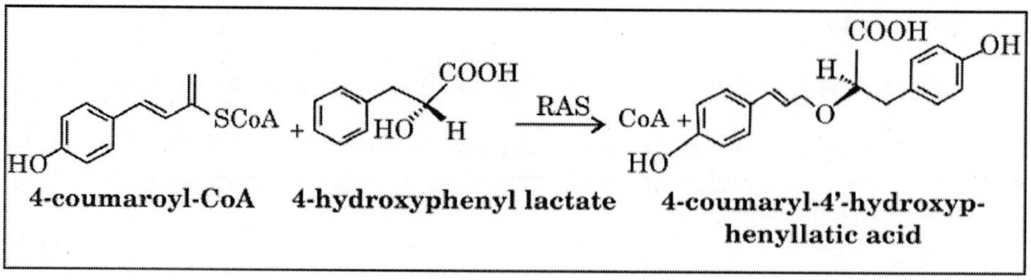

introduction of hydroxyl group in positions 3'of the aromatic ring in 4-coumaryl-4'-hydroxyphenyllactate forming 4-coumaryl-3',4'-hydroxyphenyllactate or hydroxylates caffeoyl-4'-hydroxyphenyllactate generating rosmarinic acid. The consecutive action of a corresponding 3-hydroxylase finally results either in the formation of 4-coumaryl-3', 4'-dihydroxyphenyllactate or rosmarinic acid. As these are microsomal enzymes, they requires NADPH and molecular oxygen for completing a successful hydroxylation reaction.

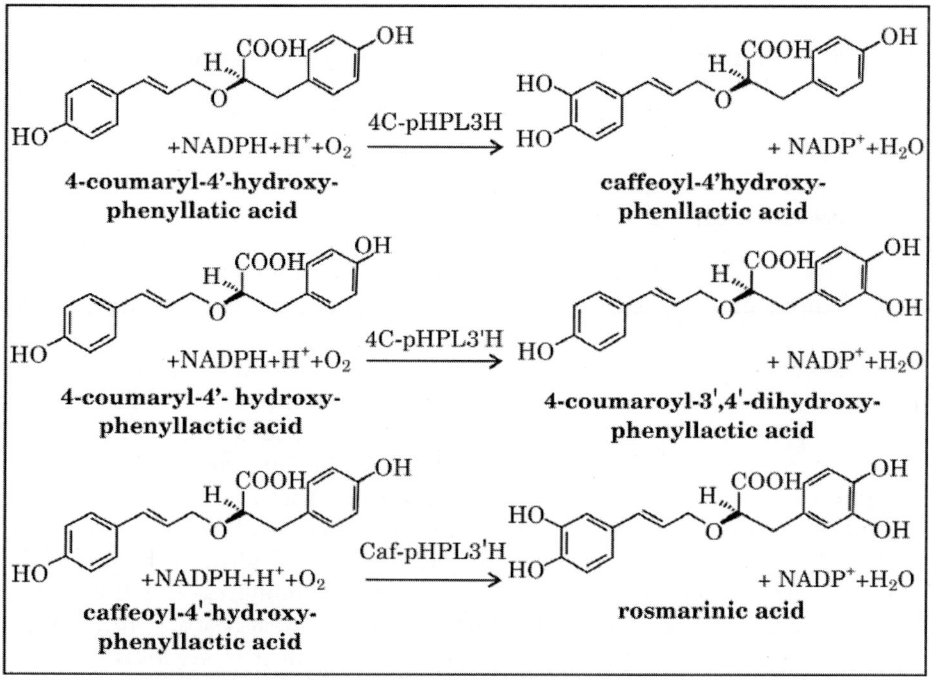

5. ROSMARINIC ACID PRODUCTION THROUGH PLANT BIOTECHNOLOGICAL TECHNIQUES

In the past few decades, plant based medicines are having high demand. However, the phytocompounds produced from wild plants is very low and cannot meet the ever increasing demand in the current market. Hence, many alternative ways including biotechnology approaches have been standardized to produce the phytocompounds. There are many successful stories regarding the production of medicinally/pharmacologically important metabolites. For example, anticancer compounds, such as paclitaxel, camptothecin, etc., (Deepthi and kumar, 2016), antidiabetic compounds, such as epigallocatechin cinchonain Ib, gallate, beta-pyrazol-1-ylalanine, etc. (Veerashree *et al.*, 2012) are derived from plant sources. Likewise, rosmarinic acid is having a huge demand due to its medicinal properties benefiting mankind. Hence, to avoid its supply crises, many plant based biotechnological approaches have been standardized for producing rosmarinic acid. In 1977, Razzaque and Ellis, for the first time established the biotechnological approach for rosmarinic acid production, which had successfully demonstrated the accumulation of 8-11% of dry weight as rosmarinic acid in stem derived suspension cultures of *Coleus blumei* Benth. From here onwards, the era of biotechnological production of rosmarinic acid has started. Later, many plant cell culture techniques have been successfully standardized. The use of elicitation strategy, precursor feeding, hairy root cultures, manipulation of nutrients and plant growth regulator concentrations in media and bioreactor cultures for scaling up rosmarinic acid production and metabolic engineering approaches have been established. For all these strategies/approaches, some examples are illustrated in Table 1 and described below.

Addition of elicitors to the plat cell cultures is one of the effective approaches for the enhancement of secondary metabolites (Rao and Ravishankar, 2002). Secondary metabolites accumulate in response to abiotic and biotic stresses; these various stress conditions have been defined as elicitors. These elicitors interact with the receptors that are present in the membrane of plant cells, and thereby further trigger the enzymes responsible for the synthesis of secondary metabolites (Giri and Zaheer, 2016). Methyl jasmonate (MeJA), salicylic acid, yeast extract are the elicitors have widely employed in the enhancement of rosmarinic acid production in plant cell cultures. For example, 3348 mg/l rosmarinic acid produced in cell suspension cultures of *Lavandula vera* after treatment with 50 µM MeJA (methyl jasmonate), which found to be 2.4 fold higher compared to control cultures (Georgiev *et al.,* 2007). Similarly in *Agastache rugosa* Kuntze suspension cultures, 4.7 folds increase of rosmarinic acid production was observed with the treatment of 50 µM MeJA compared to untreated cultures (Kim *et al.,* 2013). However, in *Mentha Xpiperita* cell suspension cultures, only 117.95 mg/g DW was produced upon elicitation with 100 µM MeJA (Krzyzanowska *et al.,* 2012), which shows that the efficacy of elicitor concentration in one plant system to other varies. 4.98 mg/g of rosmarinic acid produced in *agastache rugosa* cell cultures after treatment with yeast extract (500 mg/L) (Park *et al.,* 2016). In addition to this, the composition of medium also plays a vital role in the production of rosmarinic acid, especially the sugar composition level for example addition of 2% sucrose to the *Anthoceros agrestis* Paton cell cultures up to 5.1% DW (dry weight) of rosmarinic acid produced (Vogelsang *et al.*, 2006). *Zataria multiflora* callus cultures fed with 75 g/l glucose resulted in the production of 158 mg/g DW rosmarinic acid (Francoise *et al.,* 2007).

Table 1: Selected examples for production of rosmarinic acid in plant cell tissue cultures.

Plant name	***Culture type***	***Rosmarinic acid***	***References yield***
Salvia miltiorrhiza	Hairy roots	74.1 mg/g DW	Yan *et al.* (2006)
Coleus blumei	Hairy roots	50 mg/g DW	Bauer *et al.* (2009)
Mentha x piperita	Cell suspension cultures	117.95 mg/g DW	Krzyzanowska *et al.* (2012)
Satureja khuzistanica	Cell suspension cultures and bio-reactor	3.9 g/L3.1 g/L	Khojasteh *et al.* (2016)
Solenostemon	Organ cultures *Scutellarioides*	2.0 fold	Sahu *et al.* (2013)
Satureja khuzistanica Jamzad	Callus cultures	7.5%	Sahraroo *et al.* (2014)
Zataria multiflora Boiss	Callus cultures	158.26 mg/g DW	Françoise *et al.* (2007)
Solenostemon scutellarioides	Precursor feeding	3.1 fold	Dewanjee *et al.* (2014)
Anchusa offlcinalis	Two stage culture (Bioreactor)	94 mg/L	Su and Humphrey (1991)
Lavandula vera MM	Cell suspension cultures	3.3 g/L	Georgiev *et al.* (2007)
Agastache rugosa Kuntze	Cell suspension cultures	4.7 fold	Kim *et al.* (2013)
Agastache rugosa	Cell suspension culture	4.98 mg/g DCW	Park *et al.* (2016)
Agastache rugosa Kuntze	Hairy root cult-ures	116 mg/g DCW	Lee *et al.* (2008)
Lavandula vera MM	Cell suspension cultures	3.92 g/L	Georgiev *et al.* (2006)
Coleus blumei	Cell suspension cultures (Permeabilization)	2.85 g RA/100 g DCW	Park and Martinez (1992)
Eryngium planum L.	Callus cultures	16.24 mg/g DCW	Kikowska *et al.* (2012)
Dracocephalum forrestii W.W. Smith	Airy root cultures	19.97 mg/g DCW	Weremczuk-Jeżynaplasma *et al.* (2016)

Another effective approach for the rosmarinic acid production is the addition of plant growth regulators to the plant cell cultures. It has been reported that callus induced with 1.0 mg/L IBA (indole-3-butyric acid) + 5.0 mg/L BAP (6-benzylaminopurine) in the absence of light produced 7.5% rosmarinic acid in *Satureja khuzistanica* (Sahraroo *et al.,* 2014). In *Anchusa officinalis,* the addition of NAA (1-naphthaleneacetic acid) at 0.25 mg/L found to be the most effective for the enhancement of rosmarinic acid (De-Eknamkul and Ellis, 1987). However, in *A. rugosa* cell suspension cultures, supplementing 2 mg/L 2,4-D (2,4-dichlorophenoxyacetic acid) along with 0.1 mg/L BAP found to be more effective for the production of rosmarinic acid (11.5 mg/g DW) when compared to those cultures added with 2,4-D alone (9.5 mg/g DW) (Xu *et al.,* 2013).

Likewise, another effective approach is the addition of rosmarinic acid biosynthesis precursors (*i.e.,* intermediates involved in rosmarinic acid biosynthesis pathway) to the medium. A precursor is generally an intermediate that is enzymatically converted into a desired metabolite. Therefore, the addition of these precursors to the cell cultures may result in increasing the production of rosmarinic acid. Adding precursors to the medium activates the enzymes associated with rosmarinic acid synthesis, modulates their expression and promotes the rosmarinic acid production. For example, feeding of three precursors of rosmarinic acid biosynthetic pathway, namely phenylalanine, tyrosine and cucumber juice (rich in caffeic acid) to the *Solenostemon scutellarioides* cell cultures up regulated the enzymes of rosmarinic acid pathway and increased its synthesis. Among the studied precursors, L-tyrosine at 400 mg/l proved to be better compared to other precursors used for the rosmarinic acid production. Furthermore in the same study, a synergism was observed between the precursors, among the tried combinations, 100 mg/l phenylalanine at 400 mg/l tyrosine proved to be better for the production of rosmarinic acid (Dewanjee *et al.,* 2014).

Hairy roots in higher plants are induced by infecting any plant parts with the soil bacterium, *Agrobacterium rhizogenes* that causes the hairy root disease leading to the neoplastic growth of roots characterized by high growth rate in hormone-free media and possess the genetic stability. Hairy roots produce the same rosmarinic acid impression of the consequent wild type organ. Because of its large applications hairy roots acts as an alternative source for the production of rosmarinic acid (Khojasteh *et al.,* 2016). Hairy root cultures of *Dracocephalum moldavica* infecting with *Agrobacterium* A4 strain, about 78 mg/g DW rosmarinic acid was produced in *Dracocephalum moldavica* hairy root cultures, which was 10 folds higher compared to roots of field grown plants (Weremczuk-Je¿yna *et al.,* 2013). With *A. rhizognes* ATCC 15834 strain, 8 % rosmarinic acid content was achieved in *Hyssopus officinalis* root cultures which was 8 folds higher than in the filed grown leaves (Murakami *et al.,* 1998), and 116 mg/g DW of rosmarinic acid was produced with the strain, R 1000 in *Agastache rugosa* Kuntze. hairy root cultures (Lee *et al.,* 2008). Likewise, rosmarinic acid content production ranged from 10 to 1500 µg/g DW in hairy roots induced from LBA 9402 strain, this found to be 15 times higher compared to intact roots of *Dracocephalum kotschyi* Boiss. (Fattahi *et al.,* 2013). In addition, the elicitation strategy has also been used in hairy roots cultures to further enhance the accumulation of rosmarinic acid in both small and large scale production systems (Yan *et al.,* 2006). *Coleus forskohlii* hairy root cultures treated with 0.1 mM MeJA secreted about 9.5 mg of rosmarinic acid (Li *et al.,* 2005). Similarly in *Salvia miltiorrhiza* hairy roots, MeJA induced high amounts of rosmarinic acid production (Zhang *et al.,* 2014). Highest accumulation of rosmarinic acid was observed in an airlift bioreactor which is more potential for mass production of rosmarinic acid in *Coleus blumei* cultures (Bauer *et al.*, 2015).

Some other advanced techniques were also used to enhance the rosmarinic acid in plant cell tissue cultures. Using 5 L air-lift bioreactor, about 29 µg/g DW rosmarinic acid was produced in suspension cultures of *Ocimum basilicum* L., in three weeks (Kintzios *et al.,* 2004). In addition to this, the critical factors like, temperature, aeration and agitation also play a very important role in bioreactors. For example, in *Lavandula vera* cell suspension cultures at 30°C, the biomass and rosmarinic acid production was better compared to 26°C. In the same study, at 30% dissolved oxygen (DO) with 300 rpm of agitation, about 1870.6 mg/l DW rosmarinic acid was produced. However, the highest biomass (34.8 g/L) was obtained when agitation rate of 100 rpm supplied with 50% DO (Pavlov *et al.*, 2005a). A two fold increase in rosmarinic acid production was obtained in 3-L bioreactors compared to shake-flasks cultures with 50% DO, 400 rpm at the temperature of 29.9°C. A maximum level of rosmarinic acid (3789.4 mg/l) was achieved (Pavlov *et al.,* 2005).

Over expressing or suppressing the genes of rosmarinic acid biosynthetic pathway is another strategy to improve the rosmarinic acid production in plant cell cultures. As rosmarinic acid biosynthesis pathway enzymes (eight) have been characterized successfully, this made plant biotechnologists to establish another approach for the production of rosmarinic acid using plant cell cultures. With respect to this, genes encoding the rosmarinic acid synthesis were expressed in two *Salvia miltiorrhiza* genotypes (DS1 and DS2), and the results indicated that in DS1, the higher contents of rosmarinic acid accumulated which was correlated with the up regulation of transcript levels of the SmPAL, SmC4H, Sm4CL and SmHPPD genes. Whereas, with respect to DS2 genotype enzymes such as 4CL2, TAT and C4H had effect on the production of rosmarinic acid. The difference in rosmarinic acid accumulation was mainly due to genetic influences (Song and Li, 2015). With *Agrobacterium tumefaciens* mediated transformation in a transgenic *P. frutescens,* over expression of *PfTAT* gene was found to be 2-3 times higher than that observed in the untransformed plant lines which it led to the 1.5-2.0 fold higher accumulation of rosmarinic acid than control cultures (Lu *et al.,* 2013).

6. BIOLOGICAL ACTIVITIES OF ROSMARINIC ACID

From ancient days, plant derived products have been used to treat various diseases. The medicinal properties of the plant extracts/products is mainly due to the presence of active ingredients *i.e.,* plant secondary metabolites. The treatment of various human health issues with these plant products is highly preferred due to the fact that they are considered to be safe and have no or meager side effects. Since they have been derived from nature, they hold a great advantage over the chemical or synthetic drugs. As opposed to allopathic medicines, plant derived drugs are known to treat the diseases effectively, and aid in keeping human beings healthy, and fit in the long run. As rosmarinic acid is also one of the plant derived products, it has several advantages and is proved to be very effective in curing various ailments and diseases. Some of its important biological actions are discussed below.

6.1. Anti-inflammatory Effect

In an ototoxicity model induced by cisplatin in mice after treatment with rosmarinic acid had showed the anti-inflammatory actions by diminishing interleukin1β (IL-1β) (Jeong *et al.*, 2011). In a collagen induced murine arthritis model rosmarinic acid treatment has remarkably reduced the frequency of COX-2- expression compared to untreated mice (Youn *et al.,* 2003). In acute and chronic inflammation models administration of rosmarinic acid (100 mg/kg) which is isolated from the ethanolic extracts of *Thunbergia laurifolia* leaves has showed the anti-inflammatory properties (Boonyarikpunchai *et al.,* 2014). Anti-inflammatory effect was also observed in murine model of Japanese encephalitis after the treatment with rosmarinic acid, where 9 folds reduction in the levels of interleukin-12 (IL-12), TNF-(tumor necrosis factor-α), interferon-γ, MCP-1 (monocyte chemo attractant protein-1) and IL-6 were observed in infected animals compared to the infected animals without treatment (Swarup *et al.*, 2007). IL-6, IL-β and TNF-α levels were decreased in systemic inflammation induced rats after the treatment with *R. officinalis* extract (25 mg/kg of rosmarinic acid) (Rocha *et al.,* 2015).

6.2. Antimicrobial Effect

Rosmarinic acid, isolated from the hairy root cultures of *Ocimum basilicum* showed the antimicrobial activity against various pathogenic microorganisms, however, it was highly deleterious against *Pseudomonas aeruginosa,* an opportunistic soil bacterium, and human pathogen (Bais *et al.*, 2002). About 750 µg/ml of rosmarinic acid was found to inhibit the biofilm formation by *Aeromonas hydrophila,* a pathogenic bacterium of zebra fish. This concentration also reduced the quorum sensing mediated hemolysin, lipase and elastase production in *A. hydrophila* (Rama Devi *et al.,* 2016). Rosmarinic acid showed the antibacterial activity against *Staphylococcus aureus* and methicillin-resistant *Staphylococcus aureus* with an inhibition zone of 12.4 mm and 11.6 mm diameter, respectively. Furthermore in the same study, a synergism was observed between the rosmarinic acid and standard antibiotics (amoxicillin, ofloxacin and vancomycin). All the antibiotics along with rosmarinic acid showed the synergic effects against *S. aureus* and significantly inhibited the growth. However, only vancomycin along with rosmarinic acid showed the synergistic effect against MRSA (Ekambaram *et al.*, 2016). Antibacterial compounds, such as rosmarinic acid and its methyl ester isolated form the extract of *Hyptis atrorubens* inhibited all eight pathogenic bacteria tested at a concentration ranging from 0.3 to 1.3 mg/l (Abedini *et al.,* 2013).

6.3. Antioxidant Activity

Antioxidant therapy has been very effective in ameliorating many human diseases and to improve health conditions. With reference to this, in recent years, more interest has been given to natural antioxidants that are produced by plants. One of the most effective plant antioxidant is the rosmarinic acid, which has the antioxidant activity and scavenge reactive oxygen species (Ramanauskiene *et al.,* 2016). In an experiment, the oxidative damage induced in diabetic rats by streptozotocin (STZ) showed the decreased activities of SOD (superoxide dismutase) and catalase enzymes. However, after treatment with 10 xmg/kg of rosmarinic acid improved the SOD and catalase activities, and also it reversed the non-protein and ascorbic levels. Also, there was no variation in the glycemic levels observed after the treatment with rosmarinic acid (Mushtaq *et al.*, 2015). Similarly, rosmarinic acid reduced the β–amyloid evoked oxidative stress through activating the Nrf2-inducible cellular antioxidant defense system (Rong *et al.,* 2018). The renal ischemia reperfusion occurs during the renal surgical procedures leading to the renal injuries and acute renal failures. However, treating with rosmarinic acid reduced this condition through the inhibition of lipid peroxidation (Tavafi *et al.,* 2016).

6.4. Anticancer Activity

Rosmarinic acid inhibits proliferation of human colorectal cell lines and induces apoptosis by ERK (extracellular-signal-regulated kinase)/MAPK (mitogen activated protein kinase) pathway (Xavier *et al.,* 2009). Rosmarinic acid isolated from the extracts of *M. officinalis* (rosemary) showed the anti-proliferative activity against human colon cancer cell line HCT -116 (Encalada *et al.,* 2011). Similarly, the rosemary plant extract containing the rosmarinic acid inhibited the lung cancer cell proliferation, and survival of various non-small cell lung cancer cell lines, however the inhibition was much more effective by combining the carnosic acid along with rosmarinic acid, where anticancer activity was found to be due to altering the activity of Ak strain transforming (Akt), extra cellular-signal-regulated kinase (ERK) and AMPK(5' adenosine monophosphate-activated kinase) Akt, ERK and AMPK signaling proteins in NSCLC (non-small cell lung cancer) (Moore, 2015). More recently, rosmarinic acid administered with siRNA repressed the Hsp 27 activity and induced apoptosis in human glioma cells (Sengelen *et al.,* 2018).

6.5. Immunomodulatory Effect

Rosmarinic acid induced p56Ick-dependent apoptosis in T and NK cells *via* eliciting mitochondrial dysfunction (Hur *et al.,* 2004). Similarly, rosmarinic acid inhibited cell proliferation by altering the expression of cyclins and cyclin dependent kinase inhibitors *via* mitochondrial pathway (Kolettas *et al.,* 2006). Rosmarinic acid was found to induce apoptosis in rheumatoid arthritis patients by activating T cells *via* mitochondrial pathway (Hur *et al.,* 2007). Uptake of rosmarinic acid eases arthritis like symptoms by inhibiting the synovial tissue damage, reducing the COX2 expression, and inhibiting TCR mediated T cell activation and proliferation (Youn *et al.,* 2003).

6.6. Other Biological Activities

Apart from the above biological activities, rosmarinic acid also possess anti fibrotic effect, which is mediated by inhibiting the fibrosis of pterygium epithelial cells by down regulating type 1 collagen expression and TGF-β1/ Smad signaling (Chen *et al.,* 2018). The treatment with 100 or 200 mg/kg rosmarinic acid improved the diabetic nephropathy in uninephrectomized diabetic rats by inhibiting the glomerular hypertrophy, reducing the serum urea, creatinine levels, and loss of glomerular number and glomerulosclerosis (Tavafi *et al.,* 2011). By activating the AMPK and inhibiting the Smad3 pathways, rosmarinic acid reduced the cardiac dysfunction, and inhibited the cardiac fibrosis (Zhang *et al.,* 2018). Rosmarinic acid was found to inhibit the proliferation by inducing apoptosis in HSC-T6 (rat hepatic stellate cell line), and contributed to the setback of hepatic fibrosis (Zhang *et al.,* 2011). Rosmarinic acid also plays an important role in treatment of diabetes mellitus and obesity by inhibiting the digestive enzymes, such as α-amylase and α-glucosidase (Zhu *et al.,* 2014), and also it has anti-viral (Swarup *et al.,* 2007), neuroprotective (Fazel Nabavi *et al.,* 2015), and anti-allergic effects.

7. EXTRACTION, ISOLATION AND IDENTIFICATION OF ROSMARINIC ACID

Many extraction and isolation procedures have been tried and standardized to identify and isolate rosmarinic acid from various plants. Pertaining to the extraction, isolation and identification of rosmarinic acid, Amoah *et al.* (2016) have published a comprehensive review. Therefore, this section discusses only on some of the selected examples. In 1982, Christ and Kesselring (1982) isolated the rosmarinic acid from leaves of balmmint. Rosmarinic acid extracted and purified from leaves of *Coleus aromaticus* using a Sephadex LH-20 column (Kumaran and Karunakaran, 2007). In another study rosmarinic acid was extracted and purified from methanol extract of *Agastache rugosa* after successive column chromatography on RP-18 and Sephadex LH-20 and further finally isolated using HPLC (high performance liquid chromatography) (Kim *et al.,* 1999). Rosmarinic acid was purified from the leaves of *Melissa officinalis* using Sephadex LH-20 resin, the purity and recovery yield of rosmarinic yield were 38.8% and 43.8% respectively (Kim *et al.,* 2010). In another study, rosmarinic acid was purified from *Rabdosia serra* (Maxim) Hara leaves about 112.5 mg and 95.7 mg of rosmarinic acid obtained with HP-20 and Amberlite XAD-7HP (Lin *et al.,* 2012).

For the identification and quantification of rosmarinic acid, many analytical techniques have been standardized including TLC (thin layer chromatography), HPTLC (high-performance thin-layer chromatography), HPLC (high performance liquid chromatography), UPLC-ESIMS (ultra-performance liquid chromatography-electrospray ionization mass spectrometry), LC-MS (liquid chromatography-mass spectrometry), UV (ultraviolet-visible) spectroscopy, IR (infrared spectroscopy), NMR (nuclear magnetic resonance spectroscopy) (Amoah *et al.,* 2016).

8. CONCLUSIONS AND FUTURE PERSPECTIVES

Rosmarinic acid is a highly valued phenolic compound and possess several biological activities. It has gained more interest among researchers in various areas of knowledge due to its natural occurrence with therapeutic potentials. However, their occurrence is limited in wild plants, and hence biotechnological approaches, such as plant cell, hairy roots, and transgenic plant cell cultures have proved to be very useful in obtaining large quantity of rosmarinic acid. However, in future further studies are warranted to standardize bioreactor strategies for scale-up of rosmarinic acid production in plant cell cultures. Also, detailed molecular mechanisms must be studied for the elucidation of biological functions as discussed above. Moreover, more research should be focused on evaluating many other possible biological roles of rosmarinic acid towards its utilization as an effective drug molecule. More animal studies should be encouraged to understand the toxicity and safety aspects of rosmarinic acid before using in clinical applications. In addition, genomics, and transcriptomics studies are required to understand the involvement of genes, enzymes in the process of biosynthesis. This will facilitate in the bioengineering approach to enhance the production of rosmarinic acid. This may also improve our understanding on the biosynthesis or regulation rosmarinic acid under different conditions. Applications of genetic tools or molecular techniques would be helpful to enhance rosmarinic acid production through heterologous production in lower organisms like bacteria and yeast. This heterologous production system will be a cost effective method for the large scale production of rosmarinic acid so as to ensure their availability at low prices, and affordable to the common man.

REFERENCES

Abedini A, Roumy V, Mahieux S, Biabiany M, Standaert-Vitse A, Rivière C, Sahpaz S, Bailleul F, Neut C, Hennebelle T. Rosmarinic acid and its methyl ester as antimicrobial components of the hydromethanolic extract of *Hyptis atrorubens* Poit. (Lamiaceae). Evidence-Based Complementary and Alternative Medicine. 2013; 2013: 1-11.

Amoah SK, Sandjo LP, Kratz JM, Biavatti MW. Rosmarinic acid–pharmaceutical and clinical aspects. Planta Medica. 2016; 82(05): 388-406.

Bais HP, Walker TS, Schweizer HP, Vivanco JM. Root specific elicitation and antimicrobial activity of rosmarinic acid in hairy root cultures of *Ocimum basilicum*. Plant Physiology and Biochemistry. 2002; 40(11): 983-95.

Bauer N, Kiseljak D, Jelaska S. The effect of yeast extract and methyl jasmonate on rosmarinic acid accumulation in *Coleus blumei* hairy roots. Biologia Plantarum. 2009; 53(4): 650-6.

Bauer N, Vukoviæ R, Likiæ S, Jelaska S. Potential of different *Coleus blumei* tissues for rosmarinic acid production. Food Technology and Biotechnology. 2015; 53(1): 3.

Boonyarikpunchai W, Sukrong S, Towiwat P. Antinociceptive and anti-inflammatory effects of rosmarinic acid isolated from *Thunbergia laurifolia* Lindl. Pharmacology Biochemistry and Behavior. 2014; 124: 67-73.

Chen YY, Tsai CF, Tsai MC, Chen WK, Hsu YW, Lu FJ. Anti-fibrotic effect of rosmarinic acid on inhibition of pterygium epithelial cells. International Journal of Ophthalmology. 2018; 11(2): 189.

Christ B, Kesselring K, inventors; Natterman A, Cie GmbH, assignee. Process for isolating rosmarinic acid from plants. United States patent US 4,354,035. 1982 Oct 12.

De-Eknamkul W, Ellis BE. Purification and characterization of tyrosine aminotransferase activities from *Anchusa officinalis* cell cultures. Archives of Biochemistry and Biophysics. 1987; 257(2): 430-438.

Deepthi S, Satheeshkumar K. Enhanced camptothecin production induced by elicitors in the cell suspension cultures of *Ophiorrhiza mungos* Linn. Plant Cell, Tissue and Organ Culture. 2016; 124(3): 483-93.

Dewanjee S, Gangopadhyay M, Das U, Sahu R, Khanra R. Enhanced rosmarinic acid biosynthesis in *Solenostemon scutellarioides* culture: A precursor-feeding strategy. Natural Product Research. 2014; 28(20): 1691-1698.

Ekambaram SP, Perumal SS, Balakrishnan A, Marappan N, Gajendran SS, Viswanathan V. Antibacterial synergy between rosmarinic acid and antibiotics against methicillin-resistant *Staphylococcus aureus*. Journal of Intercultural Ethnopharmacology. 2016; 5(4): 358.

Ellis BE, Towers GH. Biogenesis of rosmarinic acid in *Mentha*. Biochemical Journal. 1970; 118(2): 291-297.

Encalada MA, Hoyos KM, Rehecho S, Berasategi I, de Ciriano MG, Ansorena D, Astiasarán I, Navarro-Blasco Í, Cavero RY, Calvo MI. Anti-proliferative effect of *Melissa officinalis* on human colon cancer cell line. Plant Foods for Human Nutrition. 2011; 66(4): 328-34.

Fattahi M, Nazeri V, Torras-Claveria L, Sefidkon F, Cusido RM, Zamani Z, Palazon J. A new biotechnological source of rosmarinic acid and surface flavonoids: Hairy root cultures of *Dracocephalum kotschyi* Boiss. Industrial Crops and Products. 2013; 50: 256-263.

Fazel Nabavi S, Carlo Tenore G, Daglia M, Tundis R, Rosa Loizzo M, Mohammad Nabavi S. The cellular protective effects of rosmarinic acid: From bench to bedside. Current Neurovascular Research. 2015; 12(1): 98-105.

Francoise B, Hossein S, Halimeh H, Zahra NF. Growth optimization of *Zataria multiflora* Boiss. tissue cultures and rosmarinic acid production improvement. Pakistan Journal of Biological Sciences. 2007; 10: 3395-3399.

Georgiev M, Kuzeva S, Pavlov A, Kovacheva E, Ilieva M. Enhanced rosmarinic acid production by *Lavandula vera* MM cell suspension culture through elicitation with vanadyl sulfate. Zeitschrift für Naturforschung C. 2006; 61(3-4): 241-244.

Georgiev MI, Kuzeva SL, Pavlov AI, Kovacheva EG, Ilieva MP. Elicitation of rosmarinic acid by *Lavandula vera* MM cell suspension culture with abiotic elicitors. World Journal of Microbiology and Biotechnology. 2007; 23(2): 301-304.

Giri, CC, Zaheer, M. Chemical elicitors versus secondary metabolite production *in vitro* using plant cell, tissue and organ cultures: Recent trends and a sky eye view appraisal. Plant Cell Tissue and Organ Culture. 2016; 126(1): 1-18.

Hausler E, Petersen M, Alfermann AW. Rosmarinsäure in Blechnum-spezies. Botanikertagung. 1992; 1992: 507.

Hur YG, Suh CH, Kim S, Won J. Rosmarinic acid induces apoptosis of activated T cells from rheumatoid arthritis patients *via* mitochondrial pathway. Journal of Clinical Immunology. 2007; 27(1): 36-45.

Hur YG, Yun Y, Won J. Rosmarinic acid induces p56lck-dependent apoptosis in Jurkat and peripheral T cells *via* mitochondrial pathway independent from Fas/Fas ligand interaction. The Journal of Immunology. 2004; 172(1): 79-87.

Jeong HJ, Choi Y, Kim MH, Kang IC, Lee JH, Park C, Park R, Kim HM. Rosmarinic acid, active component of Dansam-Eum attenuates ototoxicity of cochlear hair cells through blockage of caspase-1 activity. Plos One; 6(4): e18815.

Khojasteh A, Mirjalili MH, Hidalgo D, Corchete P, Palazon J. New trends in biotechnological production of rosmarinic acid. Biotechnology Letters. 2014; 36(12): 2393-406.

Khojasteh A, Mirjalili MH, Palazon J, Eibl R, Cusido RM. Methyl jasmonate enhanced production of rosmarinic acid in cell cultures of *Satureja khuzistanica* in a bioreactor. Engineering in Life Sciences. 2016; 16(8): 740-749.

Kikowska M, Budzianowski J, Krawczyk A, Thiem B. Accumulation of rosmarinic, chlorogenic and caffeic acids in *in vitro* cultures of *Eryngium planum* L. Acta Physiologiae Plantarum. 2012; 34(6): 2425-2433.

Kim HK, Lee HK, Shin CG, Huh H. HIV integrase inhibitory activity of *Agastache rugosa*. Archives of Pharmacology Research. 1999; 22(5): 520-523.

Kim S, Yun EJ, Bak JS, Lee H, Lee SJ, Kim CT, Lee JH, Kim KH. Response surface optimised extraction and chromatographic purification of rosmarinic acid from *Melissa officinalis* leaves. Food Chemistry. 2010; 121(2): 521-526.

Kim YB, Kim JK, Uddin MR, Xu H, Park WT, Tuan PA, Li X, Chung E, Lee JH, Park SU. Metabolomics analysis and biosynthesis of rosmarinic acid in *Agastache rugosa* Kuntze treated with methyl jasmonate. Plos One. 2013; 8(5): e64199.

Kintzios S, Kollias H, Straitouris E, Makri O. Scale-up micropropagation of sweet basil (*Ocimum basilicum* L.) in an airlift bioreactor and accumulation of rosmarinic acid. Biotechnology Letters. 2004; 26(6): 521-3.

Kolettas E, Thomas C, Leneti E, Skoufos I, Mbatsi C, Sisoula C, Manos G, Evangelou A. Rosmarinic acid failed to suppress hydrogen peroxide-mediated apoptosis but induced apoptosis of Jurkat cells which was suppressed by Bcl-2. Molecular and Cellular Biochemistry. 2006; 285(1-2): 111-1120.

Krzyzanowska J, Czubacka A, Pecio L, Przybys M, Doroszewska T, Stochmal A, Oleszek W. The effects of jasmonic acid and methyl jasmonate on rosmarinic acid production in *Mentha× piperita* cell suspension cultures. Plant Cell, Tissue and Organ Culture. 2012; 108(1): 73-81.

Kumaran A, Karunakaran RJ. Activity-guided isolation and identification of free radical-scavenging components from an aqueous extract of *Coleus aromaticus*. Food Chemistry. 2007; 100(1): 356-361.

Lee SY, Xu H, Kim YK, Park SU. Rosmarinic acid production in hairy root cultures of *Agastache rugosa* Kuntze. World Journal of Microbiology and Biotechnology. 2008; 24(7): 969-972.

Li W, Koike K, Asada Y, Yoshikawa T, Nikaido T. Rosmarinic acid production by *Coleus forskohlii* hairy root cultures. Plant Cell, Tissue and Organ Culture. 2005; 80(2): 151-155.

Lin L, Zhao H, Dong Y, Yang B, Zhao M. Macroporous resin purification behavior of phenolics and rosmarinic acid from *Rabdosia serra* (MAXIM.) HARA leaf. Food Chemistry. 2012; 130(2): 417-424.

Lu X, Hao L, Wang F, Huang C, Wu S. Molecular cloning and overexpression of the tyrosine aminotransferase (TAT) gene leads to increased rosmarinic acid yield in *Perilla frutescens*. Plant Cell, Tissue and Organ Culture. 2013; 115(1): 69-83.

Moore J. Investigation of the Biological Effects of Rosemary (*Rosmarinus officinalis* L.) Extract in Human Lung Cancer Cells. 2015. http://hdl.handle.net/10464/7223

Murakami Y, Omoto T, Asai I, Shimomura K, Yoshihira K, Ishimaru K. Rosmarinic acid and related phenolics in transformed root cultures of *Hyssopus officinalis*. Plant Cell, Tissue and Organ Culture. 1998; 53(1): 75-78.

Mushtaq N, Schmatz R, Ahmed M, Pereira LB, da Costa P, Reichert KP, Dalenogare D, Pelinson LP, Vieira JM, Stefanello N, de Oliveira LS. Protective effect of rosmarinic acid against oxidative stress biomarkers in liver and kidney of streptozotocin-induced diabetic rats. Journal of Physiology and Biochemistry. 2015; 71(4): 743-751.

Newman DJ, Cragg GM. Natural products as sources of new drugs over the 30 years from 1981 to 2010. Journal of Natural Products. 2012; 75(3): 311-335.

Park CH, Martinez BC. Enhanced release of rosmarinic acid from *Coleus blumei* permeabilized by dimethyl sulfoxide (DMSO) while preserving cell viability and growth. Biotechnology and Bioengineering. 1992; 40(4): 459-464.

Park WT, Arasu MV, Al-Dhabi NA, Yeo SK, Jeon J, Park JS, Lee SY, Park SU. Yeast extract and silver nitrate induce the expression of phenylpropanoid biosynthetic genes and induce the accumulation of rosmarinic acid in *Agastache rugosa* cell culture. Molecules. 2016; 21(4): 426.

Pavlov AI, Georgiev MI, Ilieva MP. Production of rosmarinic acid by *Lavandula vera* MM cell suspension in bioreactor: Effect of dissolved oxygen concentration and agitation. World Journal of Microbiology and Biotechnology. 2005a; 21(4): 389-392.

Pavlov AI, Georgiev MI, Panchev IN, Ilieva MP. Optimization of rosmarinic acid production by *Lavandula vera* MM plant cell suspension in a laboratory bioreactor. Biotechnology Progress. 2005; 21(2): 394-396.

Petersen M, Simmonds MS. Rosmarinic acid. Phytochemistry. 2003; 62(2): 121-5.

Petersen M. Rosmarinic acid: New aspects. Phytochemistry reviews. 2013; 12(1): 207-27.

Rama Devi K, Srinivasan R, Kannappan A, Santhakumari S, Bhuvaneswari M, Rajasekar P, Prabhu NM, Veera Ravi A. *In vitro* and *in vivo* efficacy of rosmarinic acid on quorum sensing mediated biofilm formation and virulence factor production in *Aeromonas hydrophila*. Biofouling. 2016; 32(10): 1171-1183.

Ramanauskiene K, Raudonis R, Majiene D. Rosmarinic acid and *Melissa officinalis* extracts differently affect glioblastoma cells. Oxidative Medicine and Cellular Longevity. 2016; 2016: 1-9.

Rao SR, Ravishankar GA. Plant cell cultures: Chemical factories of secondary metabolites. Biotechnol. Adv. 2002; 20(2): 101-153.

Razzaque A, Ellis BE. Rosmarinic acid production in *Coleus* cell cultures. Planta. 1977; 137(3): 287-291.

Rocha J, Eduardo Figueira M, Barateiro A, Fernandes A, Brites D, Bronze R, Duarte CM, Serra AT, Pinto R, Freitas M, Fernandes E. Anti inflammatory effect of rosmarinic acid and an extract of *Rosmarinus officinalis* in rat models of local and systemic inflammation. Basic & Clinical Pharmacology & Toxicology. 2015; 116(5): 398-413.

Rong H, Liang Y, Niu Y. rosmarinic acid attenuates β-amyloid-induced oxidative stress *via* Akt/gsk-3β/fyn-mediated Nrf2 activation in Pc12 cells. Free Radical Biology and Medicine. 2018; 120: 114-123.

Sahraroo A, Babalar M, Mirjalili MH, Moghaddam MR, Ebrahimi SN. *In-vitro* callus induction and rosmarinic acid quantification in callus culture of *Satureja khuzistanica* Jamzad (Lamiaceae). Iranian Journal of Pharmaceutical Research. 2014; 13(4): 1447.

Sahu R, Gangopadhyay M, Dewanjee S. Elicitor-induced rosmarinic acid accumulation and secondary metabolism enzyme activities in *Solenostemon scutellarioides*. Acta Physiologiae Plantarum. 2013; 35(5): 1473-1481.

Scarpati ML. Oriente G (1958) Isolation and establishment of rosmarinic acid (dal rosmarinus off.). Ric Sci. 1958; 28: 2329-33.

Sengelen A, Önay-Uçar E. Rosmarinic acid and siRNA combined therapy represses Hsp27 (HSPB1) expression and induces apoptosis in human glioma cells. Cell Stress and Chaperones. 2018; 7: 1-2.

Song Z, Li X. Expression profiles of rosmarinic acid biosynthesis genes in two *Salvia miltiorrhiza* lines with differing water-soluble phenolic contents. Industrial Crops and Products. 2015; 71: 24-30.

Su WW, Humphrey AE. Production of rosmarinic acid from perfusion culture of *Anchusa officinalis* in a membrane-aerated bioreactor. Biotechnology Letters. 1991; 13(12): 889-892.

Swarup V, Ghosh J, Ghosh S, Saxena A, Basu A. Antiviral and anti-inflammatory effects of rosmarinic acid in an experimental murine model of Japanese encephalitis. Antimicrobial agents and Chemotherapy. 2007; 51(9): 3367-3370.

Takeda R, Hasegawa J, Shinozaki M. The first isolation of lignans, megacerotonic acid and anthocerotonic acid, from non-vascular plants, Anthocerotae (hornworts). Tetrahedron letters. 1990; 31(29): 4159-62.

Tavafi M, Ahmadvand H, Khalatbari A, Tamjidipoor A. Rosmarinic acid ameliorates diabetic nephropathy in uninephrectomized diabetic rats. Iranian Journal of Basic Medical Sciences. 2011; 14(3): 275.

Tavafi M, Sameni HR, Tamjidipour A, Hasanvand A, Ashoory H. Antioxidant effect of rosmarinic acid against renal ischemia reperfusion injury in rat; A histopathological study. Annals of Research in Antioxidants. 2016; 6: 1(2).

Veerashree V, Anuradha CM, Kumar V. Elicitor-enhanced production of gymnemic acid in cell suspension cultures of *Gymnema sylvestre* R. Br. Plant Cell, Tissue and Organ Culture. 2012; 108(1): 27-35.

Vogelsang K, Schneider B, Petersen M. Production of rosmarinic acid and a new rosmarinic acid 32 -O-β-d-glucoside in suspension cultures of the hornwort *Anthoceros agrestis* Paton. Planta. 2006; 223(2): 369-373.

Weremczuk-Jeyna I, Grzegorczyk-Karolak I, Frydrych B, Królicka A, Wysokińska H. Hairy roots of *Dracocephalum moldavica*: Rosmarinic acid content and antioxidant potential. Acta Physiologiae Plantarum. 2013; 35(7): 2095-2103.

Weremczuk-Jeyna I, Ska³a E, Olszewska MA, Kiss AK, Balcerczak E, Wysokińska H, Kicel A. The identification and quantitative determination of rosmarinic acid and salvianolic acid B in hairy root cultures of *Dracocephalum forrestii* WW Smith. Industrial Crops and Products. 2016; 91: 125-131.

Xavier CP, Lima CF, Fernandes-Ferreira M, Pereira-Wilson C. *Salvia fruticosa*, *Salvia officinalis*, and rosmarinic acid induce apoptosis and inhibit proliferation of human colorectal cell lines: The role in MAPK/ERK pathway. Nutrition and Cancer. 2009; 61(4): 564-571.

Xu H, Kim YK, Jin X, Lee SY, Park SU. Rosmarinic acid biosynthesis in callus and cell cultures of *Agastache rugosa* Kuntze. Journal of Medicinal Plants Research. 2013; 2(9): 237-241.

Yan Q, Shi M, Ng J, Wu JY. Elicitor-induced rosmarinic acid accumulation and secondary metabolism enzyme activities in *Salvia miltiorrhiza* hairy roots. Plant Science. 2006; 170(4): 853-858.

Youn J, Lee KH, Won J, Huh SJ, Yun HS, Cho WG, Paik DJ. Beneficial effects of rosmarinic acid on suppression of collagen induced arthritis. The Journal of Rheumatology. 2003; 30(6): 1203-1207.

Zhang JJ, Wang YL, Feng XB, Song XD, Liu WB. Rosmarinic acid inhibits proliferation and induces apoptosis of hepatic stellate cells. Biological and Pharmaceutical Bulletin. 2011; 34(3): 343-348.

Zhang S, Yan Y, Wang B, Liang Z, Liu Y, Liu F, Qi Z. Selective responses of enzymes in the two parallel pathways of rosmarinic acid biosynthetic pathway to elicitors in *Salvia miltiorrhiza* hairy root cultures. Journal of Bioscience and Bioengineering. 2014; 117(5): 645-651.

Zhang X, Ma ZG, Yuan YP, Xu SC, Wei WY, Song P, Kong CY, Deng W, Tang QZ. Rosmarinic acid attenuates cardiac fibrosis following long-term pressure overload *via* AMPKα/Smad3 signaling. Cell Death and Disease. 2018; 9(2): 102.

Zhu F, Asada T, Sato A, Koi Y, Nishiwaki H, Tamura H. Rosmarinic acid extract for antioxidant, antiallergic, and α-glucosidase inhibitory activities, isolated by supramolecular technique and solvent extraction from Perilla leaves. Journal of Agricultural and Food Chemistry. 2014; 62(4): 885-892.

13

Electrochemistry of Phytochemicals and Natural Products

Annamalai Senthil Kumar[1,2,3,4]*, Rajagopal Desikan[2], Mansi Gandhi[1,2], Sheng-Tung Huang[4], Gaurav Verma[5], Manasa Deepa Rajagopalan[6] and Boregowda Purushotham[7]

ABSTRACT

Phytochemicals are plant based chemical products that have tremendous influence / impacts on human life well-being and suits-it-well to the proverb "let food be thy medicine and medicine be thy food". In general, soil, climate, environmental conditions, and nutrients, have significant impact on the phytochemical content which in turn determines the quality of the natural products. Conventional procedure for quality assessment of natural products is based on extraction and characterization by analytical techniques, including high performance liquid chromatography (HPLC), gas chromatography (GC), UV spectroscopy, etc. In recent times, high-importance is given to electrochemical techniques due to its low-cost, rapid analysis and easy extension to electronic systems. In addition, it provides a new route to direct

[1] Nano and Bioelectrochemistry Research Laboratory, Department of Chemistry, School of Advanced Sciences, Vellore Institute of Technology, Vellore-632014, India.

[2] Department of Chemistry, School of Advanced Sciences, Vellore Institute of Technology, Vellore-632014, India

[3] Carbon dioxide Research and Green Technology Centre, Vellore Institute of Technology, Vellore-632014, Tamil Nadu, India.

[4] Institute of Biochemical and Biomedical Engineering, National Taipei University of Technology, Taipei 10608, Taiwan (R.O.C.)

[5] Department of Chemical Engineering, Dr. S.S. Bhatnagar University, Centre for Nanoscience and Nanotechnology, Punjab University, Chandigarh, India

[6] Department of Pharmaceutics, East West College of Pharmacy, Bengaluru, India

[7] East West College of Science and Department of Biotechnology, East West College of Science, Bangalore-560091

**Corresponding authors:* askumarchem@yahoo.com; askumar@vit.ac.in *assessment of certain critical parameters like redox and anti-oxidant activities of phytochemicals in its native form. This review covers the electrochemical aspects of phytochemicals derived from natural products in the following subheadings; (i) Electrochemical antioxidant ability: In this case, electrochemical techniques were used to estimate the activity of natural products with respect to standard anti-oxidants like ascorbic acid. This approach can profoundly allow the system to detect the antioxidant potentials of various phytochemicals available in natural sources of plants including but not limited to herbs. (ii) Preparation of reduced graphene oxide and metal nanoparticles: Phytochemicals like oleuropein (olive leaf extract), gallic acid and protocatechuic acid are used as a major source for the reduction of graphene oxide (GO) to reduced form of GO. Similarly, the certain metals like M^{n+} were reduced to M^{0}-nanoparticles (M=Au and Ag). (iii) Electrochemical characterization and detection; wherein, cyclic and pulse voltammetry, electrochemical detector systems are utilized to detect the electro-active species (phytochemicals) present in the natural products. In this regards phytochemical units like canthin-6-one, trans-avicennol, coumarins, quercetin, phaeophytin betc are detected in the natural products. The literature information was collected from Scopus® with key words, phytochemicals and electrochemical from the abstract. Finally, the advantages, challenges and future application of this methodology are elaborately described.*

Key words: Phytochemicals, Natural products, Analysis, Bioactivity, Electrochemical processes.

1.0. INTRODUCTION

The medicinal features of herbs, spices and plants are attributed to the consequence of availability of phytochemical constituents (Arnason *et al.*, 1995; Da *et al.*, 2016). In general, phytochemicals such as flavonoids, tannins, alkaloids, phenolic compounds (polyphenols) and alkaloids are present in the natural systems. They confined to several biological functions such as anti-mutagenicity, anti-carcinogenicity, cardio-protective, and anti-neoplastic and are also used in the treatment of haemorrhoids and rheumatism (Liu *et al.*, 2013; Temple *et al.*, 2017). Most of the phytochemicals are electro-active in nature and hence there is an unambiguous relation found between the metabolic activity of phytonutrients and their redox activity. Quality assessment of these natural products requires standard conventional procedures and quite a number of times they are not completely understood by technicians themselves, thus chances of errors being more frequent. The chemical analysis through electrochemical methodology complements the other conventional techniques with a better understanding even for incompatible molecules.

Electrochemistry is a powerful technique related to electron-transfer behaviour of various compounds or substances or biological systems in relation to current-potential parameters (Baed *et al.*, 2000; Zen *et al.*, 2006). This technique has been used for both qualitative (electrode-kinetics and mechanism, electrochemical oxidation and reduction reactions) and quantitative purposes (Baed *et al.*, 2000). The quantitative analysis using electrochemical-techniques include cyclic-voltammetry (CV), differential pulse voltammetry (DPV), and electrochemical detectors for high-performance liquid chromatography (HPLC) and flow injection analysis (FIA) techniques etc. Fig. 1 illustrates the electrochemical experimental setup consisting of 10 mL working vial with three-electrode arrangement (i) Working electrode, any conducting system which are stable at working condition; where the electrochemical reaction are studied; (ii) Reference electrode, Ag/AgCl or Saturated Calomel Electrode, to apply potential to working electrode; (iii) Counter electrode, with respect to this electrode emf is measured, (*e.g.,* carbon or platinum electrodes). Test phytochemical extract is taken in a 10 mL cell with proper electrolyte like phosphate buffer solution (PBS) pH 7, 0.1 M KCl or KNO_3 along with three-electrode system (Fig. 1). The literature information reveals that very little attention has been paid on the electrochemistry and phytochemicals. It is noteworthy that unlike the conventional analytical techniques like HPLC coupled UV-Vis detector, Gas chromatography (GC) and simple spectroscopic technique, the electrochemical techniques offer selective and sensitive recognition of the targeted chemicals in the natural products (Zen *et al.*, 2006). This can be achieved by properly adjusting the pH of the solution and turning the working potential window. In fact, qualitative, quantitative and mechanistic (electron-transfer reaction) aspects can be probed directly without any separation technique. This book chapter covers critical aspects of the electrochemical techniques towards the phytochemicals including electrochemical bioactivity and applicability toward selected applications. The content in this chapter is discussed under four headings; (i) electrochemical estimation of antioxidant behaviour of natural products, (ii) phytochemical as reducing agent to prepare certain nanoparticle systems like reduced graphene oxide (rGO), silver (Ag) and gold (Au) nanoparticles, (iii) quantitative and qualitative analysis of phytochemicals using electrochemical techniques and (iv) phytochemicals as green-anticorrosion scaffolds.

2. ELECTROCHEMICAL ESTIMATION OF ANTIOXIDANT BEHAVIOUR OF NATURAL PRODUCTS

This is very much related to the terms, oxidative stress and antioxidant defense reactive oxygen species (ROS) which are produced during normal cellular metabolism by living organisms (Halliwell *et al.*, 1999; Stadtman *et*

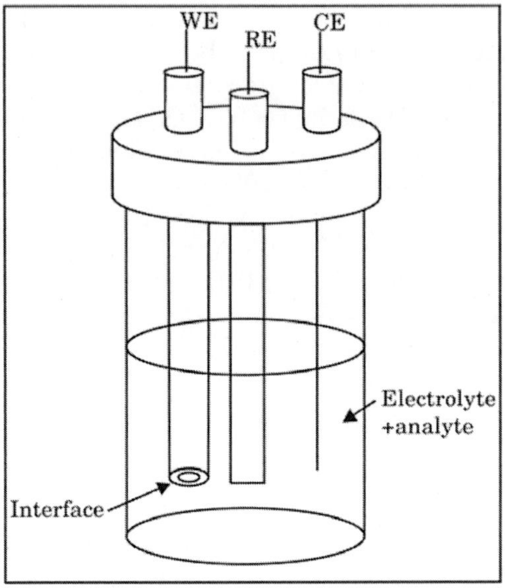

Fig. 1: Illustration of the three-electrode setup used in the electrochemical techniques. WE = Working electrode; RE= Reference electrode; CE= Counter electrode.

al., 2004; Seifried *et al.*, 2007; Ahmad *et al.*, 2008). Following are the three major ROS observed in the physiological systems; hydroxyl radical (•OH), superoxide anion ($O_2^{-\bullet}$) and hydrogen peroxide (H_2O_2). At low and moderate concentrations, these radicals exhibit normal activity in cellular-physiological processes; however at higher concentrations, they exhibit adverse effects on cellular components, such as lipids, proteins, and DNA modifications and in turn contributes to many disease/pathological conditions, such as cancer, neurological disorders, hypertension, atherosclerosis, ischemia/ perfusion, acute respiratory distress syndrome, diabetics, idiopathic pulmonary fibrosis, asthma and chronic obstructive pulmonary disease. Antioxidants are known to counter-balance the effect of oxidants in cellular systems. In general, antioxidants are categorised as: enzymatic (heme oxygenase, thioredoxins, peroxiredoxins and glutaredoxins) and non-enzymatic systems. Non-enzymatic antioxidants include low-molecular-weight compounds, such as β-carotene, vitamins (vitamins C and E), glutathione, polyphenols, and tripeptide. Many plant phytochemicals are typical example under this category (Table 1). These chemicals act as antioxidants and scavenge the ROS in the physiological system. To check the antioxidant capacity of the phytochemical, 1, 1-diphenyl-2-picryl-hydrazyl (DPPH) based assay has been widely referred (Shen *et al.*, 2010; Watson *et al.*, 2014). Shortly, 1 mL of 100 mM solution of DPPH dissolved in methanol is added to 3 mL of the test extracts in CH_3OH at different concentration

Table 1: List of the common herbs, vegetables and fruits and its important phytochemicals (polyphenols).

	Natural products	*Key phytochemical (polyphenols)*
1.	Apple	Chlorogenic acid (flesh), catechol, catechin (peel), caffeic acid, 3,4-dihydroxyphenylalanine (DOPA), 3,4-dihydroxy benzoic acid, *p*-cresol, 4-methyl catechol, leucocyanidin, *p*-coumaric acid, flavonol glycosides Isochlorogenic acid,
2.	Apricot	Caffeic acid, 4-methyl catechol, chlorogenic acid, catechin, epicatechin, pyrogallol, catechol, flavonols, *p*-coumaric acid derivatives
3.	Avocado	Catechol, dopamine, pyrogallol, catechol, 4-methyl chlorogenic acid, caffeic acid, DOPA
4.	Banana	3,4-dihydroxyphenylethylamine (Dopamine), leucodelphinidin, leucocyanidin
5.	Cacao	Catechins, leucoanthocyanidins, anthocyanins, complex tannins
6.	Coffee beans	Chlorogenic acid, caffeic acid
7.	Eggplant	Chlorogenic acid, caffeic acid, coumaric acid, cinnamic acid derivatives
8.	Grape	Catechin, chlorogenic acid, catechol, caffeic acid, DOPA, tannins, flavonols, protocatechuic acid, resorcinol, hydroquinone, phenol
9.	Lettuce	Tyrosine, caffeic acid, chlorogenic acid derivatives
10.	Mango	Dopamine-HCl, 4-methyl catechol, caffeic acid, catechol, catechin, chlorogenic acid, tyrosine, DOPA, *p*-cresol
11.	Mushroom	Tyrosine, catechol, DOPA, dopamine, adrenaline, noradrenaline
12.	Peach	Chlorogenic acid, pyrogallol, 4-methyl catechol, catechol, caffeic acid, gallic acid, catechin, dopamine
13.	Pear	Chlorogenic acid, catechol, catechin, caffeic acid, DOPA, 3,4-dihydroxy benzoic acid, *p*-cresol
14.	Plum	Chlorogenic acid, catechin, caffeic acid, catechol, DOPA
15.	Potato	chlorogenic acid, caffeic acid, catechol, DOPA, *p*-cresol, *p*-hydroxyphenyl propionic acid, *p*-hydroxyphenyl pyruvic acid, *m*-cresol
16.	Sweet potato	Chlorogenic acid, caffeic acid, caffeylamide
17.	Tea	Flavanols, catechins, tannins, cinnamic acid derivatives

(50–800) μg mL^{-1}. The mixtures were shaken and kept it aside at room temperature for 0.5 h. Then, the absorbance (l) was measured at 1=517 nm using a UV-Vis spectroscopy by using ascorbic acid (vitamin C) as a positive control. Lower intensity (absorbance) signal of the test-reaction mixture indicate higher free radical scavenging activity. The capability/performance of scavenging activity of the DPPH was calculated using the formula; Percentage inhibition = $\{(A^0 - A1)/A^0) \times 100\}$, wherein, A^0= absorbance of the control reaction, and A1 = absorbance in presence of all the extract samples and reference. The entire process is simplified and analysed the activity by electrochemical technique. Further, Table 2 provides the details of the electrochemical assays adopted for the antioxidant capacity of certain Indian

Table 2: Electrochemical detection based antioxidant assays.

Phytochemicals/ chemicals/ real sample	*Technique /medium*	*Electrode/ E(V)*	*Comment*	*References*
1. Total phenolic content/ spice plants like spice *Allium cepa*, parsley (*Petroselinum crispum*) roots and leaves, celery (*Apium graveolens*) roots and leaves and leaves of dill (*Anethum graveolens*)	HPLC-ECD/ 100 mM sodium dihydrophosphate, pH 3 acetonittrile and, methanol (30:60:10 v/ v).	GCE/0.3-0.9 V (Ag/AgCl)	*Samples are incubated with DPPH for 20 min *Compared with DPPH assay	Stankevièius *et al*. (2011)
2. Phenolic compounds, flavonoids, ascorbic acid and tocopherols/ *F. ulmaria*, flowers of Spanish broom, meadowsweet and elder	CV and DPV/ methanol/ 0.1 M $NaClO_4$	GCE/0.86 V (Ag/AgCl)	*Antioxidant capacity in terms of ascorbic acid	Barros *et al.* (2011)
3. Antioxidant activity of *Eugenia dysenterica*	CV/pH 5 phosphate buffer	Carbon paste electrode/0.3 V(Ag/AgCl)	*Estimated the redox behaviour of the various plant extract	Clementino *et al.* (2016)

spices (Stankevicius *et al.*, 2011), *F. ulmaria* flower (Barros *et al.*, 2011) and *Eugenia dysenterica* (Clementino *et al.*, 2016). In these assays, various amounts of the plant extracts were quantified (total phytochemicals) with respect to standard antioxidant like ascorbic acid. For the plant extracts, calibrations (current *versus* extract concentration) were normalized with the electrochemical calibrations of the standard system (current *versus* ascorbic acid-concentration). In fact, comparison of the DPPH assay method's result is on par with the electrochemical method (Stankevicius *et al.*, 2011; Barros *et al.*, 2011; Clementino *et al.*, 2016).

2.1. Phytochemicals as reducing agents in the chemical synthesis

In this case, certain phytochemicals like polyphenols (dihydroxy or trihydroxyl benzene derivatives) and flavonoids have been used as mild reducing agents to reduce the Au^{3+} and Ag^{2+} ions to respective nanoparticles, such as Au-nano and Ag-nano systems (Devnani *et al.,* 2015; Lee *et al.,* 2016; Chouhan *et al.,* 2017; Elemika *et al.,* 2017) (Fig. 2). Devnani *et al.*(2015) have used black rice extract, which contains anthocyanin pigments and other polyphenol reagents for the Au-nanoparticle synthesis A specific l_{max} at 560–570 nm was noticed for the Au nano-formation. In a similar way, gallic acid and protocatechuic acid (Lee *et al.*, 2016), *Trachyspermum*

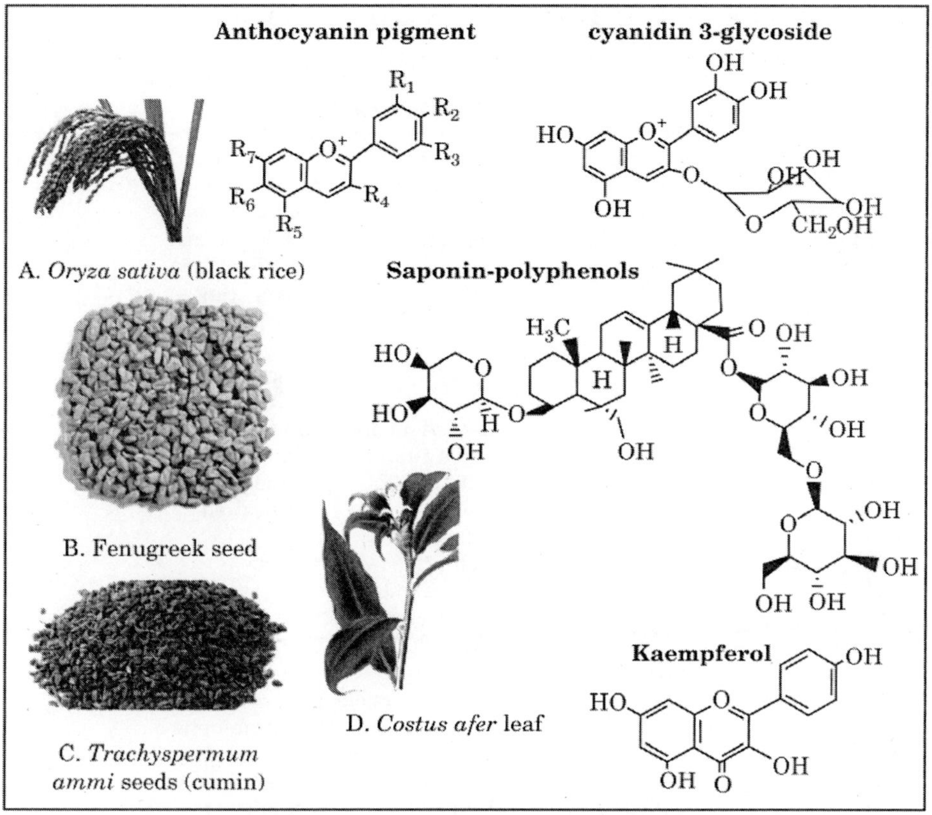

Fig. 2: Some of the natural herbs and their phytochemicals tested as reducing agents for chemical synthesis (reduced graphene oxide, Ag and Au-nanoparticles).

ammi seed extract (Chouhan *et al.*, 2017) and *Costus afer* leaf extract (Elemika *et al.*, 2017) were used for the Ag-nanoparticle synthesis. In these cases, a specific l_{max} at 405–411 nm was noticed. In continuation, in 2016, Singh *et al.*, utilized *fenugreek* seed extract that contains saponin-polyphenol ingredient for the *in-situ* reduction of Pb^{2+}/Graphene oxide system to Pd-nano/reducted Graphene oxide (Singh *et al.*, 2016). Further, this matrix has been used as a bio-electrochemical sensor platform coupled with Lipase-glutamate dehydrogenase systems for the detection of triglyceride (Table 3).

2.2. Quantitative and qualitative analysis of phytochemicals using electrochemical techniques

The oxidation and reduction ability of the phytochemicals can be exploited in the quantifications of phytochemicals and, electrochemical detectors operated at specific potential to quantify these compounds. Electrode system

Table 3: List of representative plants as reducing agents in the chemical synthesis.

	Phytochemicals/ chemicals/real sample	*Green chemical reduction*	*Electro-chemical application*	*Comment*	*References*
1	*Oryza sativa L.* - black rice extract/ anthocyanin pigments, cyanidin 3-glycoside and peonidin 3-glycoside (polyphenolic compounds)	100 mL of 0.1 M $NaAuCl_4.2H_2O$ was added drop wise to the rice extract	gold nanoparticle modified anthocyanin-based carbon paste electrode for heavy metal estimation.	*Ethanol extract of 1 g of grounded black rice was mixed with 30 ml of ethanol containing 0.1 % HCl and kept for sonication was used	Devnani *et al.* (2015)
2	Gallic acid and protocatechuic acid	5.9 mM Ag^{2+} 10 mM of the phytochemical	Ag seed mediated Ag-nano particle formation was probed using CV technique in 0.1 M KNO_3 as a electrolyte	10-20 nm sized silver nanoparticles were synthesized	Lee *et al.* (2016)
3	Phenolic compounds/ *Trachyspermum ammi* (TA, Ajwain) seeds extract	Extract obtained by mixing and soaking of 2 g seed in 20 mL of distilled water & then added to 1 mM of 25 mM $AgNO_3$.	TA consumpion on the Ag nanoparticle formation was monitoring using CV with Pt-tipped carbon elect-, rode	Catalytic reduction p-nitro phenol to p-aminophenol in excess of $NaBH_4$ was demonstrated	Chouhan *et al.* (2017)
4	*Costus afer* leaf Extract/ flavonoids such as kaempfe-, rol 3,4- di O-Me-quercetin and phenolic acids such as 2,5-dihydroxybenzoic acid, O-coumaric acid, p-hydroxybenzoic acid	2 g of dried plant power in 150 mL of water, heated at 90°C, mixed with 1 mM of Ag^{2+} again heated at 90°C	Resulting Ag-nano was modified with MWCNT and tested it conductivity using $Fe(CN)^{3-}{}_6$ redox couple.	*Antibacterial activity and antioxidant activity of the plant extract was tested.	Elemike *et al.* (2017)
5	*Fenugreek* seeds (FS)/saponin-polyphenols	5 mL of FS extract (10 g in 5 mL distilled water treated) mixed with Pb^{2+} -GO (5 mg in 1 mg in 20 mL GO solution (1 mg/mL) solution at 80°C	Lipase (LIP)-glutamate dehydrogen- ase (GLDH)-bienzyme modified on rGO/Pdnano for triglyceride detection using $Fe(CN)_6^{3-}$ as probe	*Biosensor showed detection range of 25-400 mg dL^{-1} with sensitivity of 1.3 $\mu A\ mg^{-1}$ $dLcm^{-1}$.	Singh *et al.* (2016)

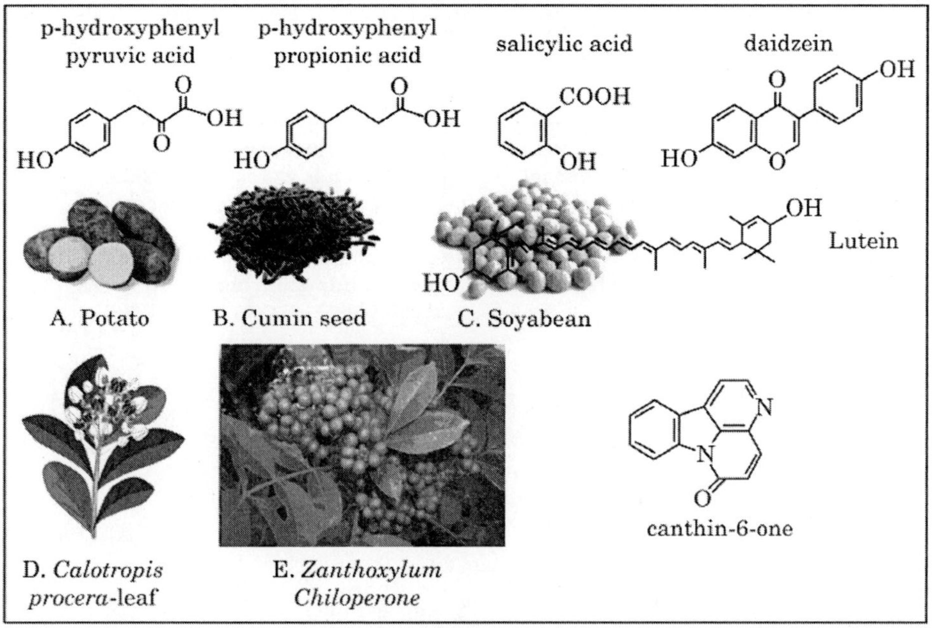

Fig. 3: Various natural products sources and their chemical structures analysed by electrochemical techniques.

accompanied with specific solvent has been used in the separation techniques like HPLC and capillary electrophoresis. Table 4 summarizes the various electrochemical detector reported so far. For instance, phytochemical-isoflavones in breast milk (Franke *et al.*, 1998), Phytoestrogens and polyphenols in body-fluid samples (Gamache *et al.*, 1998), phytonutrients like lycopene, β-carotene, -tocopherol and γ-tocopherol in tomato samples (Rozzi *et al.,* 2002) flavonoids and polyphenols in urine samples (Ouchi *et al.*, 2005), salicylic acid (aspirin) content in certain Indian herbs and species (cumin, paprika and turmeric) (Paterson *et al.*, 2006), polyphenols (c-tocopherol, lutein and daidzein) in soybean (Correa *et al.*, 2010), vitamin c in kiwi-fruit (Carr *et al.*, 2013) and flavonoids and carotenoids in *Angelica keiskei* (Correa *et al.*, 2014) have been analysed by HPLC coupled electrochemical detector technique. Similarly, photo-toxicity of the different buckwheat extract was tested by Capillary Electrophoresis (CE) coupled electrochemical and UV-Vis detection techniques (Hinneburg *et al.*, 2005). In the above case, the activity was tested in relation to oxygen consumption and generation of ROS upon irradiation with Vis-light. It has been concluded that rutin and quercetin in association with hypericin-chlorophyll causes the photo-toxicity. In all those systems, flow rate, solvents and operating potentials were properly optimized according to the test sample.

Table 4: Electrochemical characterization and electroanalysis of phytochemicals.

	Phytochemicals/ chemicals/Real sample	*Electrode/ Technique*	*Comment*	*References*
1	Isoflavones	HPLC coupled electrochemical coulometric cell detector	*Breast milk and other biological fluids were analysed	Franke *et al.* (1998)
2	Phytoestrogens (isoflavonoids, lignans, and coumestans) and Polyphenols	HPLC coupled electrochemical coulometric array detector	*Rat blood plasma, tissue, urine and human urine real samples	Gamache and Acworth (1998)
3	Lycopene (lycopene ,β-carotene, α-carotene, α-tocopherol, γ-tocopherol, andδ-tocopherol content) from Tomato	HPLC coupled electrochemical detection at an applied potential of 300-700 mV vs Ag/AgCl	*Supercritical fluid CO_2 has been used for the extraction of the phytochemicals effectively.	Rozzi *et al.* (2002)
4	Flavonoids and polyphenols	HPLC coupled electrochemical coulometric cell detector	*Urine samples were analysed.	Ouchi *et al.* (2005)
5	Salicylic acid (aspirin) in herbs and Indian spices (*cumin, paprika* and *turmeric*)	HPLC electrochemical detection	*Certain food stuffs (vegetarian) have significant content of salicylic acid (1.6 mg in 100 g of cumin)	Paterson *et al.* (2006)
6	Stability analysis of polyphenols (c-tocopherol, lutein, daidzein) in soybean	HPLC-ECD	*No significant decrease in the total polyphenol content with black soybeans stored at room temperature, 4-80°C for 14 months. *On the other hand, lutein and c-tocopherol degraded significantly within a month of storage at room temperature	Correa *et al.* (2010)
7	Comparison of bioavailability (blood serum) of synthetic and kiwifruit vitamin C	HPLC-ECD	*Pharmacokinetic and bioavailability of vitamin C is much higher in kiwifruit than synthetic sample.	Carr *et al.* (2013)
8	*Angelica keiskei* / flavonoids and carotenoids	HPLC-ECD	*Plasma ascorbic acid (ECD) and Uric acid content were measured *The plant extract increase antioxidant status.	Correa *et al.* (2014)

Table 4: (*Contd...*)

Table 4: *(Contd...)*

	Phytochemicals/ chemicals/Real sample	*Electrode/ Technique*	*Comment*	*References*
9	Phototoxicity of different buckwheat extracts and individual plant	Capillary Electrophoresis (CE) coupled with Electrochemical and UV detection	*Activity tested in terms of oxygen consumption and generation of reactive oxygen species upon irradiation with visible light* Rutin and quercetin combined with hypericin and chlorophyll caused phototoxicity	Hinneburg *et al.* (2005)
10	*Potato* polyphenol/ Caffeic acid, quinic acid and chlorogenic acid	Various in the redox potentials	*Introduced the possibility of differentiation of various polyphenols by electrochemical technique.	Friedman (1997)
11	*Turnera subulata*-chemicals (steroids, sitosterol and stigmasterol, flavonoids, Pheophytins chlorophyll-a etc)	Cyclic voltammetry with Pt as working electrode in acetonitrile containing 0.01 mol L^{-1} of lithium perchlorate as electrolyte	**Turnera subulata* Sm., possesses a macrocyclic ring structure very similar to those of phthalocyanines	De Brito Filho *et al.* (2014)
12	7-hydroxy-6-methoxycoumarin (scopoletin, a biomarker) in plants	Cyclic voltammetric technique in pH 3. A specific peak at 0.6 V corresponding to phenol oxidation was observed	*Pulse voltammetric technique was adopted for he quantification and mechanism evaluation.	Leite *et al.* (2015)
13	*Calotropis procera*-leaf/ polyphenols	Graphite/ poly (allylamine hydrochloride) /nanotubegraphene composite/ polypyrrole /de-oxy ribonucleic acid (Gr/PAH/NT-G/PPy/DNA) modified electrode with $Fe(CN)_6^{3-}$ was used for cancer cell binding	*The phytochemical extract was analysed for anticancer property against LN-18 cells using electrochemical methods.	Nalini *et al.* (2016)
14	*Zanthoxylum Chiloperone*/ leaves, seeds, fruits, roots and stem bark of *Zanthoxylum*	*Cyclic voltammetric technique using GCE was working electrode in pH 7 phosphate buffer solution	*Specific reduction and oxidation peaks at -1.28 and 0.54 V vs Ag/AgCl were noticed, which can be taken for the electroanalysis of the plant sample.	Cebrián-Torrejón *et al.* (2017)

Table 4: *(Contd...)*

Table 4: (*Contd...*)

	Phytochemicals/ chemicals/Real sample	*Electrode/ Technique*	*Comment*	*References*
	chiloperone/ canthin-6-one, 5-methoxycanthin -6-one and trans-avicennol			
15	*Ginger* plant extract/ zingibe-rene, shogaol and gingerol	Cyclic voltamme-tric technique in couple with grap-hitized mesopor-ous modified ele-ctrode was used	*Electroactive species were identified and further used for new redox active chemi-cally modified electrode preparation	Amreen *et al.* (2017)

In some cases, cyclic voltammetric technique was used for the quantitative assessment of the phytochemicals in the natural system. In 1997, Friedman, introduced the concept of redox testing of phytochemicals in natural systems, like potato (Friedman *et al.*, 1997). In 2014, de Brito Filho *et al.,* examined the *Turnera subulata* extract using Pt working electrode in acetonitrile + lithium perchlorate containing electrolyte solution and it was concluded that the electrochemical activity of the phytochemical system resembled with phthalocyanines activity (De *et al.*, 2014). In 2015, Leite *et al.* (2015) examined the phytochemical, 7-hydroxy-6-methoxycoumarin (scopoletin) using glassy carbon as a working electrode in wider pH solutions. Mechanistic activity of the phenolic site present in the compound was tested and correlated with specific natural system. In 2016, researchers tested the anticancer activity of *Calotropis procera*-leaf by electrochemical method (Nalini *et al.*, 2016). In this technique, graphite working electrode modified with poly (allylamine hydrochloride)/nanotube-graphene composite/polypyrrole/DNA and LN-18 cellular system in combination with $Fe(CN)_6^{3-}$ redox couple was used. In the same year, Cebrián-Torrejón *et al.,* tested the Zanthoxylum chiloperon-phytochemicals in certain leaves, seeds, fruits, roots and stem bank by CV technique (Cebrian *et al.*, 2017). Specific electrochemical signals at -1.28 and 0.54 V versus Ag/AgCl were noticed corresponding to the electrochemical activity of the test compound. In 2017, our group investigated the shogaol, zingiberene and gingerol (responsible for flavour and pungency) in ginger by means of cyclic voltammetric technique using graphitized mesoporous carbon nanomaterial modified glassy carbon electrode (GCE) in pH 2 KCl-HCl solution (Amreen *et al.*, 2017). It has been identified that upon heating the ginger, the methoxy functional groups in the phytochemical gets cleaved as respective phenol and then as quinone derivatives and the mechanism was verified by the electrochemical technique.

2.3. Phytochemicals as corrosion inhibitors

Corrosion is the most common electrochemical reactions that are seen in everyday activities. Destructive nature of corrosion due to chemical or microbial attack upon a base metal by its surrounding can cause huge loss. Many naturally derived chemical entities are shown to protect metallic surface by means of adsorption phenomena, wherein, the electron rich atoms like O, N and S donate its lone-pair of electron/s to the metal and can turn it to behave as cathode. These useful phytochemicals usually termed as "green corrosion inhibitors" can be either cathode or anode inhibitors depending upon the mechanism of its action on the metallic surface. Detailed list of plant based natural extracts that are investigated as corrosion inhibitors for selected base metals is given in Table 5. The method of evaluation of corrosion inhibition is largely done using electrochemical impedance spectroscopy (EIS), gravimetric method and sometime gasometrical method. Palm leaves and seed ethanol extract largely contain flavonoids and saponin as natural phenolics inhibited corrosion in carbon steel *via* adsorption mechanism (Uncoren *et al.*, 2018). Apart from this, *Chamaerops humilis* L. extract (Left *et al.*, 2018) containing tannins and terpenes, *Holoptelea integrifolia* leaf extract (HILE) (Verma *et al.*, 2018) having beta-amyrins and catechins, *neem* extract which predominantly contains *Azadirachtin* (Parthipan *et al.*, 2018) and *Solanum aethiopicum*-leaf extract (Okeniyi *et al.*, 2015) which is rich in coumarins and essential oils apart from flavonoids and saponins, have been shown to protect mild steel against corrosion. Since these natural product extracts hold a cocktail of chemical products which are predominantly phenolics and other aromatic organic molecules, often times, they follow mixed type inhibition of corrosion in the metals. Reports are also available on the anti-corrosion inhibition of natural extract in Aluminium metal. *Trigonella foenum-graecum* which predominantly contains 1-methylpyridinium-3-carboxylate, 2-isobutyl 3-methoxy pyrazine (Ladha *et al.*, 2015) and *fennel* seed extract (Ladha *et al.*, 2015) having a furfural derivative, are investigated as anti-corrosion inhibitor in Aluminium metal. Incidentally, these natural extracts seem to prevent corrosion by way of physisorption over Aluminium surface. Interestingly, *Mansoa alliacea* plant extract obtained from sodium chloride media (Suedile *et al.*, 2014) has significantly prevented the corrosion in zinc metal by means of charge-transfer and a passive layer formation. This passive mechanism holds better inhibition due to surface reactivity of chemical compounds at the interface between metals and thin layer of compounds. Furthermore, reactive nano particles offer an excellent solution to corrosion problem. Alkaloids extract from *Aniba rosaeodora* plant (Chevalier *et al.*, 2014), *Pterolobium hexapetalum, Celosia argentea* plant extracts (Pradeep *et al.*, 2014) are efficient inhibitor of corrosion in mild steel. Eco-friendly stabilized mono disperse silver nanocomposite (Atta *et al.*, 2014) has significantly

Table 5: List of naturally derived phytochemicals used as green corrosion inhibitors.

	Natural product	*Phytochem.*	*Inhibition methods*	*Corrosion metal*	*Comments*	*References*
1	*Palm* leaves and seed	Flavonoids, saponin and tannins	Using crude ethanol extract	Carbon steel	Corrosion inhibition through adsorption mechanism and follows adsorption Langmuir isotherm model.	Umoren *et al.*(2017)
2	*Chamaerops humilis L.* extract	Saponins, terpenoids, flavonoids, tannins and steroids.	EIS method and the optimal corrosion inhibition efficiency of the extract is H~60 % for 0.75 g/L.	Reinforcement steel	The extract improves the electrochemical parameters by ennobling the corrosion potential and increasing the polarization resistance.	Left *et al.* (2018)
3	*Holoptelea integrifolia* leaf extract (HILE)	Beta-amyrin, Catachins, quinones	Adsorption on metal/ electr-olyte interfaces.	Mild steel	HILE acts as mixed inhibitor and predominantly shows cathodic protection behaviour	Verma *et al.* (2018)
4	*Neem* extract	Azadirachtin, gedunin, nimbin, nimbandiol, azadirone, nimbolide, nimbinene, nimbolin, nimonol, margolone, vilasanin	Biofilm inhibition assay	Carbon steel API 5LX	Mechanism by adsorption of their organic compounds on the metal surface	Parthipan *et al.* (2017)
5	*Solanum aethiopicum*-leaf extract	Tannins, saponins, glycosides, flavonoids	Electrochemical method	Steel		Okeniyi *et al.* (2015)
6	*Trigonella foenum-graecum*	1-Methylpyridinium-3-carboxylate (Trigonelline), 2-isobutyl 3-methoxy pyrazine (IBP) and Apigenin -8-C-glucoside (Vitexin)	Gravimetric and EIS techniques	Al in 1M HCl medium	Mechanism is due to adsorption of inhibitor molecule over metal/solution interface.	Ladha *et al.* (2015a)

Table 5: (*Contd...*)

Table 5: (*Contd...*)

	Natural product	*Phytochem.*	*Inhibition methods*	*Corrosion metal*	*Comments*	*References*
7	*Fennel* seed extract	1,5-Anhydro-6-deoxyhexo-2,3-diulose; Hydroxy methyl furfural (E)-1-(4-Methoxyphenyl) propene n-Hexadecanoic acid	Gravimetric and electrochemical methods	Al in HCl	Molecules present in fennel extract was physisorbed over Al surface to inhibit the corrosion reactions occurring over Al specimen in presence of HCl solution	Ladha *et al.* (2015b)
8	*Mansoa alliacea* plant extract in sodium chloride media	Coumarins, essential oils, flavanoids	Electrochemical method, adsorption isotherm behaviour	Zinc	The impedance study presented two phenomena included a charge-transfer and a passive layer and they show same trend.	Suedile *et al.* (2014)
9	Alkaloids extract from *Aniba rosaeodora* plant	Alkaloids	EIS, XPS and adsorption isotherm	Mild steel in 1M HCl	XPS results provide direct evidence of the adsorption of extract onto the steel surface thus strongly supporting the model invoking the blocking its active sites and preventing it from being corroded easily.	Chevalier *et al.* (2014)
10	*Pterolobium hexapetalum* and *Celosia-argentea* plant extracts	Phenolics and flavanoids	Potentiodynamic polarization method, EIS	Mild steel	Adsorption method and blocking the corrosion sites	Pradeep Kumar and Mohana (2014)
11	Eco-friendly stabilized monodispzerse silver nano-composite	Nano particles	Inhibition Polarization and EIS methods.	Mild steel	The electrochemical corrosion reaction is controlled by charge transfer process.	Atta *et al.* (2014)
12	*Chlorophy tum borivili anum* root extract	Phenolics and flavanoids	EIS, polarization test,	Mild steel in HCl and H_2SO_4	Basis of molecular interaction of the inhibitor with mildsteel.	Ji *et al.* (2013)

Table 5: (*Contd...*)

Table 5: (*Contd...*)

	Natural product	*Phytochem.*	*Inhibition methods*	*Corrosion metal*	*Comments*	*References*
13	*Musa acuminata* flower extract	Terpenes	Weight loss and electrochemical method	Mild steel in H_2SO_4	Inhibition occurs due to adsorption of extract on the surface of the metal	Gunavathy and Murugavel (2013a)
14	*Lavandula dentata* aqueous extract	Phenolics, terpenes	Gravimetric method, electrochemical method.	Mild steel in 1M HCl	Mixed type as well as adsorption type of inhibition	Bouammali *et al.* (2013)
15	*Musa acuminata* fruit peel extract	Terpenoids and phenolics	Weight loss and electrochemical method	Mild steel in acid medium	Inhibition effect of the plant extract was due to physical adsorption of the nutrients present in the extract onto the active sites on thesurface of the metal.	Gunavathy and Murugavel (2013b)
16	*Pachycormus discolor* leaves ethanol extract	Polyphenols method	Polarization in 1M HCl EIS and polarization resistance	Mild steel	Mixed type inhibition	Garcia Inzunza *et al*. (2012)
17	*Piper guineense* extract	Alkaloids, tannins and saponins	Electro-chemical method	Low carbon steel	Electronic structures of specific components of the extract confirmed their inherent affinity toward adsorption on the metal surface and hence inhibit the corrosion reaction	Oguzie *et al*. (2012)
18	*Ocimum viridis, Telfairia occidentalis, Azadirachta indica and Hibiscus sabdariffa* as well as extracts from the seeds of *Garcinia kola*	Alkaloids, tepenes and phenolics	Electrochemical method	Mild steel in 2M HCl /1MH_2SO_4	Participation of both protonated and neutral species in the inhibiting action of the extracts.	Oguzie (2010)

Table 5: (*Contd...*)

Table 5: (*Contd...*)

	Natural product	*Phytochem.*	*Inhibition methods*	*Corrosion metal*	*Comments*	*References*
19	Ethanol extract of *Garcinia kola* and *Cola nitida*	Phenolics, terpenes and tannins	Gravimetry method & gasometric method	Mild Steel in H_2SO-	Adsorption models indicated that Langmuir adsorption isotherm can be used to describe the adsorption characteristics of these inhibitors.	Eddy (2010)
20	Ethanol extract of *Gongronema latifolium*	Tannins, alkaloids, carotenoids	Gasometric method	Mild steel in H_2SO_4	Due to the formation of electrostatic bond between the surface of mild steel and the inhibitor which protect the metal against further attack.	Eddy and Odiongenyi (2010)
21	Ethanol extract of *Gongronema latifolium*	Tannins, alkaloids, carotenoids	Gasometric methods	Mild steel in H_2SO_4	Inhibitive action of ethanol extract of GL is due to the presence of amino acid, tannin, alkaloid, carotenoid, flavonoid, steroid and anthocyanin in the extract.	Eddy and Ebenso (2010)

reduced the corrosion of mild steel by way of charge transfer mechanism. Other plant extracts that are reported to have efficient anticorrosion properties in mild steel in acidic medium are; *Chlorophytum borivilianum* root extract (Ji *et al.*, 2013), *Musa acuminata* flower extract (Gunavathy *et al.*, 2013), *Lavandula dentata* aqueous extract (Bouammali *et al.*, 2013), *Musa acuminata* fruit peel extract (Gunavathy *et al.*, 2013) *Pachycormus* discolor leaves ethanol extract (Garcia *et al.*, 2012), *Piper guineense* extract (Oguzie *et al.*, 2012), *Ocimum viridis, Telfairia occidentalis, Azadirachta indica* and *Hibiscus sabdariffa,* as well as extracts from the seeds of *Garcinia kola* (Oguzie *et al.*, 2010), C_2H_5OH extract of *Garcinia kola* and *Cola nitida* (Edd *et al.,* 2010), ethanol extract of *Gongronema latifolium* (Edd *et al.*, 2010) and ethanol extract of *Gongronema latifolium* (Edd *et al.*, 2010). Many of these plant extracts are getting adsorbed on the metal surface and act as passive layer and prevent the material degradation. Moreover, these natural inhibitors form strong electrostatic bond with metallic surface rendering metal being protected from corrosive environment. The plausible explanation for electrostatic bond between inhibitors and metallic surface is mainly molecular polarity due to functional groups consisting of hetero atoms, such as O, N and S which can donate electrons and aids in metal-inhibitors bonding pattern.

3. CONCLUSIONS AND FUTURE PROSPECTS

This book chapter reviewed the existing literature reports on promising and perspective results that have been obtained with the electrochemical techniques on the natural products for qualitative and quantitative aspects. Followings are the challenges and future prospective of the present approach; (i) the electrochemistry related studies are oriented with physical chemistry aspects; it needs photochemistry expert to support for the interdisciplinary studies, (ii) most of the isolated products are in organic media, which are non-conducting in nature, proper design of the electrolyte solution and working electrode are necessary for the significant success, (iii) in general, natural products are mixture of electro-active (certain phytochemicals) and electro-inactive (protein and carbohydrates units) substances, hence, enrichment of the electro-active analyt/ analytes in the test sample is a challenging task and (iv) analyzing the electro-oxidative and reductive product is another important area. Amount of product formed on the electrode or electrode/electrolyte interface is very less (~ng), it is not convenient to extend to routine characterization studies with NMR and other spectroscopic techniques. This can be solved by performing systematic bulk-electrolysis of the selective phytochemical/natural product followed by spectro-chemical analysis. In addition, several, *in-situ* characterization techniques like electrochemistry coupled with quartz crystal micro-balance and spectro-electrochemistry experiments can be adopted for the product analysis. In consideration with novel and unique approach, new direction research on *in-situ* quantification of the phytochemicals in the natural products, bio-activity and antioxidant features, mechanistic pathway of degradation and related aspects are yet to be explored in detail.

ACKNOWLEDGEMENT

The authors acknowledge the DST-SERB (DST-SERB- EMR/2016/002818) Scheme for the financial support.

REFERENCES

Ahmad P, Sarwat M, Sharma S. Reactive Oxygen Species, Antioxidants and Signaling in Plants, Journal of Plant Biology, 2008; 51:167-173.

Amreen K, Shukla VK, Shukla S, Rajagopal D, Kumar AS. Redox behaviour and surface Confinement of electro active species of ginger extract on graphitized mesoporous carbon surface and its copper complex for H_2O_2 sensing, Nano-Structures and Nano-Objects,2017; 11:56-64.

Arnason JT, Mata R, Romeo, JT. Phytochemistry of Medicinal Plants. Springer International Publishing Agency, 1995.

Atta AM, El-Mahdy GA, Al-Lohedan HA, Ezzat AO. Electrochemical behaviour of mild steel in acidic medium based on eco-friendly stabilized monodisperse silver nanocomposite, International Journal of Electrochemical Science,2014;9:8226-8238.

Bard AJ, Faulkner LR. Electroanalytical Methods: Fundamentals and Applications, 2nd Editon, Wiley VCH Publisher, 2000.

Barros L, Cabrita L, Boas MV, Carvalho AM, Ferreira ICFR. Chemical, biochemical and electrochemical assays to evaluate phytochemicals and antioxidant activity of wild plants, Food Chemistry, 2011;127(4):1600-1608.

Bouammali H, Ousslim A, Bekkouch K, Bouammali B, Aouniti A, Al-Deyab SS, Jama C, Bentiss F, Hammouti B. The anti-corrosion behavior of *Lavandula dentata* aqueous extract on mild steel in 1M HCl, International Journal of Electrochemical Science,2013;8:6005-6013.

Carr AC, Bozonet SM, Vissers MCM. A randomised cross-over pharmacokinetic bioavailability study of synthetic versus kiwifruit-derived vitamin C, Nutrients, 2013; 5: 4451-4461.

Cebrián-Torrejón G, Doménech-Carbó A, Figadère B, Poupon E, Fournet A. Phytoelectrochemical analysis of *Zanthoxylum chiloperone*, Phytochemical Analysis, 2017;28:171-175.

Clementino SE, Garcia RS, Moreira BRCC, Pagliarini BA, Cabral RB, Silveira D, De Souza GE. Voltammetric and spectrophotometric determination of antioxidant activity of *Eugenia dysenterica* DC leaves extracts, Pakistan Journal of Pharmaceutical Sciences,2016;29(2):535-540.

Chevalier M, Robert F, Amusant N, Traisnel M, Roos C, Lebrini M. Enhanced corrosion resistance of mild steel in 1 M hydrochloric acid solution by alkaloids extract from *Aniba rosaeodora* plant: Electrochemical, phytochemical and XPS studies, Electrochimica Acta, 2014;131:96-105.

Chouhan N, Ameta R, Meena RK. Biogenic silver nanoparticles from *Trachyspermum ammi* (Ajwain) seeds extract for catalytic reduction of p-nitrophenol to p-aminophenol in excess of $NaBH_4$, Journal of Molecular Liquids, 2017;230:74-84.

Correa CR, Li L, Aldini G, Carini M, Oliver Chen CY, Chun HK, Cho SM, Park KM, Russell RM, Blumberg JB, Yeum KJ. Composition and stability of phytochemicals in five varieties of black soybeans (*Glycine max*), Food Chemistry,2010;123:1176-1184.

Correa CR, Oliver Chen CY, Aldini G, Rasmussen H, Ronchi CF, Berchieri-Ronchi C, ChoSM, Blumberg JB, Yeum K. Bioavailability of plant pigment phytochemicals in *Angelica keiskei* in older adults: A pilot absorption kinetic study, Nutrition Research and Practice,2014;8:550-557.

da Silva BV, Barreira JCM, Oliveira MBPP. Natural phytochemicals and probiotics as bioactive ingredients for functional foods: Extraction, biochemistry and protected-delivery technologies, Trends in Food Science & Technology,2016;50: 144-158.

De Brito Filho SG, Fernandes MG, Chaves OS, De Oliveira Chaves MC, Araruna, FB, Eiras C, De Souza de Almeida Leite JR, De Fátima Agra M, Braz-Filho R, De Fátima Vanderlei de Souza M. Chemical constituents isolated from *Turnera subulata* sm. and electrochemical characterization of phaeophytin b, Quimica Nova, 2014;37: 603-609.

Devnani H, Satsangee SP. Green gold nanoparticle modified anthocyanin-based carbon paste electrode for voltammetric determination of heavy metals, International Journal of Environmental Science and Technology,2016;12: 1269-1282.

Eddy NO. Adsorption and inhibitive properties of ethanol extract of *Garcinia kola* and *Cola nitida* for the corrosion of mild steel in H_2SO_4, Pigment and Resin Technology, 2010;39: 348-354.

Eddy NO, Odiongenyi AO. Corrosion inhibition and adsorption properties of ethanol extract of IT *Heinsia crinita*/IT on mild steel in H_2SO_4, Pigment and Resin Technology, 2010;39:288-295.

Eddy NO, Ebenso EE. Corrosion inhibition and adsorption properties of ethanol extract of *Gongronema latifolium* on mild steel in H_2SO_4, Pigment and Resin Technology, 2010; 39: 77-83.

Elemike EE, Fayemi OE, Ekennia AC, Onwudiwe DC, Ebenso EE. Silver nanoparticles mediated by *Costus afer* leaf extract: Synthesis, antibacterial, antioxidant and electrochemical properties, Molecules,2017;22:A7.

Franke AA, Custer LJ, Tanaka Y. Isoflavones in human breast milk and other biological fluids, American Journal of Clinical Nutrition, 1998;68:1466S-1473S.

Friedman, M. Potato Polyphenols: Role in the Plant and in the Diet, ACS Symposium Series,1997;662:61-93.

Garcia Inzunza R, Valdez Salas B, Kharshan R, Furman A, Schorr Wienner M. Interesting behavior of *Pachycormus discolor* leaves ethanol extract as a corrosion inhibitor of carbon steel in 1 M HCl: A preliminary study, International Journal of Corrosion,2012; Article ID. 980654.

Gamache PH, Acworth IN. Analysis of phytoestrogens and polyphenols in plasma, tissue, and urine using HPLC with coulometric array detection, Proceedings of the Society for Experimental Biology and Medicine,1998; 217:274-280.

Gunavathy N, Murugavel SC. Study on the effect of *Musa acuminata* flower extract on the corrosion inhibition of mild steel in 1 NH_2SO_4, International Journal of Chemical Sciences, 2013;11:475-486.

Gunavathy N, Murugavel SC. Studies on corrosion inhibition of *Musa acuminata* flower extract on mild steel in acid medium, Asian Journal of Chemistry,2013;25:2483-2490.

Halliwell B, Gutteridge JMC. Free Radicals in Biology and Medicine. 3rd ed. New York: Oxford University Press,1999.

Hinneburg I, Kempe S, Rüttinger HH, Neubert RHH. A CE method for measuring phototoxicity *in vitro* Chromatographia,2005;62:325-329.

Ji G, Dwivedi P, Sundaram S, Prakash R. Inhibitive effect of *Chlorophytum borivilianum* root extract on mild steel corrosion in HCl and H_2SO_4 solutions, *Ind. Eng. Chem. Res.,* 2013; 52: 10673–10681.

Ladha DG, Wadhwani PM, Kumar S, Shah NK. Evaluation of corrosion inhibitive properties of *Trigonella foenum-graecum* for pure Aluminium in hydrochloric acid, Journal of Materials and Environmental Science,2015;6:1200-1207.

Ladha DG, Wadhwani PM, Lone MY, Jha PC, Shah NK (2015) Evaluation of fennel seed extract as a green corrosion inhibitor for pure aluminium in hydrochloric acid: An experimental and computational approach, Analytical and Bioanalytical Electrochemistry,205;7:59-74.

Lee J, Oh S, Jang M, Kim J, Lee J, Zhou, H. Synthesis of silver nanoparticles using analogous reducibility of phytochemicals, Current Applied Physics,2016;16: 738-747.

Left DB, Zertoubi M, Khoudali S, Azzi M. New application of *Chamaerops humilis* l. Extract as a green corrosion inhibitor for reinforcement steel in a simulated carbonated concrete pore solution, Portugaliae Electrochimica Acta ,2018;36: 249-257.

Leite KCS, Torres LMFC, Garcia LF, Rezende SG, de Oliveira-Neto JR, Lopes FM, Garcia TA, Verly R.M, dos Santos WTP, Gil E.S. Eletrochemical characterization of scopoletin, a 7-hydroxy-6-methoxy-coumarin, Int. J. Electrochem. Science,2015;10: 5714 – 5725.

Liu, RH. Health benefits of fruit and vegetables are from additive and synergistic combinations of phytochemicals, *The American Journal of Clinical Nutrition*, 2003;78: 517S–520S.

Nalini S, Nandini S, Suresh GS, Melo JS, Neelagund SE, NaveenKumar HN, Sanetuntikul J, Shanmugam S. An electrochemical perspective assay for anticancer activity of *Calotropis procera* against glioblastoma cell line (LN-18) using carbon nanotubes-graphene nano- conglomerate as a podium, Advanced Materials Letters, 2016;7:1003-1009.

Oguzie EE, Ogukwe CE, Ogbulie JN, Nwanebu FC, Adindu CB, Udeze IO, Oguzie, K.L., Eze, F.C. Broad spectrum corrosion inhibition: Corrosion and microbial (SRB) growth inhibiting effects of *Piper guineense* extract, Journal of Materials Science,2010;47:3592-3601.

Oguzie EE. Evaluation of the inhibitive effect of some plant extracts on the acid corrosion of mild steel, NACE - International Corrosion Conference Series,2010,10.

Okeniyi JO, Ogbiye AS, Ogunlana OO, Okeniyi ET, Ogunlana OE. Investigating *Solanum aethiopicum* leaf-extract and sodium-dichromate effects on steel-rebar corrosion in saline/marine simulating-environment: Implications on sustainable alternative for environmentally-hazardous inhibitor, TMS Annual Meeting,2015;167-175.

Ouchi K, Gamache P, Acworth I, Watanabe S. Measurement of isoflavones using liquid chromatography with multi-channel coulometric electrochemical detection, BioFactors, 2005;22:353-356.

Paterson JR, Srivastava R, Baxter GJ, Graham AB, Lawrence JR. Salicylic acid content of spices and its implications, Journal of Agricultural and Food Chemistry,2006;54:2891-2896.

Parthipan P, Narenkumar J, Elumalai P, Preethi PS, Usha Raja Nanthini A, Agrawal A, Rajasekar A. Neem extract as a green inhibitor for microbiologically influenced corrosion of carbon steel API 5LX in a hypersaline environments, Journal of Molecular Liquids,2017;240:121-127.

Pradeep Kumar CB, Mohana K.N. Phytochemical screening and corrosion inhibitive behavior of *Pterolobium hexapetalum* and *Celosia argentea* plant extracts on mild steel in industrial water medium, Egyptian Journal of Petroleum,2014;23:201-211.

Rozzi NL, Singh RK, Vierling RA, Watkins BA. Supercritical fluid extraction of lycopene from tomato processing byproducts, Journal of Agricultural and Food Chemistry,2002;50: 2638-2643.

Stadtman ER. Role of oxidant species in aging. Current Medicinal Chemistry, 2004;11: 1105–1112

Stankevièius M, Akuåeca I, Jákobsone I, Maruška A. Comparative analysis of radical scavenging and antioxidant activity of phenolic compounds present in everyday use spice plants by means of spectrophotometric and chromatographic methods, Journal of Separation Science,2011;34:1261-1267.

Seifried HE, Anderson DE, Fisher EI, Milner JA. A review of the interaction among dietary antioxidants and reactive oxygen species, The Journal of Nutritional Biochemistry, 2007;18:567-579.

Shen Q, Zhang B, Xu R, Wang Y, Ding X, Li P. Antioxidant activity *in vitro* of selenium-contained protein from the se-enriched, *Bifodobacterium animalis* 01. Anaerobe, 2010;16: 380-386.

Singh C, Ali MA, Sumana G. Green synthesis of graphene based biomaterial using fenugreek seeds for lipid detection, ACS Sustainable Chemistry and Engineering, 2016; 4:871-880.

Suedile F, Robert F, Roos C, Lebrini M. Corrosion inhibition of zinc by *Mansoa alliacea* plant extract in sodium chloride media: Extraction, characterization and electrochemical studies, Electrochimica Acta, 2014;133:631-638.

Temple NJ, Wilson T, Jacobs Jr.DR. Nutritional Health, Strategies for Disease Prevention, Springer International Publishing AG, 2017.

Umoren SA, Solomon MM, Obot I.B, Suleiman, R.K. Comparative studies on the corrosion inhibition efficacy of ethanolic extracts of date palm leaves and seeds on carbon steel corrosion in 15% HCl solution, Journal of Adhesion Science and Technology, 2018; 32: 1934-1951.

Verma C, Quraishi MA, Ebenso EE, Bahadur IA. Green and Sustainable Approach for Mild Steel Acidic Corrosion Inhibition Using Leaves Extract: Experimental and DFT Studies, Journal of Bio- and Tribo-Corrosion, 2018;4:33.

Watson RR. Polyphenols in Plants, Isolation, Purification and Extract Preparation, Elsevier Inc., 2014.

Zen JM, Kumar AS. Screen-Printed Electrochemical Sensors, in Encyclopedia of Sensors, (*eds.,*) Grimes CA, Dickey EC, Pishko MV, American Scientific Publisher, 2006.

Subject Index